Legal and Ethical Issues for Health Professionals

George D. Pozgar, MBA, CHE
Consultant
Gp Healthcare Consulting, International
Annapolis, Maryland
Surveyor
The Joint Commission
Oakbrook Terrace, Illinois

Legal Review
Nina M. Santucci, JD
General Counsel
Essex Corporation
Columbia, Maryland

JONES AND BARTLETT PUBLISHERS
Sudbury, Massachusetts
BOSTON   TORONTO   LONDON   SINGAPORE

World Headquarters
Jones and Bartlett Publishers
40 Tall Pine Drive
Sudbury, MA 01776
978-443-5000
info@jbpub.com
www.jbpub.com

Jones and Bartlett Publishers
Canada
6339 Ormindale Way
Mississauga, ON L5V 1J2
CANADA

Jones and Bartlett Publishers
International
Barb House, Barb Mews
London W6 7PA
UK

Jones and Bartlett's books and products are available through most bookstores and online booksellers. To contact Jones and Bartlett Publishers directly, call 800-832-0034, fax 978-443-8000, or visit our website at www.jbpub.com.

Substantial discounts on bulk quantities of Jones and Bartlett's publications are available to corporations, professional associations, and other qualified organizations. For details and specific discount information, contact the special sales department at Jones and Bartlett via the above contact information or send an email to specialsales@jbpub.com.

This publication is designed to provide accurate and authoritative information in regard to the Subject Matter covered. It is sold with the understanding that the publisher is not engaged in rendering legal, accounting, or other professional service. If legal advice or other expert assistance is required, the service of a competent professional person should be sought.

ISBN-13: 978-0-7637-2633-1
ISBN-10: 0-7637-2633-8

Library of Congress Cataloging-in-Publication Data

Pozgar, George D.
  Legal and ethical issues for health professionals / George D. Pozgar.—1st ed.
     p. cm.
  Includes bibliographical references and index.
  ISBN 0-7637-2633-8 (pbk.)
  1. Medical laws and legislation—Moral and ethical aspects—United States. 2. Medical personnel—Professional ethics—United States. 3. Medical ethics—United States. I. Title.
  KF3821.P68 2005
  174.2—dc22
6048   2004022164

Production Credits
Executive Editor: Jack Bruggeman
Production Director: Amy Rose
Associate Production Editor: Tracey Chapman
Editorial Assistant: Kylah Goodfellow McNeill
Senior Marketing Manager: Ed McKenna
Manufacturing Buyer: Amy Bacus

Cover Design: Kristin E. Ohlin
Composition: Paw Print Media
Text Design: Paw Print Media
Printing and Binding: Malloy, Inc.
Cover Printing: Malloy, Inc.

Printed in the United States of America
11 10 09 08   10 9 8 7 6

Acknowledgments

I am grateful to the very special people who sit on the ethics committees of the more than 600 hospitals with whom I have consulted and surveyed. Their experiences, knowledge, and methodology for resolving ethical dilemmas inspired me to write this book.

To my students in ethics and health care law classes at the New School for Social Research, Molloy College, Saint Francis College, and St. Joseph's College, and my resident while I was an on-site faculty member for the George Washington University in Washington, D.C., as well as those I have instructed through the years at various seminars including the Long Island University-CW Post College. I will always be indebted for your inspiration.

The author especially acknowledges the staff at Jones and Bartlett Publishers, Inc., whose guidance and assistance was so important in making this publication a reality. Special thanks to Jack Bruggeman, Tracey Chapman, Kylah McNeill, and Ed McKenna.

Contents

Preface

How far you go in life depends on your being tender with the young, compassionate with the aged, sympathetic with the striving and tolerant of the weak and strong. Because someday in life you will have been all of these.
GEORGE WASHINGTON CARVER

Legal and Ethical Issues for Health Professionals is a comprehensive reference dealing with the questions of right and wrong. The reader will learn how to evaluate and distinguish between the rightness and wrongness of alternative courses of action when faced with complicated problems to solve. Ethics in the health care setting is about doing the right thing. It involves recognizing ethical dilemmas and appropriately addressing them.

The purpose of this book is to provide both the student and practicing health care professional with an overview of the ethical and legal issues that face health care providers. This book:

- Presents ethical and legal concepts in an easily understood format
- Reviews the basic principles of ethics and the law
- Provides insight into how ethics and the law are intertwined
- Provides an understanding of how both ethics and the law permeate every aspect of the decision-making process in the health care setting
- Presents case studies to illustrate real-life issues
- Guides the reader to additional resources in the study of ethics and the law
- Explores the use of ethics and the law to assist the reader in resolving ethical conflicts and dilemmas
- Reviews an organization's boundaries between what is acceptable and unacceptable behavior.

This book starts with the premise that to act in an ethical manner means to engage in conduct according to acceptable principles of right and wrong. The author's objective is to provide the reader with the background knowledge necessary to understand that ethics is a manner of using integrity-based thinking to determine what actions need to be taken when faced with common health care dilemmas.

The book assumes no prior ethical or legal training. The cases presented place readers in ethical situations and guides them toward resolution of common ethical dilemmas.

When reviewing the various cases in this book, consider both the ethical and legal implications and how they intertwine with one another. Presented below is a sampling of the numerous questions that can be asked when analyzing ethical and legal issues of the various cases presented throughout the book.

SAMPLE REVIEW QUESTIONS

1. What are the relevant ethical and legal issues in the case under review?

2. Is there other information that might be helpful in the resolution of the dilemmas presented?

3. What are the pertinent breaches of ethical principles in the case?

4. What could have been done to bring more clarity to the ethical dilemma?

5. How could the legal consequences of the case have been prevented?

6. How might one's professional code of ethics have been violated in the case?

7. Describe how the principles of patient autonomy, beneficence, nonmaleficence, and justice may have been violated in the case.

8. Discuss the issues that may impact the people involved (e.g., family members, physicians, other caregivers role (e.g., nurses, chaplain, ethics committee members)).

9. If you were friendly with the patient, would it affect your ability to give an objective opinion?

10. Explain how moral values, religious beliefs, education, and life experiences of both caregivers and patients complicate the resolution of health care dilemmas.

11. Describe how financial concerns can affect the decision-making process.

SAMPLE REVIEW QUESTIONS (continued)

12. Describe how corporate culture can affect the decision-making process.

SAMPLE CASE

Caregivers who have a clear grasp of the ethical and legal concepts discussed in this book will be better equipped to make health care decisions that are ethically sound and legally correct. The following case is an example of how ethical principles and the law are intertwined.

CASE: PATIENT AUTONOMY AND THE RIGHT TO SUE

Several months after having stomach surgery, (2002), Marsingill, in *Marsingill v. O'Malley*, 58 P.3d 495, called her surgeon, Dr. O'Malley, complaining of abdominal pain and nausea. O'Malley advised Marsingill to go to the emergency room and offered to meet her there, but Marsingill said she felt better and declined to go.

O'Malley left it up to Marsingill whether to seek emergency room treatment. [Does this decision involve the principle of *autonomy*? If so, in what way?] O'Malley informed Marsingill that the doctors in the emergency room would probably take X-rays and insert a nasogastric tube to relieve the pressure in her stomach. [Is this an issue of *informed consent*? If so, what are the issues?] After hearing that she would likely need to have a nasogastric tube inserted if she went to the emergency room, Marsingill ended the call, telling O'Malley that she was feeling better. [Does this decision involve the principle of *autonomy*? If so, in what way?]

Later that night Marsingill's husband found her unconscious on the bathroom floor. Paramedics rushed her to the hospital, where an emergency operation later revealed that she had experienced an intestinal blockage. But by then the obstruction had caused Marsingill to go into shock. She suffered brain damage and partial paralysis.

Marsingill sued O'Malley, claiming that he lacked the skill and knowledge to advise her properly and that the information he gave her over the telephone did not allow her to make an intelligent treatment decision. [Does the decision to sue violate the principle of *justice*? If so, in what way?]

Section 8.08 of the AMA Code of Medical Ethics addresses the duty of disclosure, providing: "The patient's right of self-decision can be effectively exercised only if the patient possesses enough information to enable an intelligent choice." Marsingill's experts maintained that O'Malley had violated Section 8.08 by failing to give her enough information to make an intelligent choice about whether to seek emergency room treatment. O'Malley acknowledged that Section 8.08 applied to his conduct—that he did have an obligation to give Marsingill enough information so that she could make an intelligent choice as to whether she should go to the emergency room. [Is this an issue of *professional ethics*?]

Marsingill's proposed instruction by the judge to the jury would have required the jury to decide the sufficiency of O'Malley's communications from the standpoint of a reasonable patient in Marsingill's position. The trial court rejected the proposed "reasonable patient" instruction.

O'Malley acquiesced in Marsingill's decision not to go to the emergency room. In the context of a pre-existing patient/physician relationship involving post-operative care, a physician's recommendation to do nothing in the face of threatening symptoms is the equivalent of a treatment recommendation and should be accompanied by a duty of disclosure. [Does this decision involve a degree of paternalism on the part of the physician? Should O'Malley have been more insistent that Marsingill, because of her symptoms and recent medical history, go to the emergency department for care? Explain your answer.] A physician's acquiescence in a patient's decision not to seek treatment in the same circumstances should likewise be regarded as equivalent to a treatment recommendation subject to the same duty. [How do the physician's actions involve the principles of *beneficence* and *nonmaleficence*?]

The superior court deprived Marsingill of her right to have the jury decide the issue directly, from the standpoint of a reasonable patient and the case was remanded for a new trial on Marsingill's claim for breach of the duty to provide sufficient information to allow her to make an intelligent treatment choice. [Considering a patient's rights and responsibilities, what rights were violated, if any? What responsibilities, if any, did the patient not assume?]

The appellate court ruled that the jury should have been instructed to use the reasonable patient standard to decide whether O'Malley gave Marsingill sufficient information about her condition and treatment choices. On remand, the jury must be instructed to decide the claim from the standpoint of a reasonable patient. [Do you agree with the court's decision? Discuss your answer.] ■

There will always be an endless number of "what-if" scenarios. In the end, the question remains: What should one do, given the facts, knowing that whatever decision is made, there will always be some doubt as to whether the decision made is the right thing to do. This book will help the decision maker make better choices when faced with an ethical dilemma. Armed with the knowledge in this book, the reader will be a more effective caregiver and better able to make critical health care decisions.

Each life is like a novel. Filled with moments of happiness, sadness, crisis, defeat, and triumph. When the last page has been written, will you be happy or saddened by what you read?

AUTHOR UNKNOWN

Section I
Ethics

chapter one

Introduction to Ethics

I expect to pass through the world but once. Any good therefore that I can do, or any kindness I can show to any creature, let me do it now. Let me not defer it, for I shall not pass this way again.

STEPHEN GRELLET[1]

LEARNING OBJECTIVES

The reader upon completion of this chapter will be able to:

- Understand basic ethical concepts
- Understand relevant "ethical theories"
- Describe "ethical principles" relevant to patient care
- Understand the concepts of morality, virtues, and values
- Understand the concept of situational ethics

INTRODUCTION

This chapter provides the reader with an overview of ethics and moral principles. Ethics and morals are derivatives from the Greek and Latin terms (roots) for *custom*. The intent here is not to burden the reader with the philosophy and arguments surrounding ethical theories, morality, principles, virtues, and values. However, as with the study of any new subject, "words are the tools of thought." Therefore, some new vocabulary will be presented to the reader in order to apply the abstract theories and principles of ethics. One needs to understand the words and the concepts in order to make practical use of them.

Ethical dilemmas arise when values, rights, duties, and loyalties conflict, and consequently not everyone is satisfied with a particular decision. An understanding of the concepts presented here will help to reduce conflict when addressing ethical dilemmas and making difficult decisions.

ETHICS

How we perceive right and wrong is influenced by what we feed on.

AUTHOR UNKNOWN

Ethics, also referred to as moral philosophy, is the discipline concerned with what is morally good and bad, right and wrong. The term is also applied to any theoretical system of moral values or principles. Ethics is less concerned with factual knowledge than with virtues and values—namely, human conduct as it ought to be, rather than as it actually is.

Ethics is the branch of philosophy that seeks to understand the nature, purposes, justification, and founding principles of moral rules and the systems they comprise. Ethics deals with values relating to human conduct. It focuses on the rightness and wrongness of actions as well as the goodness and badness of motives and ends. Ethics encompasses the decision-making process of determining ultimate actions. It involves how individuals decide to live within accepted and desirable principles and how they live in harmony with the environment and one another.

Micro-ethics involves an individual's view of what is right and wrong based on personal life experiences. *Macro-ethics* involves a more global view of right and wrong. Although no person lives in a vacuum, solving ethical dilemmas involves consideration of ethical issues from both a micro and macro ethical perspective.

The term *ethics* is used in three different but related ways, signifying: (1) a general pattern or "way of life," such as religious ethics (e.g., Judaeo-Christian ethics); (2) a set of rules of conduct or "moral code," which involves professional ethics and unethical behavior; and (3) philosophical ethics, which involves inquiry about ways of life and rules of conduct.

The *scope of health care ethics* encompasses numerous issues, including the right to choose or refuse treatment and the right to limit the suffering one will endure. Incredible advances in technology and the resulting capability to extend life beyond what would be considered a reasonable quality of life have complicated the process of health care decision making. The scope of health care ethics is not limited to philosophical issues but embraces economic, medical, political, social, and legal dilemmas as well.

Bioethics addresses such difficult issues as the nature of life, the nature of death, what sort of life is worth living, what constitutes murder, how we should treat people who are in especially vulnerable and painful circumstances, and the responsibilities we have to other human beings. The following events are some of many that have had a significant impact on health care ethics.

1932–72   Tuskegee Study of Syphilis

The purpose of the Tuskegee study, involving African-American men, was to analyze the natural progression of untreated syphilis. The study was conducted from 1932 through the early 1970s. The participants were not warned during the study that there was a cure for syphilis (i.e., penicillin). They believed that they were receiving adequate care and unknowingly suffered unnecessarily. The Tuskegee syphilis study used disadvantaged, rural black men to investigate the untreated course of a disease, one that is by no means confined to that population. We know now that the selection of research subjects must be closely monitored to ensure that specific classes of individuals (e.g., terminally ill patients, welfare patients, racial and ethnic minorities, or persons confined to institutions) are not selected for research studies because of their easy availability, compromised position, or manipulability. Rather, they must be selected for reasons directly related to the research being conducted.

1946   Military Tribunal for War Crimes

In 1946, a military tribunal began criminal proceedings against 23 German physicians and administrators for war crimes and crimes against humanity. As a direct result of these proceedings, the Nuremberg Code was established, which made it clear that the voluntary and informed consent of human subjects is essential to research, and that benefits of research must outweigh risks to human subjects involved.[2]

1949   Nuremberg Trials: International Code of Medical Ethics

This code was adopted following numerous experiments conducted by the Nazis on prisoners in concentration camps. Prisoners were exposed to cholera, diphtheria, malaria, mustard gas, yellow fever, typhus, and other horrendous experiments, ultimately claiming thousands of lives. This exploitation of unwilling prisoners as research subjects in Nazi concentration camps was condemned as a particularly flagrant injustice.

1954   **First Kidney Transplant[3]**

The National Institutes of Health published guidelines on human experimentation. The transplantation of human organs has generated numerous ethical issues (e.g., the harvesting and selling of organs, who should have first access to freely donated human organs, how death is defined).

1960s   **Cardiopulmonary Resuscitation**

Prolonging life beyond what reasonably would be expected has generated numerous ongoing ethical dilemmas. Should limited resources, for example, be spent on those who have been determined to be in a comatose vegetative state with no hope of recovery? Or should limited resources be spent on preventative medicine that would improve the quality of life for all?

1968   **Harvard Medical School Report on Brain Death Criteria**

How does one determine when brain death occurs? In 1968 the Harvard Ad Hoc Committee on Brain Death published a report describing the following characteristics of a permanently nonfunctioning brain, a condition it referred to as "irreversible coma," now known as brain death:

1. Patient shows total unawareness to external stimuli and unresponsiveness to painful stimuli.
2. No movements or breathing: All spontaneous muscular movement, spontaneous respiration, and response to stimuli are absent.
3. No reflexes: Fixed, dilated pupils; no eye movement even when hit or turned, or when ice water is placed in the ear; no response to noxious stimuli; no tendon reflexes.

In addition to these criteria, a flat electroencephalogram was recommended.[4]

1964   **World Medical Association[5]**

In 1964, the World Medical Association established guidelines for medical doctors doing biomedical research involving human subjects. The Declaration of Helsinki is the basis for good clinical practices today.[6]

1970   **The Patient as a Person by Paul Ramsey:
"Paternalism" Questioned**

As physicians are faced with many options for saving lives, transplanting organs, and furthering research, they also must wrestle with new and troubling choices—for example, who should receive scarce and vital treatment, how to determine when life ends, and what limits should be placed on care for the dying.

1971   Kennedy Institute of Ethics at Georgetown University

The Joseph P. and Rose F. Kennedy Institute of Ethics was established at Georgetown University in 1971 by a generous grant from the Joseph P. Kennedy, Jr. Foundation. Today it is the world's oldest and most comprehensive academic bioethics center. The Institute and its library serve as an unequaled resource for those who research and study ethics, as well as those who debate and make public policy. The Kennedy Institute is home to scholars who engage in research, teaching, and public service on issues that include protection of research subjects, reproductive and feminist bioethics, end-of-life care, health care justice, intellectual disability, cloning, gene therapy, eugenics, and other major bioethical issues. Institute scholars figure prominently among the pioneers of the discipline. They are extending the boundaries of the field to incorporate emerging issues of racial and gender equality, international justice and peace, and other policies affecting the world's most vulnerable populations.[7]

1972   Informed Consent

Canterbury v. Spence, 464 F.2d 772 (D.C. Cir. 1972).

This case set the "reasonable man" standard requiring informed consent for treatment. Patients must be informed of the risks, benefits, and alternatives associated with recommended treatments.

1974   National Research Act

Due to publicity from the Tuskegee Syphilis Study, the National Research Act of 1974 was passed. This Act created the National Commission for the Protection of Human Subjects of Biomedical and Behavioral Research. One of the Commission's charges was to identify the basic ethical principles that should underlie the conduct of biomedical and behavioral research involving human subjects, and to develop guidelines to ensure that such research is conducted in accordance with those principles.[8]

The Commission was directed to consider:

- the boundaries between biomedical and behavioral *research* and the accepted and routine *practice* of medicine,
- the role of assessment of risk-benefit criteria in determining the appropriateness of research involving human subjects,
- appropriate guidelines for the selection of human subjects for participation in such research, and
- the nature and definition of informed consent in various research settings.[9]

The Food and Drug Administration and the National Institutes of Health internal policy guidelines became federal regulation. As a result of the National Research Act, the National Commission for the Protection of Human Subjects in Biomedical and Behavioral Research was established.

1976 Substituted Judgment

In the Matter of Karen Ann Quinlan, 70 N.J. 10 (1976):

The Supreme Court rendered a unanimous decision providing for the appointment of Joseph Quinlan as personal guardian of his daughter Karen, with full power to make decisions regarding the identity of her treating physicians. Upon the concurrence of the guardian and family, if Karen's physicians concluded that there was no reasonable possibility of her emerging from her comatose condition to a cognitive, sapient state and that her life support apparatus should be withdrawn, they were to consult with the ethics committee of the institution where Karen was then hospitalized. If that consultative body concurred in the prognosis, the life support system could be withdrawn without any civil or criminal liability on the part of any participant, whether it be the guardian, physician, hospital, or others. In addressing itself to the question of possible homicide, the Court concluded that there is a valid distinction between withdrawing life support systems in cases such as Karen's and the infliction of deadly harm either on one's self or another. It saw a difference between Karen's situation and the unlawful killing that is condemned in statutory law. The court denied that the death following withdrawal of treatment would be homicidal. Rather, it would be the result of previously existing natural causes, not from the withdrawal of treatment; and, even if it were considered homicide, it could not be unlawful if done pursuant to the exercise of an explicitly recognized constitutional right.

1978 Establishment of the President's Commission for Study of Ethical Problems in Medicine

The duties of the commission include conducting studies of the ethical and legal implications of the requirements for informed consent to participate in research projects and to otherwise undergo medical procedures; the matter of defining death, including the advisability of developing a uniform definition of death; voluntary testing, counseling, and information and education programs with respect to genetic diseases and conditions, taking into account the essential equality of all human beings, born and unborn; the differences in the availability of health services as determined by the income or residence of the persons receiving the services; current procedures and mechanisms designed to safeguard the privacy of human subjects of behavioral and biomedical research, to ensure the confidentiality of individually identifiable patient records, and to ensure appropriate access of patients to information; and such other matters relating to medicine or biomedical or behavioral research as the President may designate for study by the Commission.[10]

1990 Physician-Assisted Suicide

Jack Kevorkian, a physician, assisted terminally ill patients in suicide outside the boundaries of the law.

1990   Patient Self-Determination Act

The Patient Self-Determination Act of 1990[11] was enacted to ensure that patients are informed of their rights to execute advance directives and accept or refuse medical care.

1994   Oregon's Death with Dignity Act

Physician-assisted suicide became a legal medical option for terminally ill Oregonians. The Oregon Death with Dignity Act allows terminally ill Oregon residents to obtain from their physicians and use prescriptions for self-administered, lethal medications.

1996   Health Insurance Portability and Accountability Act

The "Health Insurance Portability and Accountability Act" of 1996 (Public Law 104-191) was designed to protect the privacy, confidentiality, and security of patient information.

2001   President's Council on Bioethics

The President's Council on Bioethics was created by President George W. Bush in 2001. The Council was charged with advising the President on bioethical issues that may emerge as a consequence of advances in biomedical science and technology. [http://www.bioethics.gov/reports/past_commissions/index.html].

2003   Human Genome Became Fully Sequenced

The human genome system became fully sequenced, allowing molecular genetics and medical research to accelerate at an unprecedented rate. The ethical implications of human genome research are as immense as the undertaking of the totality of the research that was conducted to map the human genome system (e.g., cloning of humans).[12]

ETHICAL THEORIES

Ethics, too, are nothing but reverence for life. This is what gives me the fundamental principle of morality, namely, that good consists in maintaining, promoting, and enhancing life, and that destroying, injuring, and limiting life are evil.

ALBERT SCHWEITZER[13]

Ethics seeks to understand and to determine how human actions can be judged as right or wrong. Ethical judgments can be made based upon our own experiences or based upon the nature of or principles of reason. Those who study ethics believe that ethical decision making is based upon theory. *Ethical theories* attempt to introduce order into the way people think about life and action. The following paragraphs provide a review of the more commonly discussed ethical theories.

Normative Ethics

Normative ethics is the attempt to determine what moral standards should be followed so that human behavior and conduct may be morally right. Normative ethics is primarily concerned with establishing standards or norms for conduct and is commonly associated with general theories about how one ought to live. One of the central questions of modern normative ethics is whether human actions are to be judged right or wrong solely according to their consequences.

General normative ethics is the critical study of major moral precepts of such matters as what things are right, what things are good, and what things are genuine. General normative ethics is the determination of correct moral principles for all autonomous rational beings.

Applied ethics is the application of normative theories to practical moral problems. It attempts to explain and justify specific moral problems such as abortion, euthanasia, and assisted suicide.

Consequential or Teleological Ethics

The consequential or *teleogical* ethical theory emphasizes that the morally right action is whatever action leads to the maximum balance of good over evil. From a contemporary standpoint, theories that judge actions by their consequences have been referred to as consequentialism. *Consequential* ethical theories revolve around the premise that the rightness or wrongness of an action depends upon the consequences or effects of an action. The theory of *consequentialism* is based on the view that the value of an action derives solely from the value of its consequences. The goal of a consequentialist is to achieve the greatest good for the greatest number. It involves asking:

- What will be the effects of each course of action?
- Will they be positive or negative?
- For whom?
- What will do the least harm?

Nonconsequential Ethics

The *nonconsequential* ethical theory denies that the consequences of an action or rule are the only criteria for determining the morality of an action or rule. In this theory, the rightness or wrongness of an action is based on properties intrinsic to the action, not on its consequences.

Deontological Ethics

Deontological theory focuses on one's duties to others. It includes telling the truth and keeping your promises. *Deontology* involves ethical analysis according to a moral code or rules, religious or secular, as presented below.

Religious Ethics

The Great Physician

Dear Lord, You are the Great Physician, I turn to you in my sickness asking for your help.
I place myself under your loving care, praying that I may know your healing grace and wholeness.
Help me to find love in this strange world and to feel your presence by my bed both day and night.
Give my doctors and nurses wisdom that they may understand my illness.
Steady and guide them with your strong hand.
Reach out your hand to me and touch my life with your peace. Amen.
UNIVERSITY OF PENNSYLVANIA HEALTH SYSTEM

Religious ethics, as it relates to character and morality, varies from person to person based on one's religious beliefs. Religious beliefs are heavily influenced by the family within which one is born. The more dogmatic the belief, the more likely one will adopt the family's religious beliefs and values.

Often one's religious beliefs can change as circumstances change. What is troublesome to one individual may not be to another. One's need to survive can change his or her moral character. The extent to which one will adapt in order to survive can take on the extremes of who we really are and how far we will go in order to survive.

Religious codes of ethics are based on a particular religion. Biblical ethics, for example, is God centered. Judaism is based on Old Testament scriptures. Christianity is based on both Old and New Testament scriptures. The notion of right and wrong is not so much an object of philosophical inquiry as an acceptance of divine revelation. Moses, for example, received a list of ten laws directly from God. These laws were known as the Ten Commandments. Some of the Commandments are related to the basic principles of justice that have been adhered to by society since they were first proclaimed and published. For some societies, the Ten Commandments were a turning point where essential commands such as "thou shalt not kill" or "thou shalt not commit adultery" were accepted as law.

The Ten Commandments

1. I am the Lord thy God, which have brought thee out of the land of Egypt, out of the house of bondage. Thou shalt have no other gods before me.
2. Thou shalt not take the name of the Lord thy God in vain.
3. Thou shalt not make unto thee any graven image, or any likeness of anything that is in heaven above, or that is in the earth beneath, or

that is in the water under the earth. Thou shalt not bow down thyself to them, nor serve them.

4. Remember the sabbath day, to keep it holy.
5. Honor thy father and thy mother: that thy days may be long.
6. Thou shalt not kill.
7. Thou shalt not commit adultery.
8. Thou shalt not steal.
9. Thou shalt not bear false witness against thy neighbor.
10. Thou shalt not covet thy neighbor's house, thou shalt not covet thy neighbor's wife, nor his manservant, nor his maidservant, nor his ox, nor his ass, nor anything that is thy neighbor's.

Spirituality in the religious sense implies that there is purpose and meaning to life; spirituality generally refers to faith in a higher being. For a patient, injury and sickness is a frightening experience. This fear is often heightened when the patient is admitted to a health care facility. Health care organizations can help reduce patient fears by making available to them appropriate emotional and spiritual support and coping resources. It is a well-proven fact that patients who are able to draw upon their spirituality and religious beliefs tend to have a more comfortable and often improved healing experience. To assist both patients and caregivers in addressing spiritual needs, patients should be provided with information as to how their spiritual needs can be addressed.

Difficult questions regarding a patient's spiritual needs and how to meet those needs are best addressed upon admission by first collecting information about the patient's religious or spiritual preferences. Caregivers often find it difficult to discuss spiritual issues for fear of offending a patient who may have beliefs different from their own. If caregivers know from admission records a patient's religious beliefs, the caregiver can share with the patient those religious and spiritual resources available in the hospital and community.

Secular Ethics

Unlike religious ethics, *secular ethics* are based on codes developed by societies that have relied on customs to formulate their codes. The Code of Hammurabi, for example, carved on a black Babylonian column, eight feet high, now located in the Louvre in Paris, depicts a mythical sun god presenting a code of laws to Hammurabi, a great military leader and ruler of Babylon (1795–1750 BC). Hammurabi's code of laws is an early example of a ruler proclaiming to his people an entire body of laws. The following excerpts are from the Code of Hammurabi.

CODE OF HAMMURABI

5

If a judge try a case, reach a decision, and present his judgment in writing; if later error shall appear in his decision, and it be through his own fault, then he shall pay twelve times the fine set by him in the case, and he shall be publicly removed from the judge's bench, and never again shall he sit there to render judgment.

194

If a man give his child to a nurse and the child die in her hands, but the nurse unbeknown to the father and mother nurse another child, then they shall convict her of having nursed another child without the knowledge of the father and mother and her breasts shall be cut off.

215

If a physician make a large incision with an operating knife and cure it, or if he open a tumor (over the eye) with an operating knife, and saves the eye, he shall receive ten shekels in money.

217

If he be the slave of some one, his owner shall give the physician two shekels.

218

If a physician make a large incision with the operating knife, and kill him, or open a tumor with the operating knife, and cut out the eye, his hands shall be cut off.

219

If a physician make a large incision in the slave of a freed man, and kill him, he shall replace the slave with another slave.

221

If a physician heal the broken bone or diseased soft part of a man, the patient shall pay the physician five shekels in money.

PRINCIPLES OF HEALTH CARE ETHICS

> *You cannot by tying an opinion to a man's tongue, make him the representative of that opinion; and at the close of any battle for principles, his name will be found neither among the dead, nor the wounded, but the missing.*
>
> E.P. WHIPPLE (1819–1886)[14]

Ethical principles are universal rules of conduct that identify what kinds of actions, intentions, and motives are valued. *Ethical principles core to the ethical practice of medicine* are discussed next. These principles assist caregivers in making choices based on moral principles that have been identified as standards considered worthwhile in addressing health care-related ethical dilemmas. Ethical principles provide a generalized framework within which particular ethical dilemmas can be analyzed. Caregivers, in the study of ethics, will find that difficult decisions often involve choices between conflicting ethical principals.

Autonomy

> *. . . no right is held more sacred, or is more carefully guarded, by the common law, than the right of every individual to the possession and control of his own person.*
>
> UNION PACIFIC RY. CO. V. BOTSFORD[15]

The principle of *autonomy* involves recognizing the right of a person to make one's own decisions. Auto comes from a Greek word meaning "self" or the "individual." In this context it means recognizing an individual's right to make his or her own decisions about what is best for him or herself. Autonomy is not an absolute principle. The autonomous actions of one person must not infringe upon the rights of another.

Respect for autonomy has been recognized in the 14th amendment to the Constitution of the United States. The law upholds an individual's right to make his or her own decisions about health care. A patient has the right to refuse to receive health care even if it is beneficial to saving his or her life. Patients can refuse treatment, refuse to take medications, refuse blood or blood by-products, and refuse invasive procedures regardless of the benefits that may be derived from them. They have a right to have their decisions followed by family members who may disagree simply because they are unable to "let go."

What has been mandated by law has been reflected in bioethical thinking. Although patients have a right to make their own decisions, they also have a concomitant right to know the risks, benefits, and alternatives to recommended procedures.

When analyzing an ethical dilemma, caregivers must consider how autonomy and the respect for a patient's wishes affect the caregivers' decision-making processes. Is, for example, the patient's right to self-determination being compromised because of a third party's wishes for the patient?

The caregiver respects the mentally competent decision-making capabilities of autonomous persons and that right of an individual to make his or her own decisions. The eminent Justice Cardozo, in *Schloendorff v. Society of New York Hospital*, stated:

> Every human being of adult years and sound mind has a right to determine what shall be done with his own body and a surgeon who performs an operation without his patient's consent commits an assault, for which he is liable in damages, except in cases of emergency where the patient is unconscious and where it is necessary to operate before consent can be obtained.[16]

What happens when the right to autonomy conflicts with other moral principles, such as beneficence and justice? Conflict can arise, for example, when a patient refuses a blood transfusion considered necessary to save his or her life while the caregiver's principal obligation is to do no harm.

Autonomous decision making can be affected by one's disabilities, mental status, maturity, or incapacity to make decisions. Although the principle of autonomy may be inapplicable in certain cases, one's autonomous wishes may be carried out through an advance directive and/or an appointed health care agent in the event of one's inability to make decisions.

Beneficence

Beneficence describes the principle of doing good, demonstrating kindness, showing compassion, and helping others. In the health care setting, caregivers demonstrate beneficence by providing benefits and balancing benefits against risks. Beneficence requires one *to do good*. Doing good requires knowledge of the beliefs, culture, values, and preferences of the patient— what one person may believe to be good for a patient may in reality be harmful. For example, a caregiver may decide that a patient should be told frankly, "there is nothing else that I can do for you." This could be injurious to the patient if the patient really wants encouragement and information about care options from the caregiver. Compassion here requires the caregiver to tell the patient, "I am not aware of new treatments for your illness; however, I have some ideas about how I can help treat your symptoms and make you more comfortable. In addition, I will keep you informed as to any significant research that may be helpful in treating your disease processes."

Paternalism is a form of beneficence. People, often believing that they know what is best for another, often make decisions that they believe are in that person's best interest. It may involve, for example, withholding information from someone, believing that the person would be better off that way. Paternalism can occur due to one's age, cognitive ability, and level of dependency.

Medical paternalism involves making choices for (or forcing choices on) patients who are capable of choosing for themselves. This directly violates patient autonomy. Physicians are often in situations where they can influence a patient's health care decision simply by selectively telling the patient what he or she prefers based on personal beliefs. The problem of paternalism involves a conflict between principles of autonomy and beneficence, each of which is conceived by different parties as the overriding principle in cases of conflict. Conflict between the demands of beneficence and autonomy underlies a broad range of controversies.

Can the Physician "Change His Mind"?

Walls had a condition that caused his left eye to be out of alignment with his right eye. Walls discussed with Shreck, his physician, the possibility of surgery on his left eye to bring both eyes into alignment. Walls and Shreck agreed that the best approach to treating Walls was to attempt surgery on the left eye. Prior to surgery, Walls signed an authorization and consent form that included the following language:

a. I hereby authorize Dr. Shreck . . . to perform the following procedure and/or alternative procedure necessary to treat my condition . . . of the left eye.
b. I understand the reason for the procedure is to straighten my left eye to keep it from going to the left.
c. It has been explained to me that conditions may arise during this procedure whereby a different procedure or an additional procedure may need to be performed, and I authorize my physician and his assistants to do what they feel is needed and necessary.

During surgery, Shreck encountered excessive scar tissue on the muscles of Walls' left eye and elected to adjust the muscles of the right eye instead. When Walls awoke from the anesthesia, he expressed anger at the fact that both of his eyes were bandaged. The next day, Walls went to Shreck's office for a follow-up visit and adjustment of his sutures. Walls asked Shreck why he had operated on the right eye, and Shreck responded that "he reserved the right to change his mind" during surgery.

Walls filed a lawsuit. The trial court concluded that Walls had failed to establish that Shreck had violated any standard of care. It sustained Shreck's motion for directed verdict, and Walls appealed. The court stated that the consent form that had been signed indicated that there can be extenuating circumstances when the surgeon exceeds the scope of what was discussed pre-surgery. Walls claims that it was his impression that Shreck was talking about surgeries in general.

Roussel, an ophthalmologist, had testified on behalf of Walls. Roussel stated that it was customary to discuss with patients the potential risks of a surgery, benefits, and the alternatives to surgery. Roussel testified that *medical ethics requires informed consent.*

Shreck claimed that he had obtained the patient's informed consent not from the form but from what he discussed with the patient in his office. The court found that the form itself does not give or deny permission for anything. Rather, it is evidence of the discussions that occurred and during which informed consent was obtained. Shreck therefore asserted that he obtained informed consent to operate on both eyes based on his office discussions with Walls.

Ordinarily, in a medical malpractice case, the plaintiff must prove the physician's negligence by expert testimony. One of the exceptions to the requirement of expert testimony is the situation whereby the evidence and the circumstances are such that the recognition of the alleged negligence may be presumed to be within the comprehension of laymen. This exception is referred to as the "common knowledge exception."

The evidence showed that Shreck did not discuss with Walls that surgery might be required on both eyes during the same operation. There is evidence that Walls specifically told Shreck he did not want surgery performed on the right eye.

Expert testimony was not required to establish that Walls did not give express or implied consent for Shreck to operate on his right eye. Absent an emergency, it is common knowledge that a reasonably prudent health care provider would not operate on part of a patient's body if the patient told the health care provider not to do so.

On appeal, the trial court was found to have erred in directing a verdict in favor of Shreck. The evidence presented established that the standard of care in similar communities requires health care providers to obtain informed consent before performing surgery. In this case, the applicable standard of care required Shreck to obtain Walls' express or implied consent to perform surgery on his right eye.[17]

1. Discuss the conflicting ethical principles in this case.
2. Did the physician's actions in this case involve medical paternalism? Explain your answer.

Nonmaleficence

Nonmaleficence is an ethical principle that requires caregivers to avoid causing patients harm. Nonmaleficence is not concerned with improving others' well-being but rather with avoiding the infliction of harm. Medical ethics require health care providers to "first, do no harm." *In re Conroy*, 464 A.2d 303, 314 (N.J. Super. Ct. App. Div. 1983), "the physician's primary obligation is . . . First do no harm."). Telling the truth, for example, can sometimes cause harm. If there is no cure for a patient's disease, you may have a dilemma. Do I tell the patient and possibly cause serious psychological harm, or do I give the patient what I consider false hopes? Is there a middle ground? If so, what is it? To avoid causing harm, alternatives may need to be considered in solving the ethical dilemma.

The caregiver, realizing that he or she cannot help a particular patient, attempts to avoid harming the patient. This is done as a caution against taking a serious risk with the patient, or doing something that has no immediate or long-term benefits.

The principle of nonmaleficence is broken when a physician is placed in the position of ending life by removing respirators, giving lethal injections, or by writing prescriptions for lethal doses of medication. Helping patients die violates the physician's duty to save lives. In the final analysis there needs to be a distinction between killing patients and letting them die.

Justice

Justice is the obligation to be fair in the distribution of benefits and risks. Justice demands that persons in similar circumstances be treated similarly. A person is treated justly when he or she is receives what is due, is deserved, or can legitimately be claimed. Justice involves how people are treated when their interests compete with one another.

Distributive justice is a principle requiring that all persons be treated equally and fairly. No one person, for example, should get a disproportional share of society's resources or benefits. There are many ethical issues involved in the rationing of health care. This is often due to limited or *scarce resources, limited access* due to geographic remoteness, or a patient's inability to pay for services combined with many physicians who are unwilling to accept patients who are perceived as "no pays" with high risks for legal suits.

Justice and Government Spending

Scarce resources are challenging to the principles of justice. Justice involves equality. Yet equal access to health care, for example, across the United States does not exist. How do you think the government should spend a trillion dollars? With 45 million Americans without health care insurance, describe the value of the one-time $300 to $600 per household give back from the United States treasury under the Bush administration. Consider the following questions:

- Should the money be distributed equally among families?
- Should the money be distributed equally among all citizens?
- Should the money be invested and saved for a rainy day?
- Should the money be used to improve educational programs, build libraries, build state-of-the-art hospitals, or fund after-school programs for disadvantaged youths?

- Should the money include *both* savings for that rainy day and funding for the programs described above?
- What would be the greater good for all?

Injustice for the Insured

Even if you're insured, getting ill could bankrupt you. Hospitals are garnishing wages, putting liens on homes and having patients who can't pay arrested. It's enough to make you sick.

SELF, *THINK YOU'RE COVERED? THINK AGAIN,*
BY SARA AUSTIN, OCTOBER 2004, AT 247.

Hospitals are receiving between 4 and 60 million dollars annually in charity funds in New York alone according to Elizabeth Benjamin, director of the health law unit of the Legal Aid Society of New York City. However, even the insured face injustice. In 2003, almost one million Americans declared bankruptcy because of medical issues, accounting for nearly half of all of the bankruptcies in the country. When an insured patient gets ill and exhausts his or her insurance benefits, should the hospital be able to:

- garnish the patient's wages?
- place liens on homes?
- arrest patients who cannot pay?
- block patients from applying for the hundreds of millions of dollars in government funds designated to help pay for care for those who need it?

Age and Justice

- Should an 89-year-old patient get a heart transplant because he or she is higher on the waiting list to receive a heart transplant than a ten-year-old girl?
- Should a 39-year-old single patient get a heart transplant because he or she is higher on the waiting list to receive a heart transplant than a ten-year-old boy?
- Should a 29-year-old mother of three get a heart transplant because she is higher on the waiting list to receive a heart transplant than a ten-year-old girl?
- Should a 29-year-old pregnant mother with two children get a heart transplant because she is higher on the waiting list to receive a heart transplant than a ten-year-old boy?

Emergency Care

When two patients arrive in the emergency department in critical condition, consider who should get treated first. Should the caregiver base his or her decision on the

- first patient who walks through the door?
- age of the patients?

- likelihood of survival?
- ability of the patient to pay for services rendered?
- condition of the patient?

Patients are to be treated justly, fairly, and equally. Yet what happens when resources are scarce and only one patient can be treated at a time? What happens if caregivers decide that age should be the determining factor as to who is treated first? One patient is saved and another dies. What happens if the patient saved is terminal and has an advance directive in his wallet requesting no heroic measures to save his life? What are the legal issues intertwined with the ethical issues in this case?

Justice describes how people are treated when their interests compete. *Distributive justice* implies that all are treated fairly; no one person is to get a disproportional share of society's resources or benefits. This principle raises numerous issues, including how limited resources should be allocated.

When there is a reduction in staff, managers are generally asked to eliminate "nonessential" personnel. In the health care industry this translates to those individuals not directly involved in patient care (e.g., environmental services employees). Is this fair? Is this justice? Is this the right thing to do?

MORALITY

Aim above morality. Be not simply good; be good for something.

HENRY DAVID THOREAU

Morality implies the quality of being in accord with standards of right and good conduct. Morals are deeply ingrained into a culture or religion and are often part of its identity. Morals are ideas about what is right and what is wrong; as examples, killing is wrong, helping the poor is right, easing pain is right, and causing pain is wrong. Morals should not be confused with cultural habits or customs, such as wearing a certain style of clothing. Morality is a code of conduct. It is a guide to behavior that all rational persons would put forward for governing their behavior.

It is important not only to examine what one considers the right thing to do in a given situation, but why it is the right thing to do. Being morally responsible requires that a person look inward and question his or her own values.

Morality describes a class of rules held by society to govern the conduct of its individual members. A moral dilemma occurs when moral ideas of right and wrong conflict.

Moral judgments are those judgments concerned with what an individual or group believes to be the right or proper behavior in a given situation. It involves assessing another person's moral character based on how he or she conforms to the moral convictions established by the individual and/or group. Lack of conformity typically results in moral censure, condemnation, and possibly derision of the violator's character. What is considered right varies from nation to nation, culture to culture, religion to religion, and person to person. There is no "universal morality."

When it is important that disagreements be settled, *morality is often legislated*. Law is distinguished from morality by having explicit rules and penalties, and officials who interpret the laws and apply the penalties. There is often considerable overlap in the conduct governed by morality and that governed by law. Laws are created to set boundaries for societal behavior. They are enforced to ensure that the expected behavior happens.[18]

VIRTUES AND MORAL VALUES

The term *virtue* is normally defined as some sort of moral excellence or beneficial quality. In traditional ethics, virtues are those characteristics that differentiate good people from bad people. Virtues, such as honesty and justice, are abstract moral principles. Properly understood, virtues serve as indispensable guides to our actions. However, they aren't ends in themselves. Virtues are merely abstract means to concrete ends. The ends are values: the things in life that we aim to gain or keep. Most individuals have a tendency to focus on values and not virtues. Simply stated, most individuals find it difficult to make the connection between abstract principles (virtues) and that which has value. The relationship between means and ends, principles (virtues) and practice (values) is often difficult to grasp.

A moral *value* is the relative worth placed on some virtuous behavior. What has value to one person may not have value to another. A value is a standard of conduct. Values are used for judging the goodness or badness of some action. Ethical values imply standards of worth. They are the standards by which we measure the goodness in our lives. *Intrinsic value* is something that has value in and of itself. *Instrumental value* is something that helps to give value to something else (e.g., money is valuable for what it can buy).

Values may change as needs change. If one's basic needs for food, water, clothing, and housing have not been met, one's values may change such that a friendship, for example, might be sacrificed if one's basic needs can be better met as a result of the sacrifice. If mom's estate is being squandered at the end of her life, the financially well-off family member may want to take more aggressive measures to keep mom alive despite the financial drain on her estate. Another family member who is struggling financially may more readily see the futility of expensive medical care and find it easier to let go. Values give purpose to each life. They make up one's moral character.

All people make value judgments and make choices among alternatives. The values one so dearly proclaims may change as needs change. Values are the motivating power of a person's actions and necessary to survival, both psychologically and physically.

We begin our discussion here with an overview of those virtues commonly accepted as having value when addressing difficult health care dilemmas. The reader should not get overly caught up in the philosophical morass of how virtues and values differ, but be aware that virtues and values have been used by many interchangeably. Whether we call compassion a virtue or a value or both, the importance for our purposes in this text is to understand what compassion is and how it is applied in the health care setting.

Commitment

I know the price of success: dedication, hard work, and an unremitting devotion to the things you want to see happen.

FRANK LLOYD WRIGHT

Commitment is the act of binding oneself (intellectually or emotionally) to a course of action. It is an agreement or pledge to do something. It can be ongoing or a pledge to do something in the future.

Compassion

Compassion is the basis of morality.

ARNOLD SCHOPENHAUER

Compassion in the health care setting means a deep awareness of and sympathy for another's suffering. The ability to show compassion is a true mark of moral character. There are those who argue that compassion will blur one's judgment. Detachment, or lack of concern for the patient's needs, however, is what often translates into mistakes that often result in patient injuries. Caregivers need to show the same compassion for others as they would expect for themselves or their loved ones. Those who have excessive emotional involvement in a patient's care may be best suited to work in those settings where patients are most likely to recover and have good outcomes (e.g., maternity units). As with all things in life, there needs to be a comfortable balance between compassion and detachment.

Never apologize for showing feeling.
When you do so,
You apologize for the truth.

BENJAMIN DISRAELI

Who Makes the Rules?

Mr. Jones was trying to get home from a long trip to see his ailing wife. Mrs. Jones had been ill for several years, suffering a great deal of pain. His flight was to leave at 7:00 PM. Upon arrival at the airport in New York at 4:30 PM, he inquired at the ticket counter, "Is there an earlier flight that I can take to Washington?" The counter agent responded, "There is plenty of room on the 5:00 PM flight but you will have pay a $200 change fee." The passenger inquired, "Could you please waive the change fee? I need to get home to my ailing wife." The ticket agent responded, "Sorry, your ticket does not allow me to make the change."

The passenger made a second attempt at the gate to get on an earlier flight but the manager at the gate was unwilling to authorize the change, saying "I don't make the rules."

Mr. Jones decided to give it one more try. He called the airline's customer service center. The customer service agent responded to Mr. Jones' plea: "We cannot overrule the agent at the gate. Sorry, you just got the wrong supervisor. He is going by the book."

1. Should rules be broken for a higher good?
2. Who decides?

Conscientiousness

A *conscientious* person is one who has moral integrity and a strict regard for doing what is considered the right thing to do. An individual acts *conscientiously* if he or she is motivated to do what is right, believing it is the right thing to do. *Conscience* is a form of self-reflection on and judgment about whether one's actions are right or wrong, good or bad. It is an internal sanction that comes into play through critical reflection. This sanction often appears as a bad conscience in the form of painful feelings of remorse, guilt, shame, disunity, or harmony as the individual recognizes that his or her acts were wrong. Although a person may conscientiously object and/or refuse to participate in some action (e.g., abortion), that person must not obstruct others from performing the same act if he or she has no moral objection to it.

Cooperativeness

Cooperativeness is the willingness and ability to work with others. In the health care setting, it is important that caregivers work cooperatively as a team.

Courage

Courage is the greatest of all virtues, because if you haven't courage, you may not have an opportunity to use any of the others.

SAMUEL JOHNSON

Courage is the mental or moral strength to persevere and withstand danger. "Courage is the ladder on which all the other virtues mount."[19]

Discernment

> *Get to know two things about a man—how he earns his money and how he spends it—and you have the clue to his character, for you have a searchlight that shows up the innermost recesses of his soul. You know all you need to know about his standards, his motives, his driving desires, and his real religion.*
>
> Robert J. McCracken

The virtue of *discernment* is the ability to make a good decision without personal biases, fears, and undue influences from others. A person who has discernment has the wisdom to decide the best course of action when there are many possible actions to choose from.

Fairness

> *Do all the good you can,*
> *By all the means you can,*
> *In all the ways you can,*
> *In all the places you can,*
> *At all the times you can,*
> *To all the people you can,*
> *As long as you ever can.*
>
> John Wesley[20]

In ethics, *fairness* means being objective, unbiased, dispassionate, impartial, and consistent with the principles of ethics. Fairness is the ability to make judgments free from discrimination, dishonesty, or one's own bias.

Fidelity

> *Nothing is more noble, nothing more venerable, than fidelity. Faithfulness and truth are the most sacred excellences and endowments of the human mind.*
>
> Cicero

Fidelity is the virtue of faithfulness, being true to our commitments and obligations to others. A component of fidelity, *veracity*, implies that we will be truthful and honest in all our endeavors. It involves being faithful and loyal to obligations, duties, or observances. The opposite of fidelity is infidelity, meaning unfaithfulness.

Freedom

Freedom is the quality of being free to make choices for oneself within the boundaries of law. Freedoms enjoyed by citizens of the United States include the freedom of speech, freedom of religion, freedom from want, and freedom from physical aggression.

Honesty/Trustworthiness/Truth-Telling

Lies or the appearance of lies are not what the writers of our Constitution intended for our country—it's not the America we salute every Fourth of July, it's not the America we learned about in school, and it is not the America represented in the flag that rises above our land.

MESSAGE FROM THE INTERNET

The virtue of *honesty* is possessed by those who do not lie, resulting in their being "good." *Trust* involves confidence that a person will act with the right motives. It is the assured reliance on the character, ability, strength, or truth of someone or something. To tell the truth, to have integrity, and to be honest are most honorable virtues. *Veracity* is devotion to and conformity with what is truthful. It involves an obligation to be truthful.

Truth-telling involves providing enough information so that a patient can make an informed decision about his or her health care. Intentionally misleading a patient to believe something that the caregiver knows to be untrue may give the patient false hopes. There is always apprehension when one must share bad news; the temptation is to gloss over the truth for fear of being the bearer of bad news. To lessen the pain and the hurt is only human. But in the end, truth must win over fear.

At the end of our days, the most basic principles of life, trust and survival, are on trial.

AUTHOR UNKNOWN

Health Care Morass

The declining trust in the nation's ability to deliver quality health care is evidenced by a system caught up in the morass of managed care companies, which have in some instances inappropriately devised ways to deny health care benefits to their constituency. In addition, the continuing reporting of numerous medical errors serves only to escalate distrust in the nation's political leadership and the providers of health care.

Physicians find themselves vulnerable to lawsuits, often because of misdiagnosis. As a result, patients are passed from specialist to specialist in an effort to leave no stone unturned. Fearful to step outside the boundaries of their own specialities, physicians escalate the problem by ineffectively communicating with the primary care physician responsible for managing the patient's overall health care needs. This can also be problematic if no one physician has taken overall responsibility to coordinate and manage a patient's care.

Politics and Discerning Truth

Truthfulness is just one measure of one's moral character. Unfortunately, politicians don't always set good examples for the people they serve. The following are but a few examples of how political decisions have caused, or have given the appearance of causing, division to the detriment of unity. Discuss the following political decisions and how they have helped to divide the nation by political party.

1963: JFK Assassination
Was President Kennedy killed by a small group of powerful members of the CIA, military intelligence, FBI, and Mafia?[21]

1964: Gulf of Tonkin
Did President Johnson order U.S. bombers to "retaliate" for a North Vietnamese torpedo attack that never happened?[22]

2003: Persian Gulf War
Did President Bush have legitimate reasons to believe that Saddam Hussein had weapons of mass destruction? If so, was there a real threat that he would use them against the United States?

2004: Prescription Drugs
Unless senior citizens are assured of prescription drug coverage through Medicare, many will find that needed medications are unaffordable. Has this issue been honestly and effectively addressed by our government, or must many of the nation's aging population substitute drugs for food?

Hopefulness

Hope is the last thing that dies in man; and though it be exceedingly deceitful, yet it is of this good use to us, that while we are traveling through life, it conducts us in an easier and more pleasant way to our journey's end.
FRANS DE LA ROCHEFOUCAULD

Hopefulness in the patient care setting involves looking forward to something with the confidence of success. Caregivers have a responsibility to balance truthfulness while promoting hope. The caregiver must be sensitive to each patient's needs and provide hope.

Integrity

Integrity involves a steadfast adherence to a strict moral or ethical code and a commitment to not compromise this code. A person with integrity has a staunch belief in and faithfulness to, for example, his or her religious beliefs, values, and moral character. Patients and professionals alike often make health care decisions based on their integrity and their strict moral beliefs. For example, a Jehovah's Witness will refuse a blood transfusion because it is against his or her religious beliefs, even if such refusal may result in death. A provider of health care may refuse to participate in an abortion because it is against his or her moral beliefs. A person without personal integrity lacks sincerity and moral conviction, and may fail to act on professed moral beliefs.

Preservation of Life

Medical ethics do not require that a patient's life be preserved at all costs and in all circumstances. The ethical integrity of the profession is not threatened by allowing competent patients to decide for themselves whether a particular medical treatment is in their best interests. If the doctrines of informed consent and right of privacy have as their foundations the right to bodily integrity and control of one's own fate, then those rights are superior to the institutional considerations of hospitals and their medical staffs. A state's interest in maintaining the ethical integrity of a profession does not outweigh, for example, a patient's right to refuse blood transfusions.

Kindness

When you carry out acts of kindness, you get a wonderful feeling inside. It is as though something inside your body responds and says, yes, this is how I ought to feel.

HAROLD KUSHNER

Kindness involves the quality of being considerate and sympathetic to another's needs.

Respect

Respect for ourselves guides our morals; respect for others guides our manners.

LAURENCE STERNE

To give and show *respect* is to show special regard to someone or something. Caregivers who demonstrate respect for their patients will be more effective in helping them cope with the anxiety of their illness. Respect helps to develop trust between the patient and caregiver, and improve healing processes. If caregivers respect the family of a patient, cooperation and understanding will be the positive result, encouraging a team effort to improve patient care.

SITUATIONAL ETHICS

A person's moral values and moral character can be compromised when faced with difficult choices. Why do good people behave differently in different situations? Why do good people sometimes do bad things? The answer is fairly simple: One's moral character can sometimes change as circumstances change; thus the term *situational ethics*.

> Situational ethics refers to a particular view of ethics, in which absolute standards are considered less important than the requirements of a particular situation. The standards used may, therefore, vary from one situation to another, and may even contradict one another."[23]

For example, a decision not to use extraordinary means to sustain the life of an unknown 84-year-old may result in a different decision if the 84-year-old is one's mother. To better understand this concept, consider the desire to live, and the extreme measures one will take in order to do so. Remember that ethical decision making is the process of determining the right thing to do in the event of a moral dilemma. For example, those who survived the crash of a Fairchild FH-227 twin turboprop airplane on Friday, October 13, 1972, crossing the Andes Mountains carrying 40 passengers and 5 crew were faced with some difficult survival decisions. The plane would disappear from the modern world and everyone on board was thought to be dead, but 72 days later, 16 would emerge alive and tell their story. [http://members.aol.com/porkinsr6/alive.html]. They chose to live by feeding off of those who did not live. A gruesome picture indeed, but it illustrates to what lengths one may go in certain situations (*situational ethics*) in order to survive.

Here are some situational issues to think about:

1. Describe how what you believe to be the right thing to do might change as circumstances change.
2. Describe how your consultative advice might change based on a patient's needs, beliefs, and family influences.

THE FINAL ANALYSIS

People are often unreasonable, illogical and self-centered;
Forgive them anyway.
If you are kind, people may accuse you of selfish, ulterior motives.
Be kind anyway.
If you are successful, you will win some false friends and some true
enemies;
Succeed anyway.
What you spend years building, someone may destroy overnight;
Build anyway.
The good you do today, people will often forget tomorrow;
Do good anyway.
Give the world the best you have, and it may never be enough;
Give the world the best you have anyway.
You see, in the final analysis, it is between you and God;
It was never between you and them anyway.

AUTHOR UNKNOWN

SUMMARY CASE: HONESTY

Annie, a 23-year-old woman with two children, began experiencing severe pain in her abdomen while visiting her family in May 2002. After complaining of pain to Mark, her husband, in June 2002, he scheduled an appointment with Dr. Roberts, a gastroenterologist, who ordered a series of tests. While conducting a barium scan, a radiologist at Community Hospital noted a small bowel obstruction. Dr. Roberts recommended surgery, and Annie agreed.

Following surgery on July 7, Dr. Brown, the operating surgeon, paged Mark over the hospital intercom as he walked down a corridor on the ground floor. Mark, hearing the page, picked up a house phone and dialed zero for an operator. The operator inquired, "May I help you?" "Yes," Mark replied. "I was just paged." "Oh, yes. Dr. Brown would like to talk to you. I will connect you with him. Hang on. Don't hang up." Mark's heart began to pound. "Mark?" "Yes." "Well surgery is over. Your wife is recovering nicely in the recovery room." Mark was relieved but for a moment. "That's good." Dr. Brown continued, "I am sorry to say that she has carcinoma of the colon." Mark replied, "Did you get it all?" "I am sorry, but the cancer has spread to her lymph nodes and surrounding organs," the doctor said. Mark asked, "Can I see her?" Dr. Brown replied, "She is in the recovery room but I am sure it will be okay to see her." Before hanging up, Mark told Dr. Brown, "Please do not tell Annie that she has cancer. I want her to always have hope." Dr. Brown agreed, "Don't worry, I won't tell her. You can tell her that she had a narrowing of the colon."

Mark hung up the phone and proceeded to the recovery room. Upon entering the recovery room, he spotted his wife. His heart sank into his stomach. Tubes seemed to be running out of every part of her body. He walked to her bedside. His immediate concern was to see her wake up and have the tubes pulled out so that he could take her home.

Later in a hospital room, Annie asked Mark, "What did the doctor find?" Mark replied, "He found a narrowing of the colon." "Am I going to be okay?" "Yes, but it will take a while to recover." "Oh, that's good. I was so worried," said Annie. "You go home and get some rest." "I'll see you in the morning."

Mark left the hospital and went to see his friends, Jerry and Helen, who had invited him for dinner. As Mark pulled up to Jerry and Helen's home, he got out of his car and just stood there looking up a long stairway leading to Jerry and Helen's home. They were standing there looking down at Mark. It was early evening, the sun was setting, a warm breeze was blowing, and Helen's eyes were watering. But for a few moments, it seemed like a lifetime. Mark discovered a new emotion as he stood there speechless. He knew then that he was losing a part of himself. Things would never be the same.

Annie had one more surgery two months later in a futile attempt to extend her life.

By November 2002, Annie was admitted to the hospital for the last time. Annie was so ill that even during her last moments she was unaware that she was dying. Dr. Brown entered the room and asked Mark, "Can I see you for a few moments?" "Yes," Mark replied. He followed Dr. Brown into the hallway. "Mark, I can keep Annie alive for a few more days or we can let her go." Mark, not responding, went back into the room. He was now alone with Annie. Shortly thereafter a nurse walked into the room and gave Annie an injection. Mark asked, "What did you give her?" The nurse replied, "Something to make her more comfortable." Annie had been asleep; she awoke, looked at Mark, and said, "Could you please cancel my appointment at the University? I will have to reschedule my appointment. I don't think I will be well enough to go tomorrow." Mark replied, "Okay, try to get some rest." Annie closed her eyes, never to open them again.

Ethical and Legal Issues

1. Do you agree with Mark's decision not to tell Annie about the seriousness of her illness? Explain your answer.
2. Should the physician have spoken to Annie as to the seriousness of her illness? Explain your answer.
3. Describe the ethical dilemmas in this case (e.g., how Annie's rights were violated). Place yourself in Annie's shoes, the physician's shoes, and Mark's shoes, and then discuss how the lives of each may have been different if the physician had informed Annie as to the seriousness of her illness.
4. In the final analysis, is it possible to say who is right? ■

CHAPTER REVIEW

1. Ethics is referred to as moral philosophy, the discipline concerned with what is morally good and bad, right and wrong.
   - Micro-ethics involves an individual's view of what is right and wrong based on his or her life experiences.
   - Macro-ethics involves a more generalized view of right and wrong.
2. Ethics signifies a general pattern or way of life, such as religious ethics; a set of rules of conduct or "moral code," which involves professional ethics and unethical behavior; or philosophical ethics, which involves inquiry about ways of life and rules of conduct.
3. Ethical theories
   - Normative ethics is the attempt to determine what moral standards should be followed so that human behavior and conduct may be morally right.
     - General normative ethics is the critical study of major moral precepts of such matters as what things are right, what things are good, and what things are genuine.
     - Applied ethics is the application of normative theories to practical moral problems. It is the attempt to explain and justify specific moral problems such as abortion, euthanasia, and assisted suicide.
   - The consequential or teleological ethical theory emphasizes that the morally right action is whatever action leads to the maximum balance of good over evil. The consequential theory is based on the view that the value of an action derives solely from the value of its consequences.
   - The nonconsequential ethical theory denies that the consequences of an action or rule are the only criteria for determining the morality of an action or rule. Deontological theory focuses on one's duties to others. It includes telling the truth and keeping your promises. Deontology is an ethical analysis according to a moral code or rules.
     - Religious ethics are based on religious codes.
     - Secular ethics are based on codes developed by societies that have relied on customs to guide their behavior.
4. Ethical Principles
   - Autonomy involves recognizing the right of a person to make one's own decisions.
   - Beneficence describes the principle of doing good, demonstrating kindness, showing compassion, and helping others.
     - Paternalism is a form of beneficence. It may involve withholding information from a person because of the belief that doing so is in the best interest of that person.

   – Medical paternalism involves making choices for (or forcing choices on) patients who are capable of choosing for themselves. It directly violates patient autonomy.
   - Nonmaleficence is an ethical principle that requires caregivers to avoid causing harm to patients.
   - Justice is the obligation to be fair in the distribution of benefits and risks.
     – Distributive justice is a principle that requires treatment of all persons equally and fairly.
5. Morality is a code of conduct. It is a guide to behavior that all rational persons would put forward for governing the behavior of all moral agents.
   - Moral judgments are those judgments concerned with what an individual or group believes to be the right or proper behavior in a given situation.
   - There is no "universal morality." Whatever guide to behavior that an individual regards as overriding and wants to be universally adopted is considered that individual's morality.
   - Morality is often legislated when differences cannot be resolved because of conflicting moral codes with varying opinion as to what is right and what is wrong (e.g., abortion). Laws are created to set boundaries for societal behavior, and they are enforced to ensure that the expected behavior is followed.
6. The term virtue is normally defined as some sort of moral excellence or beneficial quality. In traditional ethics, virtues are characteristics that differentiate good people from bad people.
7. A value is something that has worth. Values are used for judging the goodness or badness of some action. Ethical values imply standards of worth.
   - Intrinsic value is something that has value in and of itself.
   - Instrumental value is something that helps to give value to something else (e.g., money is valuable for what it can buy). Values may change as needs change. Commonly accepted virtues include commitment, compassion, conscientiousness, cooperativeness, courage, discernment, fairness, faith, fidelity, freedom, happiness, honesty, veracity, hopefulness, humility, integrity, kindness, and respect.
8. In situational ethics, a particular situation may influence how one's reaction and values may change in order to cope with changing circumstances.
9. The reason one studies ethical and legal issues is to understand and help guide others through the decision-making process as it relates to ethical dilemmas.

TEST YOUR UNDERSTANDING

Terminology

ethics	justice	faith
ethical theories	distributive justice	fidelity
normative ethics	morality	freedom
consequential ethics	virtues	happiness
nonconsequential ethics	moral values	honesty
religious ethics	commitment	hopefulness
secular ethics	compassion	humility
autonomy	conscientiousness	integrity
beneficence	cooperativeness	kindness
paternalism	courage	respect
medical paternalism	discernment	veracity
nonmaleficence	fairness	situational ethics

REVIEW QUESTIONS

1. What is ethics?

2. Describe the ethical theories reviewed in this chapter.

3. Describe the various ethical principles reviewed in this chapter and how they might be helpful in resolving health care dilemmas.

4. Discuss how the principle of justice can raise ethical issues.

5. Discuss the meaning of virtues and values.

6. Describe an ethical dilemma (e.g., abortion) and how the ethical theories and principles reviewed in this chapter apply.

7. Why do good people behave differently in different situations?

8. Discuss the ethical dilemmas involved in the allocation of scarce resources. How would the ethical principles, virtues, and values discussed in this chapter affect how you would allocate scarce resources?

NOTES

1. French/American religious leader (1773–1855).
2. http://www.rcr.emich.edu/module1/a_7part1.html.
3. http://www.pbs.org/wgbh/aso/databank/entries/dm54ki.html.
4. http://www.ascensionhealth.org/ethics/public/issues/harvard.asp.
5. http://www.wma.net/e/history/index.htm.

6. http://www.rcr.emich.edu/module1/a_7part1.html.
7. http://www.georgetown.edu/research/kie/site/index.htm.
8. http://dor.ncat.edu/compliance/compliance-ed/ethics3F.html.
9. *Id.*
10. United States Code, Title 42—The Public Health and Welfare, Chapter 6A—Public Health Service, Subchapter XVI—President's Commission for the Study of Ethical Problems in Medicine and Biomedical and Behavior Research, Section 300v-1. http://caselaw.lp.findlaw.com/casecode/uscodes/42/chapters/6a/subchapters/xvi/sections/section_300v-1.html.
11. 42 U.S.C. 1395cc(a)(1).
12. http://bioresearch.ac.uk/browse/mesh/C0020125L0020125.html.
13. *Civilization and Ethics,* 1949.
14. American essayist.
15. 141 U.S. 250, 251 (1891).
16. 105 N.E. 92, 93 (N.Y. 1914).
17. Walls v. Shreck, 658 N.W.2d 686 (2003).
18. http://plato.stanford.edu/entries/morality-definition/.
19. Clare Booth Luce (1903–1987) in *Reader's Digest,* 1979.
20. Evangelist and founder of Methodism (1703–1791).
21. http://www.totse.com/en/conspiracy/dead_kennedys/jfklyfor.html.
22. http://www.fair.org/media-beat/940727.html.
23. http://en.wikipedia.org/wiki/Situational_ethics.

chapter *two*

Contemporary Ethical Dilemmas

No right is held more sacred, or is more carefully guarded, by the common law, than the right of every individual to the possession and control of his own person, free from all restraint or interference of others, unless by clear and unquestioned authority of law.[1]

LEARNING OBJECTIVES

The reader upon completion of this chapter will be able to:

- Better understand the concept of ethical dilemmas and the decision-making process.
- Understand the following common ethical dilemmas:
  - Abortion
  - AIDS
  - Artificial insemination
  - Organ donations
  - Research, experimentation, clinical trials
  - Sterilization
  - Wrongful birth, wrongful life, and wrongful conception

INTRODUCTION

An *ethical dilemma* arises in situations where a choice must be made between unpleasant alternatives. It can occur whenever a choice involves giving up something good and suffering something bad, no matter what course of action is taken. *Ethical dilemmas* often require caregivers to make decisions that may break some ethical norm or contradict some ethical value. For example, should I choose life knowing that an unborn child will be born with severe disabilities, or should I choose abortion and thus prevent pain for both parent and child? Should I adhere to my spouse's wishes not to be placed on a respirator, or should I choose life over death, disregarding her wishes and right to self-determination? Should I encourage the abortion my pregnant daughter—the victim of a gang rape—wants, or should I choose life and "do no harm" to the unborn child? Such dilemmas give rise to conflict.

There is a wide range of ethical and legal issues impacting the health care system. This chapter focuses on some of the more common ethical and legal dilemmas facing the providers of health care. In reviewing this chapter, the reader should apply the ethical theories, principles, and values discussed in Chapter 1.

ABORTION

We shall have to fight the politician, who remembers only that the unborn have no votes and that since posterity has done nothing for us we need do nothing for posterity.

William Ralph Inge (1860–1954)[2]

A consensus about when life begins has not been reached. There has been no final determination as to the proper interplay among a mother's liberty, the interests of an unborn child, and the state's interests in protecting life. In abortion cases, the law presupposes a theory of ethics and morality, which in turn presupposes deeply personal ideas about being and existence. Answers to such questions as when life begins define ethical beliefs, and these ethical beliefs should determine how we govern ourselves. Abortion in this context is less a question about constitutional law and more about who we are as a people. This is a decision the Supreme Court cannot make. Taking these issues out of the public discourse threatens to foment hostility, stifle the search for answers, distance people from their Constitution, and undermine the credibility of that document.[3]

With more than one million abortions performed annually in the United States, it is certain that the conflict between "pro-choice" and "pro-life" advocates will continue to pervade America's landscape. When does life begin? Who decides? Who protects the unborn fetus? What are the rights of the individual, the spouse, the parent, society, and the State? Should the principles of autonomy and the right to self-determination prevail? This is the ethical dilemma.

United States Supreme Court Decisions

Abortion is the premature termination of pregnancy. It can be classified as spontaneous or induced. It may occur as an incidental result of a medical procedure, or it may be an elective decision on the part of the patient. In addition to having substantial ethical, moral, and religious implications, abortion has proven to be a major political issue and will continue as such in the future. More laws will be proposed, more laws will be passed, and more lawsuits will wind their way up to the Supreme Court.

1973: Roe v. Wade

Roe v. Wade gave strength to a woman's right to privacy in the context of matters relating to her own body, including how a pregnancy would end.[4] However, the Supreme Court also has recognized the interest of the states in protecting potential life and has attempted to spell out the extent to which the states may regulate and even prohibit abortions.

In *Roe v. Wade*, the United States Supreme Court held the Texas penal abortion law unconstitutional, stating: "[s]tate criminal abortion statutes . . . that except from criminality only a lifesaving procedure on behalf of the mother, without regard to the stage of her pregnancy and other interests involved, is violating the Due Process Clause of the Fourteenth Amendment."[5]

First Trimester. During the first trimester of pregnancy, the decision to undergo an abortion procedure is between the woman and her physician. A state may require that abortions be performed by a physician licensed pursuant to its laws. However, a woman's right to an abortion is not unqualified because the decision to perform the procedure must be left to the medical judgment of her attending physician. "For the stage prior to approximately the end of the first trimester, the abortion decision and its effectuation must be left to the medical judgment of the pregnant woman's attending physician."[6]

Second Trimester. In *Roe v. Wade*, the Supreme Court stated, "[f]or the stage subsequent to approximately the end of the first trimester, the State, in promoting its interest in the health of the mother, may, if it chooses, regulate the abortion procedure in ways that are reasonably related to maternal health."[7] Thus, during approximately the fourth to sixth months of pregnancy, the state may regulate the medical conditions under which the procedure is performed. The constitutional test of any legislation concerning abortion during this period would be its relevance to the objective of protecting maternal health.

Third Trimester. The Supreme Court reasoned that by the time the final stage of pregnancy has been reached, the state has acquired a compelling interest in the product of conception, which would override the woman's right to privacy and justify stringent regulation even to the extent of prohibiting abortions. In the *Roe* case, the Court formulated its ruling as to the last trimester in the following words: "[f]or the stage subsequent to viability, the State in promoting its interest in the potentiality of human life, may, if it chooses, regulate, and even proscribe, abortion except where it is necessary, in appropriate medical judgment for the preservation of the life or health of the mother."[8]

Thus, during the final stage of pregnancy, a state may prohibit all abortions except those deemed necessary to protect maternal life or health. The state's legislative powers over the performance of abortions increase as the pregnancy progresses toward term.

1973: Doe v. Bolton

The Supreme Court then went on to delineate what regulatory measures a state lawfully may enact during the three stages of pregnancy. In the companion decision, *Doe v. Bolton*,[9] where the Court considered a constitutional attack on the Georgia abortion statute, further restrictions were placed on state regulation of the procedure. The provisions of the Georgia statute establishing residency requirements for women seeking abortions and requiring that the procedure be performed in a hospital accredited by the Joint Commission on Accreditation of Healthcare Organizations were declared constitutionally invalid. In considering legislative provisions establishing medical staff approval as a prerequisite to the abortion procedure, the Court decided that "interposition of the hospital abortion committee is unduly restrictive of the patient's rights and needs that . . . have already been medically delineated and substantiated by her personal physician. To ask more serves neither the hospital nor the State."[10]

The Court was unable to find any constitutionally justifiable rationale for a statutory requirement of advance approval by the abortion committee of the hospital's medical staff. Insofar as statutory consultation requirements are concerned, the Court reasoned that the acquiescence of two co-practitioners has no rational connection with a patient's needs and, further, unduly infringes on the physician's right to practice.

Thus, by using a test related to patient needs, the Court in *Doe v. Bolton* struck down four pre-abortion procedural requirements commonly imposed by state statutes: (1) residency, (2) performance of the abortion in a hospital accredited by the Joint Commission, (3) approval by an appropriate committee of the medical staff, and (4) consultations.

1976: Danforth v. Planned Parenthood

The Supreme Court ruled in *Danforth v. Planned Parenthood*[11] that it is unconstitutional to require all women younger than the age of 18 years to obtain parental consent in writing prior to obtaining an abortion. The Court, however, failed to provide any definitive guidelines as to when and how parental consent may be required if the minor is too immature to fully comprehend the nature of the procedure.

1977: Maher v. Roe

In *Maher v. Roe,*[12] the Supreme Court considered the Connecticut statute that denied Medicaid benefits for first-trimester abortions that were not medically necessary. The Court rejected the argument that the state's subsidy of medical expenses incident to pregnancy and childbirth created an obligation on the part of the state to subsidize the expenses incident to nontherapeutic abortions. The Supreme Court voted six to three that the states may refuse to spend public funds to provide nontherapeutic abortions for women.

1979: Colautti v. Franklin

The Supreme Court in *Colautti v. Franklin*[13] voted six to three that the states may seek to protect a fetus that a physician has determined could survive outside the womb. Determination of whether a particular fetus is viable is, and must be, a matter for judgment of the responsible attending physician. State abortion regulations that impinge on this determination, if they are to be constitutional, must allow the attending physician the room that he or she needs to make the best medical judgment.

1979: Bellotti v. Baird—Parental Consent

The Supreme Court in *Bellotti v. Baird*[14] ruled eight to one that a Massachusetts statute requiring parental consent before an abortion could be performed on an unmarried woman younger than the age of 18 years was held to be unconstitutional. Justice Stevens, joined by Justices Brennan, Marshall, and Blackmun, concluded that the Massachusetts statute was unconstitutional, because under that statute as written and construed by the Massachusetts Supreme Judicial Court, no minor, no matter how mature and capable of informed decision making, could receive an abortion without the consent of either both parents or a superior court judge, thus making the minor's abortion subject in every instance to an absolute third-party veto.

1980: Harris v. McRae

In *Harris v. McRae,*[15] the Supreme Court upheld in a five to four vote the Hyde Amendment, which restricts the use of federal funds for Medicaid abortions. Under this case, the different states are not compelled to fund Medicaid recipients' medically necessary abortions for which federal reimbursement is unavailable, but may choose to do so.

1981: H. L. v. Matheson

The Supreme Court in *H. L. v. Matheson,*[16] by a six to three vote, upheld a Utah statute that required a physician to "notify, if possible" the parents or guardian of a minor on whom an abortion was to be performed. In this case, the physician advised the patient that an abortion would be in her best medical interest but, because of the statute, refused to perform the abortion without notifying her parents. The Supreme Court ruled that although a state may not constitutionally legislate a blanket, unreviewable power of parents to veto their daughter's abortion, a statute setting out a mere requirement of parental notice when possible does not violate the constitutional rights of an immature, dependent minor.

1983: City of Akron v. Akron Center for Reproductive Health

The Supreme Court in *City of Akron v. Akron Center for Reproductive Health*[17] decided that the different states cannot (1) mandate what information physicians give abortion patients or (2) require that abortions for women more than three months pregnant be performed in a hospital. With respect to a requirement that the attending physician must inform the woman of specified information concerning her proposed abortion, it was found unreasonable for a state to insist that only a physician is competent to provide information and counseling relative to informed consent. A state may not adopt regulations to influence a woman's informed choice between abortion and childbirth.

With regard to a second-trimester hospital requirement, this could significantly limit a woman's ability to obtain an abortion. This is especially so in view of the evidence that a second-trimester abortion may cost more than twice as much in a hospital as in a clinic.

1989: Webster v. Reproductive Health Services

Webster v. Reproductive Health Services[18] began the Court's narrowing of abortion rights by upholding a Missouri statute providing that no public facilities or employees should be used to perform abortions and that physicians should conduct viability tests before performing abortions.

1991: Rust v. Sullivan

Federal regulations that prohibit abortion counseling and referral by family planning clinics that receive funds under Title X of the Public Health Service Act were found not to violate the constitutional rights of pregnant women or Title X grantees in a decision by the Supreme Court in *Rust v. Sullivan*.[19] Proponents of abortion counseling argue that the regulations impermissibly burden a woman's privacy right to abortion. Prohibiting the delivery of abortion information, even as to where such information could be obtained, the regulations deny a woman her constitutionally protected right to choose under the First Amendment. The question arises: How can a woman make an informed choice between two options when she cannot obtain information as to one of them? In *Sullivan*, however, the Supreme Court found that there was no violation of a woman's or provider's First Amendment rights.

The Court here found that government need not subsidize the exercise of the fundamental rights to free speech. The plaintiff had argued that the government may not condition receipt of a benefit on the relinquishment of constitutional rights.

1992: Planned Parenthood v. Casey

In *Planned Parenthood v. Casey,*[20] the Supreme Court affirmed Pennsylvania law restricting a woman's right to abortion. The Court was one vote shy of overturning *Roe v. Wade.* The Supreme Court ruling, as enunciated in *Roe v. Wade,* reaffirmed:

- the constitutional right of women to have an abortion before viability of the fetus, as first enunciated in *Roe v. Wade,*
- the state's power to restrict abortions after fetal viability, so long as the law contains exceptions for pregnancies that endanger a woman's life or health, and
- the principle that the state has legitimate interests from the outset of the pregnancy in protecting the health of the woman and the life of the fetus.

The Supreme Court rejected the trimester approach in *Roe v. Wade,* which limited the regulations states could issue on abortion depending on the development stage of the fetus. In place of the trimester approach, the Court will evaluate the permissibility of state abortion rules based on whether they unduly burden a woman's ability to obtain an abortion. A rule is an undue burden if its purpose or effect is to place a substantial obstacle in the path of a woman seeking an abortion before the fetus attains viability. The Supreme Court ruled that it is "not an undue burden" to require that a woman be informed of the nature of the abortion procedure and the risks involved, offered information on the fetus and alternatives to abortion, and given informed consent before the abortion procedure. In addition, it is not an undue burden to require parental consent for a minor seeking an abortion, providing for a judicial bypass option if the minor does not wish or cannot obtain parental consent, and requiring a 24-hour waiting period before any abortion can be performed.

1998: Women's Medical Professional Corp. v. Voinovich

The Supreme Court in *Women's Medical Professional Corp. v. Voinovich*[21] denied *certiorari* for the first partial-birth case to reach the federal appellate courts. This case involved an Ohio statute that banned the use of the intact dilation and extraction (D&X) procedure in the performance of any pre- or post-viability abortion. The Sixth Circuit Court of Appeals held that the statute banning any use of the D&X procedure was unconstitutionally vague. It is likely that a properly drafted statute will eventually be judged constitutionally sound.

2000: Stenberg v. Carhart

On June 28, 2002, the United States Supreme Court struck down a Nebraska ban on "partial birth abortion," finding it an unconstitutional violation of *Roe v. Wade*. The court found these types of bans to be extreme descriptive attempts to outlaw abortion—even early in pregnancy—that jeopardizes women's health [192 F.3d 1142 (8th Cir. 1999), 120 S. Ct. 2597 (2000)].

2003: Partial Birth Abortion Ban Made Law

President Bush, on November 6, signed the first federal restrictions banning late-term partial-birth abortions. (The partial-birth abortion, also referred to as the D&X procedure, is a late-term abortion involving partial delivery of the baby prior to it being aborted.) Both houses of Congress passed the ban. The ban permits no exceptions when a woman's health is at risk or the fetus has life-threatening disabilities. A U.S. District Court in Nebraska has already issued a restraining order on the ban. Additional restraining orders are anticipated by other courts.

2004: Hundreds of Thousands March to Support Abortion Rights

Hundreds of thousands of both men and women from more than 60 countries marched in Washington, D.C. on April 25, 2004, supporting women's reproductive rights. The slogans at the rally included slogans such as "Pro Choice—Pro Child," "It's Your Choice . . . Not Theirs," "My Family My Choice," "My Body My Choice," "Justice for All," "Who Decides?", and "Keep Abortion Legal."

State Abortion Statutes

The effect of the Supreme Court's 1973 decisions in *Roe* and *Doe* was to invalidate all or part of almost every state abortion statute then in force. The responses of state legislatures to these decisions were varied, but it is clear that many state laws had been enacted to restrict the performance of abortions as much as possible. Although *Planned Parenthood v. Casey* was expected to clear up some issues, it is evident that the states have been given more power to regulate the performance of abortions.

24-Hour Waiting Period Not Burdensome

The 1993 Utah Abortion Act Revision, Senate Bill 60, provides for informed consent by requiring that certain information be given to the pregnant woman at least 24 hours prior to performing an abortion. The law allows for exceptions to this requirement in the event of a medical emergency. The Utah Women's Clinic, in *Utah Women's Clinic, Inc. v. Leavitt*,[22] filed a 106-page complaint challenging the constitutionality of the new Utah law. It was determined that the 24-hour waiting period did not impose an undue burden on the right to an abortion. On appeal, a U.S. District Court held that the Utah abortion statute's 24-hour waiting period and informed consent requirements do not render the statute unconstitutionally vague.

In 1992, the Supreme Court in *Planned Parenthood of Southeastern Pennsylvania v. Casey*[23] determined that in asserting an interest in protecting fetal life, a state may place some restrictions on pre-viability abortions, so long as those restrictions do not impose an "undue burden" on the woman's right to an abortion. The Court determined that the 24-hour waiting period, the informed consent requirement, and the medical emergency definitions did not unduly burden the right to an abortion and were therefore constitutional.

"The abortion issue is obviously one that invokes strong feelings on both sides. Individuals are free to urge support for their cause through debate, advocacy, and participation in the political process. The subject also might be addressed in the courts so long as there are valid legal issues in dispute. Where, however, a case presents no legitimate legal arguments, the courthouse is not the proper forum. Litigation, or the threat of litigation, should not be used as economic blackmail to strengthen one's hand in the political battle."[24]

Consent

Spousal Consent

Provisions of the Florida Therapeutic Abortion Act, which required a married woman to obtain the husband's consent prior to abortion was found to be unconstitutional. The state's interest was found not to be sufficiently compelling to limit a woman's right to abortion. The husband's interest in the baby was held to be insufficient to force his wife to face the mental and physical risks of pregnancy and childbirth.[25]

In *Doe v. Zimmerman*,[26] the court declared unconstitutional the provisions of the Pennsylvania Abortion Control Act, which required that the written consent of the husband of a married woman be secured before performing an abortion. The court found that these provisions impermissibly permitted the husband to withhold his consent either because of his interest in the potential life of the fetus or for capricious reasons. The natural father of an unborn fetus in *Doe v. Smith*[27] was found not to be entitled to an injunction to prevent the mother from submitting to an abortion. Although the father's interest in the fetus was legitimate, it did not outweigh the mother's constitutionally protected right to an abortion, particularly in light of evidence that the mother and father had never married.

In the 1992 decision of *Planned Parenthood v. Casey*, the Supreme Court ruled that spousal consent would be an undue burden on the woman.

Incompetent Persons' Consent

An abortion was found to have been authorized properly by a family court in *In re Doe*[28] for a profoundly retarded woman. She had become pregnant during her residence in a group home as a result of a sexual attack by an unknown person. The record had supported a finding that if the woman had been able to do so, she would have requested the abortion. The court properly chose welfare agencies and the woman's *guardian ad litem* (a guardian appointed to prosecute or defend a suit on behalf of a party incapacitated by infancy, mental incompetence, etc.) as the surrogate decision makers.

Parental Consent

The trial court in *In re Anonymous*[29] was found to have abused its discretion when it refused a minor's request for waiver of parental consent to obtain an abortion. The record indicated that the minor lived alone, was within one month of her 18th birthday, lived by herself most of the time, and held down a full-time job.

Parental Notification

The issue in *Planned Parenthood v. Owens*[30] is whether the Colorado Parental Notification Act,[31] which requires a physician to notify the parents of a minor prior to performing an abortion upon her, violates the minor's rights protected by the United States Constitution. The Act, a citizen-initiated measure, was approved at Colorado's general election. The Act generally prohibits physicians from performing abortions on an unemancipated minor until at least 48 hours after written notice has been delivered to the minor's parent, guardian, or foster parent.

The United States District Court decided that the Act violated the rights of minor women protected by the Fourteenth Amendment. The Supreme Court, for more than a quarter of a century, has required that any abortion regulation except from its reach an abortion medically necessary for the preservation of the mother's health. The Act fails to provide such a health exception.

Continuing Controversy

Right-to-Life advocates argue that life comes from God and that no one has a right to deny the right to life. Upon review, the court of appeals concluded that the Patient Notification Act was unconstitutional because it failed to provide a health exception as required by the U.S. Constitution.[31b]

CASE: BILL BANNING ABORTION

March 9, 2004: Gov. Rounds of South Dakota vetoed legislation that would have all but banned abortion in the state. The two houses of South Dakota's state legislature had voted overwhelmingly for the bill, which called for abortions to be banned in all cases except when a woman's life was in danger.

Ethical and Legal Issues

1. What are the ethical and legal issues in this case?
2. Are limited state funds being spent wisely, considering the financial difficulties many states are already facing and the high cost of legal fees in pursuing such issues?

3. Does the fact that this bill challenges the 1973 *Roe v. Wade* Supreme Court ruling influence your thinking?

Pro choice advocates argue that a woman has a right to choose preservation and protection of her health, and therefore, in many cases, her life is at least as compelling as the state's interest in promoting childbirth. The protection of a fetus and promotion of childbirth cannot be considered so compelling as to outweigh a woman's fundamental right to choose and the state's obligation to be evenhanded in the design and application of its health care policies. ■

CASE: UTAH WOMAN REFUSES C-SECTION

March 12, 2004: A 28-year-old Utah woman refused a C-section and was charged with criminal homicide after one of her twins died prior to delivery. The charge claimed that the mother showed a depraved indifference to human life by ignoring medical advice to deliver her twins by C-section. It is alleged that a nurse told police that the patient said she would rather lose one of the babies than be cut.

Ethical and Legal Issues

1. If convicted, what should happen to mothers who smoke, drink, or don't follow their physician's orders for diet and exercise? Explain your answer.
2. Is it okay to charge this mother for murder because some do not like the choices she made? Discuss your answer.

There will most likely be a continuing stream of court decisions, as well as political and legislative battles, well into the 21st century. Given the emotional, religious, and ethical concerns, as well as those of women's rights groups, it is unlikely that this matter will be resolved anytime soon. ■

Morality of Abortion

The morality of abortion is not a legal or constitutional issue; it is a matter of philosophy, of ethics, and of theology. It is a subject upon which reasonable people can, and do, adhere to vastly divergent convictions and principles. Rather, our obligation is to define the liberty of all, not to mandate our own moral code.[32]

ACQUIRED IMMUNE DEFICIENCY SYNDROME

The epidemic of acquired immune deficiency syndrome (AIDS) is considered to be the deadliest epidemic in human history. The first case appeared in the literature in 1981.[33] It has been estimated that more than 21 million people have died from AIDS.[34] AIDS, generally, is accepted as a syndrome—a collection of specific, life-threatening, opportunistic infections and manifestations that are the result of an underlying immune deficiency. AIDS is caused by the human immunodeficiency virus (HIV) and is the most severe form of the HIV infection. HIV is a highly contagious bloodborne virus. It is a fatal disease that destroys the body's capacity to ward off bacteria and viruses that ordinarily would be fought off by a properly functioning immune system. Although there is no effective long-term treatment of the disease, indications are that proper management of the disease can improve the quality of life and delay progression of the disease. Internationally, AIDS is posing serious social, ethical, economic, and health problems.

CASE: FALSE POSITIVE TEST RESULTS

The patient-plaintiff had a blood specimen drawn and sent to a laboratory for testing for HIV. The laboratory informed the physician that his patient tested positive for HIV. The patient was informed that he had AIDS. Not believing that his symptoms mimicked those of an individual with AIDS, the patient was retested for HIV. On three separate occasions involving two separate laboratories, the patient tested negative for the virus. The patient-plaintiff filed a lawsuit against his physician and laboratory for the negligent interpretation and reporting of his blood samples as being HIV positive.

The West Virginia Supreme Court of Appeals ruled that the plaintiff had stated a claim for the negligent infliction of emotional distress. "Given the well-known fact that AIDS had replaced cancer as the *most feared disease in America* and, as defendant . . . candidly acknowledges, a diagnosis of AIDS is a death sentence, conventional wisdom mandates that fear of AIDS triggers genuine—not spurious—claims of emotional distress."[35]

Ethical and Legal Issues

1. Do you agree with the court's finding? Explain your answer.
2. If this same reasoning applied to hundreds of cases at one hospital laboratory, how would you determine awards? Consider what effect the awards granted might have on the hospital's financial viability, as well as the quality of services provided to the community. Discuss your answer.
3. Review the news article at the end of this section on AIDS. Further discuss your thoughts as to right and wrong, and how the theories and principles of ethics might apply. ■

Spread of AIDS

AIDS is spread by direct contact with infected blood or body fluids, such as vaginal secretions, semen, and breast milk. At the present time there is no evidence that the virus can be transmitted through food, water, or casual body contact. HIV does not survive well outside the body. Although there is presently no cure for AIDS, early diagnosis and treatment with new medications can help HIV-infected persons remain healthy for longer periods. High-risk groups include unprotected sexual encounters, intravenous drug users, and those who require transfusions of blood and blood products, such as hemophiliacs.

Blood Transfusions

The administration of blood is considered to be a medical procedure. It results from the exercise of professional medical judgment that is composed of two parts: (1) diagnosis, deciding the need for blood, and (2) therapy, the actual administration of blood.

Suits often arise as a result of a person with AIDS claiming that he or she contracted the disease as a result of a transfusion of contaminated blood or blood products. In blood transfusion cases, the standards most commonly identified as having been violated concern blood testing and donor screening. An injured party generally must prove that a standard of care existed, that the defendant's conduct fell below the standard, and that this conduct was the proximate cause of the plaintiff's injury.

The most common occurrences that lead to lawsuits in the administration of blood involve

- transfusion of mismatched blood,
- improper screening and transfusion of contaminated blood,
- unnecessary administration of blood, and
- improper handling procedures (i.e., inadequate refrigeration and storage procedures).

The risk of HIV infection and AIDS through a blood transfusion has been reduced significantly through health history screening and blood donations testing. All blood donated in the United States has been tested for HIV antibodies since May 1985. Blood units that do test positive for HIV are removed from the blood transfusion pool.

AIDS and Health Care Workers

Although transmission of HIV from an infected physician to his or her patient during invasive surgery may be unlikely, it is a theoretical possibility and therefore foreseeable. Because of the potentially deadly consequence of such transmission, infected physicians should not engage in activity that creates a risk of transmission.

The ever-increasing likelihood that health care workers will come into contact with persons carrying the AIDS virus demands that health care workers comply with approved safety procedures. This is especially important for those who come into contact with blood and body fluids of HIV-infected persons.

An AIDS-infected surgeon in New Jersey was unable to recover on a discrimination claim when the hospital restricted his surgical privileges. In *Estate of Behringer v. Medical Center at Princeton*,[36] the New Jersey Superior Court held that the hospital acted properly in initially suspending a surgeon's surgical privileges, thereafter imposing a requirement of informed consent and ultimately barring the surgeon from performing surgery. The Court held that in the context of informed consent, the risk of a surgical accident involving an AIDS-positive surgeon and implications thereof would be a legitimate concern to a surgical patient that would warrant disclosure of the risk. "The 'risk of harm' to the patient includes not only the actual transmission of HIV from the surgeon to patient but the risk of a surgical accident, i.e., a scalpel cut or needle stick, which may subject the patient to post-surgery HIV testing."[37]

Confidentiality

Guidelines drafted by the Centers for Disease Control and Prevention call on health care workers who perform "exposure-prone" procedures to undergo tests voluntarily to determine whether they are infected. The guidelines also recommend that patients be informed. Both health care workers and patients claim mandatory HIV testing violates their Fourth Amendment right to privacy. The dilemma is how to balance these rights against the rights of the public in general to be protected from a deadly disease.

State laws have been developed that protect the confidentiality of HIV-related information. Some states have developed informational brochures and consent, release, and partner notification forms. The unauthorized disclosure of confidential HIV-related information can subject an individual to civil and/or criminal penalties.

Information regarding a patient's diagnosis as being HIV positive must be kept confidential and should be shared with other health care professionals only on a need-to-know basis. Each person has a right to privacy as to his or her personal affairs. The plaintiff surgeon, in *Estate of Behringer v. Medical Center at Princeton*,[38] was entitled to recover damages from the hospital and its laboratory director for the unauthorized disclosure of his condition during his stay at the hospital. The hospital and the director had breached their duty to maintain confidentiality of the surgeon's medical records by allowing placement of the patient's test results in his medical chart without limiting access to the chart, which they knew was available to the entire hospital community. "The medical center breached its duty of confidentiality to the plaintiff, as a patient, when it failed to take reasonable precautions regarding the plaintiff's medical records to prevent the patient's AIDS diagnosis from becoming a matter of public knowledge."[39]

The hospital in *Tarrant County Hospital District v. Hughes*[40] was found to have properly disclosed the names and addresses of blood donors in a wrongful death action alleging that a patient contracted AIDS from a blood transfusion administered in the hospital. The physician-patient privilege expressed in the Texas Rules of Evidence did not apply to preclude such disclosure because the record did not reflect that any such relationship had been established. The disclosure was not an impermissible violation of the donors' right of privacy. The societal interest in maintaining an effective blood donor program did not override the plaintiff's right to receive such information. The order prohibited disclosure of the donors' names to third parties.

In *Doe v. University of Cincinnati*,[41] a patient who was infected with HIV-contaminated blood during surgery brought an action against a hospital and a blood bank. The trial court granted the patient's request to discover the identity of the blood donor, and the defendants appealed. The court of appeals held that the potential injury to a donor in revealing his identity outweighed the plaintiff's modest interest in learning of the donor's identity. A blood donor has a constitutional right to privacy not to be identified as a donor of blood that contains HIV. At the time of the plaintiff's blood transfusion in July 1984, no test had been developed to determine the existence of AIDS antibodies. By May 27, 1986, all donors donating blood through the defendant blood bank were tested for the presence of HIV antibodies. Patients who received blood from donors who tested positive were to be notified through their physicians. In this case, the plaintiff's family was notified because of the plaintiff's age and other disability.

Any new HIV-related regulations must continue to address the rights and responsibilities of both patients and health care workers. Although this will require a delicate balancing act, it must not be handled as a low-priority issue by legislators.

CASE: DISCLOSURE OF PHYSICIAN'S HIV STATUS

The physician, Doe, was a resident in obstetrics and gynecology at a Medical Center. In 1991, he cut his hand with a scalpel while he was assisting another physician. Because of the uncertainty that blood had been transferred from Doe's hand wound to the patient through an open surgical incision, he agreed to have a blood test for HIV. His blood tested positive for HIV, and he withdrew himself from participation in further surgical procedures. The Medical Center and Harrisburg Hospital, where Doe also participated in surgery, identified those patients who could be at risk. The Medical Center identified 279 patients and Harrisburg identified 168 patients who fell into this category. Because hospital records did not identify those surgeries in which physicians may have accidentally cut themselves, the hospitals filed petitions in the Court of Common Pleas, alleging that there was, under the Confidentiality of HIV-Related Information Act [35 P.S. § 7608(a)(2)], a "compelling need" to disclose information regarding Doe's condition to those patients who conceivably could have been exposed to HIV. Doe argued that there was no compelling need to disclose the information and that he was entitled to confidentiality under the Act.

The Pennsylvania Supreme Court held that a compelling need existed for at least a partial disclosure of the physician's HIV status.

The medical experts who testified agreed that there was some risk of exposure and that some form of notice should be given to the patients at risk. Even the expert witness presented by Doe agreed that there was at least some conceivable risk of exposure and that giving a very limited form of notice would not be unreasonable. Failure to notify the patients at risk could result in the spread of the disease to other noninfected individuals through sexual contact and through exposure to other body fluids. Doe's name was not revealed to the patients, only the fact that a resident physician who participated in their care had tested HIV-positive. "No principle is more deeply embedded in the law than that expressed in the maxim *Salus populi suprema lex, . . .* (the welfare of the people is the supreme law), and a more compelling and consistent application of that principle than the one presented would be quite difficult to conceive."[42]

Ethical and Legal Issues

1. Do you agree that there was a need for a partial disclosure of the physician's HIV status?
2. If "the welfare of the people is the supreme law," did the court fall short of its responsibility by not allowing disclosure of the physician's name? Discuss your answer. ■

AIDS: The Right to Treatment

More and more health care organizations are expressing in their ethics statements that HIV-infected patients have a right not to be discriminated against in the provision of treatment. The Ethics Committee of the American Academy of Dermatology, for example, states that "it is unethical for a physician to discriminate against a class or category of patients and to refuse the management of a patient because of medical risk, real or imagined."[43] Patients with HIV infection, therefore, should receive the same compassionate and competent care given to other patients.

News Media and Confidentiality

The Pennsylvania Superior Court in *Stenger v. Lehigh Valley Hospital Center*[44] upheld the court of common pleas' order denying the petition of The Morning Call, Inc., which challenged a court order closing judicial proceedings to the press and public in a civil action against a hospital and physicians. A patient and her family had all contracted AIDS after the patient received a blood transfusion. The access of the media to pretrial discovery proceedings in a civil action is subject to reasonable control by the court in which the action is pending. The protective order limiting public access to pretrial discovery material did not violate the newspaper's First Amendment rights. The discovery documents were not judicial records to which the newspaper had a common-law right of access. Good cause existed for nondisclosure of information about the intimate personal details of the plaintiffs' lives, disclosure of which would cause undue humiliation.

CASE: ADMINISTRATION OF THE WRONG BLOOD

The patient-plaintiff, in *Bordelon v. St. Francis Cabrini Hospital*,[45] was admitted to the hospital to undergo a hysterectomy. Prior to surgery, she provided the hospital with her own blood in case it was needed during surgery. During surgery the patient did indeed need blood but was administered donor blood other than her own. The patient filed a lawsuit claiming that the hospital's failure to provide her with her own blood resulted in her suffering mental distress.

The Court of Appeal held that the plaintiff stated a cause of action for mental distress. It is well established in law that a claim for negligent infliction of emotional distress unaccompanied by physical injury is a viable claim of action. It is indisputable that HIV can be transmitted through blood transfusions even when the standard procedure for screening for the virus is in place. The plaintiff's fear was easily associated with receiving someone else's blood, and therefore a conceivable consequence of the defendant's negligent act. The hospital had a "duty" to administer the plaintiff's own blood. The hospital breached that duty by administering the wrong blood.

Ethical and Legal Issues

1. Do you agree with the court's decision? Explain your answer.
2. In cases such as this, do you believe that financial awards are effective in preventing future incidents? Explain your answer. ▪

CASE: ERRORS POSSIBLE IN HIV TESTS

Over 400 patients may have received incorrect HIV and hepatitis test results. Some patients might have been told they were HIV-negative when in fact they were positive and vice versa, and the hospital failed to notify the patients of the problem. A complaint had apparently been filed by a former hospital employee. State health officials discovered in January that the hospital's laboratory personnel overrode controls in the testing equipment that showed the results might be in error, then mailed them to patients anyway.[46]

Ethical and Legal Issues

1. What ethical theories and principles were violated in this case?
2. What are the legal concerns for the hospital? ▪

CASE: HIV AUTONOMY AND CONFIDENTIALITY

Jones, a divorcee with two children, was sentenced to ten years in prison for repeated robberies of three banks. He has been in prison for eight years. His wife, Nora, disappeared shortly after he was sentenced. Five of his close inmate friends at Sing Prison had tested positive for the HIV virus and have since passed away. Prison officials are planning to test Jones for the HIV virus. He objects and has sought legal counsel. Meanwhile, local school officials have been informed of the death of Mr. Jones' friends and his refusal to be tested for the HIV virus. Strangely, the community at large became aware of Jones' situation and the fact that his children are attending school with their children. The parents are insisting that the Jones' kids either be removed from school or they will remove their children from class. Meanwhile, Nora showed up at a local navy recruiting station posing as a single woman with no children. She admitted to being bisexual several years ago but claims that she is now straight. The navy learned of this situation and requires HIV testing. She objects and seeks legal counsel.

Ethical and Legal Issues

1. What are Mr. Jones' rights?
2. What are the rights of other prisoners?
3. What are the rights of the children?
4. What are the rights of the parents?
5. Is there a legitimate need for a physician to disclose otherwise confidential testing data to the spouse and other intimate sexual partners of an HIV-infected patient? ■

ARTIFICIAL INSEMINATION

Generally, *artificial insemination* is the injection of seminal fluid into a woman to induce pregnancy. The term also may encompass insemination that takes place outside of the woman's body, as with so-called test-tube babies. If the semen of the woman's husband is used to impregnate her, the technique is called homologous artificial insemination; but if the semen comes from a donor other than the husband, the procedure is identified as heterologous artificial insemination.

The absence of answers to many questions concerning heterologous artificial insemination may discourage couples from seeking to use the procedure and physicians from performing it. Some of the questions concern the procedure itself; others concern the status of the offspring and the effect of the procedure on the marital relationship.

Consent

The Oklahoma heterologous artificial insemination statute specifies that husband and wife must consent to the procedure.[47] It is obvious that the wife's consent must be obtained; without it, the touching involved in the artificial insemination would constitute a battery. Besides the wife's consent, it is important to obtain the husband's consent to ensure against liability accruing if a court adopted the view that without the consent of the husband, heterologous artificial insemination was a wrong to the husband's interest, for which he could sustain a suit for damages.

The Oklahoma statute also deals with establishing proof of consent. It requires the consent to be in writing, and it must be executed and acknowledged by the physician performing the procedure and by the local judge who has jurisdiction over the adoption of children, as well as by the husband and wife.

In states without specific statutory requirements, medical personnel should attempt to avoid such potential liability by establishing the practice of obtaining the written consent of the couple requesting the heterologous artificial insemination procedure.

Confidentiality

Another problem that directly concerns medical personnel involved in heterologous artificial insemination birth is preserving confidentiality. This problem is met in the Oklahoma heterologous artificial insemination statute, which requires that the original copy of the consent be filed pursuant to the rules for filing adoption papers and is not to be made a matter of public record.[48]

ORGAN DONATIONS

Federal regulations require that hospitals have, and implement, written protocols regarding their organ procurement responsibilities. The regulations impose specific notification duties, as well as other requirements concerning informing families of potential donors. It encourages discretion and sensitivity in dealing with the families and in educating hospital staff on a variety of issues involved with donation matters, in order to facilitate timely donation and transplantation.

Organ transplantation is done to treat patients with end-stage organ disease who face organ failure. Developments in medical science have enabled physicians to take tissue from persons immediately after death and use it to replace or rehabilitate diseased or damaged organs or other parts of living persons. Interest in organ transplantation began about 25 years ago when attempts were made to transplant kidneys between twins.[49] Success rates have improved because of better patient selection, improved clinical and operative management and skills, and immunosuppressant drugs that aid in decreasing the incidence of tissue rejection (e.g., cyclosporin A, which acts to suppress the production of antibodies that attack transplanted tissue). Yet this progress has created the problem of obtaining a sufficient supply of replacement body parts. There is a corresponding cry for more organs as the success rate in organ transplantation increases. Because of the fear of people buying and selling organs, the National Organ Procurement Act was enacted in 1984, making it illegal to buy or sell organs. Throughout the country, there are tissue banks and other facilities that store and preserve organs and tissue that can be used for transplantation and other therapeutic services.

The ever-increasing success of organ transplants and the demand for organ tissue require the close scrutiny of each case, to make sure that established procedures have been followed in the care and disposal of all body parts. Section 1138, Title XI, of the Omnibus Budget Reconciliation Act of 1986 requires hospitals to establish organ procurement protocols or face a loss of Medicare and Medicaid funding. Physicians, nurses, and other paramedical personnel assigned with this responsibility often are confronted with several legal issues. Liability can be limited by complying with applicable regulations. Organs and tissues to be stored and preserved for future use must be removed almost immediately after death. Therefore, it is imperative that an agreement or arrangement for obtaining organs and tissue from a body be completed before death, or very soon after death, to enable physicians to remove and store the tissue promptly.

There is a shortage of cadavers needed for medical education and transplantation. Some people may wish to make arrangements for the use of their bodies after death for such purposes. A surviving spouse may, however, object to such disposition. In such cases, the interest of the surviving spouse or other family member could supersede that of the deceased.

Uniform Anatomical Gift Act

The American Bar Association has endorsed a Uniform Anatomical Gift Act drafted by the Commission on Uniform State Laws. This statute has been enacted by all 50 states and has many detailed provisions that apply to the wide variety of issues raised in connection with the making, acceptance, and use of anatomic gifts. The Act allows a person to make a decision to donate organs at the time of death and allows potential donors to carry an anatomical donor card. State statutes regarding donation usually permit the donor to execute the gift during his or her lifetime.

The right to privacy of the donor and his or her family must be respected. Information should not be disseminated regarding transplant procedures that publish the names of the donor or donee without adequate consent.

States have enacted legislation to facilitate donation of bodies and body parts for medical uses. Virtually all the states have based their enactments on the Uniform Anatomical Gift Act, but it should be recognized that in some states there are deviations from this Act or additional laws dealing with donation.

Individuals who are of sound mind and 18 years of age or older are permitted to dispose of their own bodies or body parts by will or other written instrument for medical or dental education, research, advancement of medical or dental science, therapy, or transplantation. Among those eligible to receive such donations are any licensed, accredited, or approved hospitals; accredited medical or dental schools; surgeons or physicians; tissue banks; or specified individuals who need the donation for therapy or transplantation. The statute provides that when only a part of the body is donated, custody of the remaining parts of the body shall be transferred to the next of kin promptly after removal of the donated part.

A donation by will becomes effective immediately on the death of the testator, without probate, and the gift is valid and effective to the extent that it has been acted on in good faith. This is true even if the will is not probated or is declared invalid for testimonial purposes.

Failure to Obtain Consent

Although failure to obtain consent for removal of body tissue can give rise to a lawsuit, not all such claims are successful. In *Nicoletta v. Rochester Eye & Human Parts Bank*,[50] emotional injuries resulted from the removal of Nicoletta's son's eyes for donation after a fatal motorcycle accident. The hospital was immune from liability under the provisions of the Uniform Anatomical Gift Act because the hospital had neither actual nor constructive knowledge that the woman who had authorized the donation was not the decedent's wife. The hospital was entitled to the immunity afforded by the "good-faith" provisions of Section 4306(3) of the act in which its agents had made reasonable inquiry as to the status of the purported wife, who had resided with the decedent for 10 years and was the mother of their two children. The hospital had no reason to believe that any irregularity existed. The father, who was present at the time his son was brought to the emergency department, failed to object to any organ donation and failed to challenge the authority of the purported wife to sign the emergency department authorization.

There are several methods by which a donation may be revoked. If the document has been delivered to a named donee, it may be revoked by

- a written revocation signed by the donor and delivered to the donee,
- an oral revocation witnessed by two persons and communicated to the donee,
- a statement to the attending physician during a terminal illness that has been communicated to the donee, or
- a written statement that has been signed and on the donor's person or in the donor's immediate effects.

If the written instrument of donation has not been delivered to the donee, it may be revoked by destruction, cancellation, or mutilation of the instrument. If the donation is made by a will, it may be revoked in the manner provided for revocation or amendment of wills. Any person acting in good-faith reliance on the terms of an instrument of donation will not be subject to civil or criminal liability unless there is actual notice of the revocation of the donation.

RESEARCH, EXPERIMENTATION, AND CLINICAL TRIALS

A research study is designed to answer specific questions, sometimes about a drug or device's safety and its effectiveness. Being in a research study is different from being a patient. As a patient, one's personal physician has a great deal of freedom in making health care decisions. As a research subject, the Protocol Director and the research staff follow the rules of the research study (protocol) as closely as possible, without compromising the patient's health.[51]

Ethical principles relevant to the ethics of research involving human subjects include respect for person, beneficence, and justice. These principles cannot always be applied to resolve ethical problems beyond dispute. The objective in applying ethical principles is to provide an analytical framework that will guide the resolution of ethical problems arising from research involving human subjects.

Ethical considerations that must be addressed when conducting research on human subjects include personal autonomy; self-determination; the ethical considerations involved in using persons as subjects of research; the Hippocratic maxim of "do no harm" and the Hippocratic oath's requirement that physicians benefit their patients "according to their best judgment"; research involving subjects; and various meanings of the term "justice," such as whether burdens are to be distributed to each person equally, to each according to his needs, to each according to his societal contribution, or to each according to merit.

The science of medicine, by the very nature of that which it studies, the human body, is often prevented from making progress through direct experimentation. It must resort to necessary tests in laboratories and on animals, whose reactions are similar to humans. But most of all, it advances by observing how the body functions in health and in disease. It is natural that much of this laboratory experimentation and clinical observation should be done in the hospital. To increase the possibility of advancement by observation, clinical records must be accurate and complete in every case, no matter how trivial, and they should be preserved in such a manner as to be available for the study of similar cases. New remedies of all kinds should be tried out under conditions that favor accurate observation. Laboratories should be available under the direction of scientific physicians, and results of examinations should be carefully compiled and studied. Systematized research is possible only when directed by a physician with a scientific specialty, and it is rare not to find one such individual working in every hospital.

Medical progress and improved patient care are dependent on advances in medicine made through research. The basic principle of research is honesty, which must be ensured through institutional protocols. Fraud in research is not uncommon, and it must be condemned and punished. Honesty and integrity must govern all stages of research.

The Nuremberg Code and the Declaration of Helsinki is an international code of ethics that governs human research and experimentation. It was set in place after the discovery of Nazi medical atrocities of World War II. The code requires that human subjects be fully informed as to the nature and societal benefits of the research being undertaken. The code provides guidelines for the development of federal regulations for medical research and the protection of human subjects. Federal regulations control federal grants that apply to experiments involving new drugs, new medical devices, or new medical procedures. Generally, a combination of federal and state guidelines and regulations ensures proper supervision and control over experimentation that involves human subjects. For example, federal regulations require hospital-based researchers to obtain the approval of an institutional review board. This board functions to review proposed research studies and conduct follow-up reviews on a regular basis.

Informed Consent

Physicians have a clear duty to warn patients as to the risks and benefits of an experimental procedure, as well as the alternatives to a proposed experimental procedure.

Written consent should be obtained from each patient who participates in a clinical trial. Consent should include the risks, benefits, and alternatives to the proposed treatment protocol. The consent form must not contain any coercive or exculpatory language through which the patient is forced to waive his or her legal rights, including the release of the investigator, sponsor, or organization from liability for negligent conduct.

Organizations conducting clinical trials on human subjects, at the very least, must:

- fully disclose to the patient the inherent risks, benefits, and treatment alternatives to the proposed research protocol/s
- determine the competency of the patient to consent
- obtain written consent from the patient
- educate the staff as to the potential side effects, implementation of, and ongoing monitoring of protocols
- require financial disclosure issues associated with the protocols
    - promote awareness of ethical issues
    - promote education in regard to ethical decision making
    - increase nurse participation in ethical decision making
    - have ongoing monitoring of approved protocols

The following is a bill of rights developed by the Veterans Administration system for patients involved in research studies.

Experimental Subject's Bill of Rights

As a human subject, you have the following rights. These rights include, but are not limited to, the subject's right to:

- be informed of the nature and purpose of the experiment;
- be given an explanation of the procedures to be followed in the medical experiment, and any drug or device to be utilized;
- be given a description of any attendant discomforts and risks reasonably to be expected;
- be given an explanation of any benefits to the subject reasonably to be expected, if applicable;
- be given a disclosure of any appropriate alternatives, drugs, or devices that might be advantageous to the subject, their relative risks, and benefits;
- be informed of the avenues of medical treatment, if any, available to the subject after the experiment if complications should rise;
- be given an opportunity to ask questions concerning the experiment or the procedures involved;
- be instructed that consent to participate in the medical experiment may be withdrawn at any time and the subject may discontinue participation without prejudice;
- be given a copy of the signed and dated consent form; and
- be given the opportunity to decide to consent or not to consent to a medical experiment without the intervention of any element of force, fraud, deceit, duress, coercion, or undue influence on the subject's decision.[52]

Medical Research: Duty to Warn

About 5,000 patients at Michael Reese Hospital and Medical Center, located in Chicago, Illinois, were treated with X-ray therapy for some benign conditions of the head and neck from 1930 to 1960. Among them was Joel Blaz, now a citizen of Florida, who received this treatment for infected tonsils and adenoids while a child in Illinois from 1947 through 48. He has suffered various tumors, which he now attributes to this treatment. Blaz was diagnosed with a neural tumor in 1987.

In 1974, Michael Reese set up a Thyroid Follow-Up Project to gather data and conduct research among the people who had been subjected to the X-ray therapy. In 1975, the Program notified Blaz by mail that he was at increased risk of developing thyroid tumors because of the treatment. In 1976, someone associated with the Program gave him similar information by phone and invited him to return to Michael Reese for evaluation and treatment at his own expense, which he declined to do.

Dr. Arthur Schneider was put in charge of the Program in 1977. In 1979, Schneider and Michael Reese submitted a research proposal to the National Institutes of Health stating that a study based on the Program showed "strong evidence" of a connection between X-ray treatments of the sort administered to Blaz and various sorts of tumors: thyroid, neural, and other. In 1981, Blaz received but did not complete or return a questionnaire attached to a letter from Schneider in connection with the Program. The letter stated that the purpose of the questionnaire was to "investigate the long-term health implications" of childhood radiation treatments and to "determine the possible associated risks." It did not say anything about "strong evidence" of a connection between the treatments and any tumors.

In 1996, after developing neural tumors, Blaz sued Michael Reese's successor, Galen Hospital in Illinois, and Dr. Schneider, alleging, among other things, that they failed to notify and warn him of their findings that he might be at greater risk of neural tumors in a way that might have permitted their earlier detection and removal or other treatment. There is a clear duty to warn the subject of previously administered radiation treatments when there is a strong connection between those treatments and certain kinds of tumors. The harm alleged, neural and other tumors, would here be reasonably foreseeable as a likely consequence of a failure to warn, and was in fact foreseen by Schneider. A reasonable physician, indeed any reasonable person, could foresee that if someone were warned of "strong evidence" of a connection between treatments to which he had been subjected and tumors, he would probably seek diagnosis or treatment and perhaps avoid these tumors, and if he were not warned he probably would not seek diagnosis or treatment, increasing the likelihood that he would suffer from such tumors. Other things being equal, therefore, a reasonable physician would warn the subject of the treatments.[53]

Food and Drug Administration

Clinical trials for investigational drugs are regulated by the Food and Drug Administration (FDA). The FDA, after much criticism over the years because of the red tape involved in the approval of new drugs, issued rules to speed up the approval process. The rules permit the use of experimental drugs outside a controlled clinical trial if the drugs are used to treat a life-threatening condition. However, clinical trials of new drugs and medical devices have been referred to as endangered because manufacturers have been taking their devices overseas for faster approvals.

Patients participating in research studies should fully understand the implications of their participation. Health care organizations involved in research studies should have appropriate protocols in place that protect the rights of patients. Consent forms should describe both the risks and benefits involved in the research activity.

Institutional Review Board

Each organization conducting medical research must have a mechanism in place for approving and overseeing the use of investigational protocols. This is accomplished through the establishment of an Institutional Review Board (IRB). An IRB is a committee designated by an institution to provide initial approval and periodic monitoring for biomedical research studies. The IRB should include community representation. The IRB's primary responsibilities include:

- protecting the rights and welfare of human subjects
- ensuring protocols are presented by the sponsor(s)
- ensuring sponsor(s) of a protocol discloses
  - areas of concern that might give the impression of a conflict of interest in the outcome of the clinical research
  - financial interests that might occur should the clinical trials prove to be successful or give the impression of success, including stock options and cash payouts
- reviewing, monitoring, and approving clinical protocols for investigations of drugs and medical devices involving human subjects
- ensuring that the rights, including the privacy and confidentiality, of each individual are protected
- ensuring that all research is conducted within appropriate state and federal guidelines (e.g., FDA guidelines)

Nursing Facilities

The Centers for Medicare and Medicaid Services survey process includes a review of the rights of any nursing facility residents participating in experimental research. Surveyors will review the records of residents identified as participating in a clinical research study. They will determine whether informed consent forms have been executed properly. The form will be reviewed to determine whether all known risks have been identified. Appropriate questions may be directed to both the staff and residents or the residents' guardians.

Possible questions to ask staff include:

- Is the facility participating in any experimental research?
- If yes, what residents are involved? (Interview a sample of these residents.)[54]
- Residents or guardians may be asked questions such as:
  - Are you participating in the study?
  - Was this explained to you well enough so that you understand what the study is about and any risks that might be involved?[55]

Patients participating in research studies should fully understand the implications of their participation. Health care organizations involved in research studies should have appropriate protocols in place that protect the rights of patients. Consent forms should describe both the risks and benefits involved in the research activity.

> My . . . husband participated in a clinical trial involving both an autologus (self) and allogeneic (donor) transplant for a hopeful cure of the disease. We both understood the risks involved and the no-promise guarantee, as such is the nature of a clinical trial. The ultimate responsibility for whatever the outcome rested with us, as we were the ones who voluntarily entered into the program. Three years

later, we have just learned of the disease's progression, but we continue to look forward, remain optimistic, and support those who dedicate their lives for the betterment of those afflicted with these cursed cancers.

• • •

The reality is that someday, probably sooner than later, my husband will lose the battle with this tenacious enemy, but we are still thankful for the compassionate and learned members of the Fred Hutchinson Cancer Research Center who helped and are still helping us to navigate a most challenging road.[56]

STERILIZATION

Sterilization is the termination of the ability to produce offspring. Sterilization often is accomplished by either a vasectomy for men or a tubal ligation for women. A *vasectomy* is a surgical procedure in which the vas deferens is severed and tied to prevent the flow of the seminal fluid into the urinary canal. A *tubal ligation* is a surgical procedure in which the fallopian tubes are cut and tied, preventing passage of the ovum from the ovary to the uterus. Sterilizations are often sought because of

- economic necessity, to avoid the additional expense of raising a child
- therapeutic purposes, to prevent harm to a woman's health (e.g., to remove a diseased reproductive organ)
- genetic reasons, to prevent the birth of a defective child

Elective Sterilization

Voluntary or elective sterilizations on competent individuals present few legal problems, so long as proper consent has been obtained from the patient and the procedure is performed properly. Civil liability for performing a sterilization of convenience may be imposed if the procedure is performed in a negligent manner.

Regulation of Sterilization

Like abortion, voluntary sterilization is the subject of many debates concerning its moral and ethical propriety. Some health care institutions have adopted policies restricting the performance of such operations at their facilities.

Therapeutic Sterilization

If the life or health of a woman may be jeopardized by pregnancy, the danger may be avoided by terminating her ability to conceive or her husband's ability to impregnate. Such an operation is a therapeutic sterilization—one performed to preserve life or health. The medical necessity for sterilization renders the procedure therapeutic. Sometimes a diseased reproductive organ has to be removed to preserve the life or health of the individual. The operation results in sterility, although this was not the primary reason for the procedure. Such an operation technically should not be classified as a sterilization because the sterilization is incidental to the medical purpose.

Eugenic Sterilization

The term *eugenic sterilization* refers to the involuntary sterilization of certain categories of persons described in statutes, without the need for consent by, or on behalf of, those subject to the procedures. Persons classified as mentally deficient, feebleminded, and, in some instances, epileptic are included within the scope of the statutes. Several states also have included certain sexual deviates and persons classified as habitual criminals. Such statutes ordinarily are said to be designed to prevent the transmission of hereditary defects to succeeding generations, but several statutes also have recognized the purpose of preventing procreation by individuals who would not be able to care for their offspring.

Although there have been many judicial decisions to the contrary, the United States Supreme Court in *Buck v. Bell*[57] specifically upheld the validity of such eugenic sterilization statutes, provided that certain procedural safeguards are observed.

Several states have laws authorizing eugenic sterilization. The decision in *Wade v. Bethesda Hospital*[58] strongly suggests that in the absence of statutory authority, the state cannot order sterilization for eugenic purposes. At the minimum, eugenic sterilization statutes provide the following: a grant of authority to public officials supervising state institutions for the mentally ill or prisons and to certain public health officials to conduct sterilizations; a requirement of personal notice to the person subject to sterilization and, if that person is unable to comprehend what is involved, notice to the person's legal representative, guardian, or nearest relative; a hearing by the board designated in the particular statute to determine the propriety of the prospective sterilization; at the hearing, evidence may be presented, and the patient must be present or represented by counsel or the nearest relative or guardian; and an opportunity to appeal the board's ruling to a court.

The procedural safeguards of notice, hearing, and the right to appeal must be present in sterilization statutes to fulfill the minimum constitutional requirements of due process. An Arkansas statute was found to be unconstitutional in that it did not provide for notice to the incompetent patient and opportunity to be heard, or for the patient's entitlement to legal counsel.[59]

WRONGFUL BIRTH, WRONGFUL LIFE, AND WRONGFUL CONCEPTION

There is substantial legal debate regarding the impact of an improperly performed sterilization. Suits have been brought on such theories as wrongful birth, wrongful life, and wrongful conception. Wrongful life suits are generally unsuccessful, primarily because of the court's unwillingness, for public policy reasons, to permit financial recovery for the "injury" of being born into the world.

However, some success has been achieved in litigation by the patient (and his or her spouse) who allegedly was sterilized and subsequently proved fertile. Damages have been awarded for the cost of the unsuccessful procedure; pain and suffering as a result of the pregnancy; the medical expense of the pregnancy; and the loss of comfort, companionship services, and consortium of the spouse. Again, as a matter of public policy, the courts have indicated that the joys and benefits of having the child outweigh the cost incurred in the rearing process.

There have been many cases in recent years involving actions for wrongful birth, wrongful life, and wrongful conception. Such litigation originated with the California case in which a court found that a genetic testing laboratory can be held liable for damages from incorrectly reporting genetic tests, leading to the birth of a child with defects.[60] Injury caused by birth had not been previously actionable by law. The court of appeals held that medical laboratories engaged in genetic testing owe a duty to parents and their unborn child to use ordinary care in administering available tests for the purpose of providing information concerning potential genetic defects in the unborn. Damages in this case were awarded on the basis of the child's shortened life span.

Wrongful Birth

In a *wrongful birth* action, the plaintiffs claim that but for a breach of duty by the defendant(s) (e.g., improper sterilization), the child would not have been born. A wrongful birth claim can be brought by the parent(s) of a child born with genetic defects against a physician who or a laboratory that negligently fails to inform them, in a timely fashion, of an increased possibility that the mother will give birth to such a child, therefore precluding an informed decision as to whether to have the child.

In a New Jersey case, *Canesi ex rel. v. Wilson*,[61] the New Jersey Supreme Court reviewed the dismissal of an action for wrongful birth on the claim of the parents that, had the mother been informed of the risk that a drug, Provera, which she had been taking before she learned that she was pregnant, might cause the fetus to be born with congenital anomalies, such as limb reduction, she would have decided to abort the fetus. It was alleged that the physicians failed to disclose the risks associated with the drug. The physicians argued that the informed consent doctrine requires that the plaintiffs establish that the drug in fact caused the birth anomalies. The court rejected the argument and distinguished the wrongful birth action from one based on informed consent:

> In sum, the informed consent and wrongful birth causes of action are similar in that both require the physician to disclose those medically accepted risks that a reasonably prudent patient in the plaintiff's

position would deem material to her decision. What is or is not a medically acceptable risk is informed by what the physician knows or ought to know of the patient's history and condition. These causes of action, however, have important differences. They encompass different compensable harms and measures of damages. In both causes of action, the plaintiff must prove not only that a reasonably prudent patient in her position, if apprised of all material risks, would have elected a different course of treatment or care. In an informed consent case, the plaintiff must additionally meet a two-pronged test for proximate causation: She must prove that the undisclosed risk actually materialized and that it was medically caused by the treatment. In a wrongful birth case, on the other hand, a plaintiff need not prove that the doctor's negligence was the medical cause of her child's birth defect. Rather, the test of proximate causation is satisfied by showing that an undisclosed fetal risk was material to a woman in her position; the risk materialized, was reasonably foreseeable and not remote in relation to the doctor's negligence; and, had plaintiff known of that risk, she would have terminated her pregnancy. The emotional distress and economic loss resulting from this lost opportunity to decide for herself whether or not to terminate the pregnancy constitute plaintiff's damages.[62]

With the increasing consolidation of hospital services and physician practices, a case could be made for finding a hospital liable for the physician's failure to obtain informed consent where the hospital actually owns or controls the physician's practice or where both the hospital and the physician's practice are owned or controlled by another corporation that sets policy for both the hospital and the physician's practice.

Wrongful Life

A *wrongful life* claim is brought by the parent(s) or child who claims to have suffered harm as a result of being born. The plaintiffs generally contend that the physician or laboratory negligently failed to inform the child's parents of the risk of bearing a genetically defective infant and hence prevented the parents' right to choose to avoid the birth.[63] Because there is no recognized legal right not to be born, wrongful life cases are generally not successful.

[L]egal recognition that a disabled life is an injury would harm the interests of those most directly concerned, the handicapped. Disabled persons face obvious physical difficulties in conducting their lives. They also face subtle yet equally devastating handicaps in the attitudes and behavior of society, the law, and their own families and friends. Furthermore, society often views disabled persons as burdensome misfits. Recent legislation concerning employment, education, and building access reflects a slow change in these attitudes. This change evidences a growing public awareness that the handicapped can be valuable and productive members of society. To characterize the life of a disabled person as an injury would denigrate both this new awareness and the handicapped themselves.[64]

A cause of action for wrongful life was not cognizable under Kansas law in *Bruggeman v. Schimke*.[65] Human life is valuable, precious, and worthy of protection. Not to be born rather than to be alive with deformities cannot be recognized. The Kansas Supreme Court held that there was no recognized cause for wrongful life.

In *Kassama v. Magat*,[66] Kassama alleged that Dr. Magat failed to advise her of the results of an alpha-fetoprotein blood test that indicated a heightened possibility that her child, Ibrion, might be afflicted with Down syndrome. Had she received that information, Kassama contends, she would have undergone amniocentesis, which would have confirmed that prospect. Kassama claims, if that occurred, she would have chosen to terminate the pregnancy through an abortion.

The Supreme Court of Maryland decided that for purposes of tort law, an impaired life was not worse than non-life, and, for that reason, life itself was not, and could not be considered an injury. There was no evidence that Ibrion was not deeply loved and cared for by her parents or that she did not return that love. Studies have shown that people afflicted with Down syndrome can lead productive and meaningful lives. They can be educated, employed, form friendships, and get along in society. Allowing a recovery of extraordinary life expenses on some theory of fairness—that the physician or his or her insurance company should pay not because the physician caused the injury or impairment but because the child was born—ignores that fundamental issue.

Wrongful birth is based on the premise that being born, and having to live, with the affliction is a disadvantage and thus a cognizable injury. The injury sued upon is the fact that Ibrion was born; she bears the disability and will bear the expenses only because, but for the alleged negligence of Magat, her mother was unable to terminate the pregnancy and avert her birth. The issue here is whether Maryland law is prepared to recognize that kind of injury—the injury of life itself.

The child has not suffered any damage cognizable at law by being brought into existence. One of the most deeply held beliefs of our society is that life, whether experienced with or without a major physical handicap, is more precious than nonlife. No one is perfect, and each person suffers from some ailments or defects, whether major or minor, that make impossible participation in all the activities life has to offer. Our lives are not thereby rendered less precious than those of others whose defects are less pervasive or less severe. Despite their handicaps, the Down syndrome child is able to love and be loved and to experience happiness and pleasure—emotions that are truly the essence of life and that are far more valuable than the suffering that may be endured.

The right to life and the principle that all are equal under the law are basic to our constitutional order. To presume to decide that a child's life is not worth living would be to forsake these ideals. To characterize the life of a disabled person as an injury would denigrate the handicapped themselves. Measuring the value of an impaired life as compared to nonexistence is a task that is beyond mortals.

Unless a judgment can be made on the basis of reason rather than the emotion of any given case, that nonlife is preferable to impaired life—that the child-plaintiff would, in fact, have been better off had he or she never been born—there can be no injury; and, if there can be no injury, whether damages can or cannot be calculated becomes irrelevant.

The crucial question, a value judgment about life itself, is too deeply immersed in each person's own individual philosophy or theology to be subject to a reasoned and consistent community response, in the form of a jury verdict.

Wrongful Conception

Wrongful conception or *wrongful pregnancy* refers to a claim for damages sustained by the parents of an unexpected child based on an allegation that conception of the child resulted from negligent sterilization procedures or a defective contraceptive device.[67] Damages sought for a negligently performed sterilization might include

- pain and suffering associated with pregnancy and birth
- expenses of delivery
- lost wages
- father's loss of consortium
- damages for emotional or psychological pain
- suffering resulting from the presence of an additional family member in the household
- the cost and pain and suffering of a subsequent sterilization
- damages suffered by a child born with genetic defects

The most controversial item of damages claimed is that of raising a normal healthy child to adulthood. The mother in *Hartke v. McKelway*[68] had undergone a sterilization for therapeutic reasons to avoid endangering her health from pregnancy. The woman became pregnant as a result of a failed sterilization. She delivered a healthy child without injury to herself. It was determined that "the jury could not rationally have found that the birth of this child was an injury to this plaintiff. Awarding child-rearing expense would only give Hartke a windfall."[69]

The cost of raising a healthy newborn child to adulthood was recoverable by the parents of the child conceived as a result of an unsuccessful sterilization by a physician employee at Lovelace Medical Center. The physician in *Lovelace Medical Center v. Mendez*[70] found and ligated only one of the patient's two fallopian tubes and then failed to inform the patient of the unsuccessful operation. The court held that:

the Mendezes' interest in the financial security of their family was a legally protected interest which was invaded by Lovelace's negligent failure properly to perform Maria's sterilization operation (if proved at trial), and that this invasion was an injury entitling them to recover damages in the form of the reasonable expenses to raise Joseph to majority.[71]

Some states bar damage claims for emotional distress and the costs associated with the raising of healthy children but will permit recovery for damages related to negligent sterilizations. In *Butler v. Rolling Hills Hospital*,[72] the Pennsylvania Superior Court held that the patient stated a cause of action for the negligent performance of a laparoscopic tubal ligation. The patient was not, however, entitled to compensation for the costs of raising a normal healthy child. "In light of this Commonwealth's public policy, which recognizes the paramount importance of the family to society, we conclude that the benefits of joy, companionship, and affection which a normal, healthy child can provide must be deemed as a matter of law to outweigh the costs of raising that child."[73]

As the Court of Common Pleas of Lycoming County, Pennsylvania, in *Shaheen v. Knight*, stated:

> Many people would be willing to support this child were they given the right of custody and adoption, but according to plaintiff's statement, plaintiff does not want such. He wants to have the child and wants the doctor to support it. In our opinion, to allow such damages would be against public policy.[74]

CASE: NEGLIGENT STERILIZATION

Chaffee performed a partial salpingectomy on Seslar. The purpose of the procedure was to sterilize Seslar, who had already borne four children, so that she could not become pregnant again. After undergoing the surgery, however, Seslar conceived and delivered a healthy baby. Seslar sued Chaffee.

The Court of Appeals held that damages for the alleged negligent sterilization procedure could not include the costs of raising a normal healthy child. Although raising an unplanned child is costly, all human life is presumptively invaluable. A child, regardless of the circumstances of birth, does not constitute *harm* to the parents so as to permit recovery for the costs associated with raising and educating the child. As with a majority of jurisdictions, the court held that the value of a child's life to the parents outweighs the associated pecuniary burdens as a matter of law. Recoverable damages may include pregnancy and childbearing expenses, but not the ordinary costs of raising and educating a normal, healthy child conceived following an allegedly negligent sterilization procedure.[75]

Ethical and Legal Issues

1. Do you agree with the court's decision?
2. Under what circumstances would you not agree with the court's decision?
3. Describe the ethical issues in this case. ■

CHAPTER REVIEW

1. An ethical dilemma arises whenever a choice has to be made in which something good has to be given up or something bad has to be suffered no matter what is chosen.
2. Abortion is the premature termination of a pregnancy, either spontaneous or induced.
3. The morality of abortion is not a legal or constitutional issue; it is a matter of philosophy, of ethics, and of theology. It is a subject upon which reasonable people can, and do, adhere to vastly divergent convictions and principles.
4. A partial birth abortion is a late-term abortion that involves partial delivery of the baby prior to its being aborted.
5. Acquired immune deficiency syndrome is a fatal disease that destroys the body's ability to fight bacteria and viruses.
6. Artificial insemination most often takes the form of the injection of seminal fluid into a woman to induce pregnancy. Homologous artificial insemination is when the husband's semen is used in the procedure. Heterologous artificial insemination is when the semen is from a donor other than the husband.
7. Federal regulations require that hospitals have, and implement, written protocols regarding the organization's organ procurement responsibilities.
8. Organ transplantation is the result of the need for treating patients with end-stage organ disease and who face organ failure.
9. The Uniform Anatomical Gift Act has many provisions that apply to the wide variety of issues raised in connection with the making, acceptance, and use of anatomic gifts. The Act allows a person to make a decision to donate organs at the time of death and allows potential donors to carry an anatomical donor card.
10. Ethical principles that are relevant to the ethics of research involving human subjects include respect for person, beneficence, and justice. These principles cannot always be applied to resolve ethical problems beyond dispute. The objective in applying ethical principles is to provide an analytical framework that will guide the resolution of ethical problems arising from research involving human subjects.
11. Sterilization is defined as the termination of the ability to produce offspring.

12. As long as proper consent is obtained and the procedure is performed properly, elective sterilizations present few legal problems. A therapeutic sterilization is performed to preserve life or health.

13. Wrongful birth actions claim that, but for breach of duty by the defendant, a child would not have been born. Wrongful life suits—those in which a parent or child claims to have suffered harm as a result of being born—are generally unsuccessful. Wrongful conception/pregnancy actions claim that damages were sustained by the parents of an unexpected child based on the allegation that the child's conception was the result of negligent sterilization procedures or a defective contraceptive device.

TEST YOUR UNDERSTANDING

Terminology

ethical dilemma	institutional review board
abortion	sterilization
Roe v. Wade	elective sterilization
partial birth abortion	therapeutic sterilization
AIDS	eugenic sterilization
artificial insemination	wrongful birth
Uniform Anatomical Gift Act	wrongful life

REVIEW QUESTIONS

1. What ethical principles are involved in performing an abortion? Does performing an abortion break any of the principles discussed in Chapter 1? If yes, which ones? Discuss your answer.

2. Do you agree that individual states should be able to place reasonable restrictions or waiting periods for abortion? Who should determine what is reasonable?

3. Should a married woman be allowed to abort without her husband's consent?

4. Discuss the arguments for and against partial birth abortions.

5. Why is the medical issue of abortion an example of legislating morality?

6. Describe the concerns of confidentiality and nonmaleficence as it relates to AIDS patients.

REVIEW QUESTIONS (continued)

7. Why is it important that a written consent be obtained from each patient who participates in a clinical trial?

8. Do you agree that eugenic sterilization should be allowed? Explain your answer.

9. Describe the distinctions among wrongful birth, wrongful life, and wrongful conception. Discuss the moral dilemmas of these concepts.

WEB SITES

American Association of Tissue Banks
www.aatb.org
Association of Organ Procurement Organizations
www.aopo.org
American Society of Transplantation
www.a-s-t.org
Coalition on Donation
www.shareyourlife.org
Eye Bank Association of America
www.restoresight.org
HHS Health Resources and Services Administration
www.hrsa.gov/osp/dot
Michigan Electronic Library Health Info
mel.org/health/health-disease-cancer-bo.html
Minority Organ Tissue Transplant Education Program
www.nationalmottep.org
National Marrow Donor Program
www.marrow.org
Scientific Registry of Transplant Recipients
www.organdonor.gov
United Network for Organ Sharing
www.unos.org
VA Consent Form
http://humansubjects.stanford.edu/medical/VASampCons.html

NOTES

1. Union Pac. Ry. Co. v. Botsford, 141 U.S. 250, 251 (1891).
2. English Clergy, Dean of Westminster.
3. Causeway Medical Suite v. Ieyoub, 109 F.3d 1096 (1997).
4. 410 U.S. 113 (1973).

5. *Id.* at 164.
6. *Id.*
7. *Id.*
8. *Id.*
9. 410 U.S. 179 (1973).
10. *Id.* at 198.
11. 428 U.S. 52 (1976).
12. 432 U.S. 464 (1977).
13. 99 S. Ct. 675 (1979).
14. 443 U.S. 622 (1979).
15. 448 U.S. 297 (1980).
16. 101 S. Ct. 1164 (1981).
17. 103 S. Ct. 2481 (1983).
18. 492 U.S. 490 (1989).
19. 111 S. Ct. 1759 (1991).
20. Planned Parenthood v. Casey, 112 S. Ct. 2792 (1992).
21. 118 S. Ct. 1347 (1998)..
22. 844 F. Supp. 1482 (D. Utah 1994).
23. 112 S. Ct. 2791 (1992).
24. 844 F. Supp. 1482 (D. Utah 1994) at 1494.
25. Poe v. Gerstein, 517 F.2d 787 (5th Cir. 1975).
26. 405 F. Supp. 534 (M.D. Pa.1975).
27. 486 U.S. 1308 (1988).
28. 533 A.2d 523 (R.I. 1987).
29. 515 So. 2d 1254 (Ala. Civ. App. 1987).
30. 107 F. Supp. 2d 1271 (2000).
31. COLO. REV. STAT. § 12-37.5-101 et seq. (1998).
31b. Planned Parenthood of the Rocky Mts. Servs. Corp. v. Owens, 287 F.3d 910   (10th Cir. 2002).
32. American Acad. of Pediatrics v. Lungren, 940 P.2d 797 (1997).
33. Cantwell, *AIDS: The Mystery and the Solutions*, L.A. (1986), at 54.
34. JOINT UNITED NATIONS PROGRAMME ON HIV/AIDS, AIDS EPIDEMIC UPDATE: DECEMBER 2000, UNAIDS/00.44E—WHO/CDS/CSR/EDC/2000.9. http://www.unaids.org.
35. Bramer v. Dotson, 437 S.E.2d 775 (W. Va. 1993).
36. 592 A.2d 1251 (N.J. Super. Ct. Law Div. 1991).
37. *Id.* at 1255.
38. 592 A.2d 1251 (N.J. Super. Ct. Law Div. 1991).
39. *Id.* at 1255.
40. 734 S.W.2d 675 (Tex. Ct. App. 1987).
41. 538 N.E.2d 419 (Ohio Ct. App. 1988).
42. Application of Milton S. Hershey Med. Ctr., 639 A.2d 159, 163 (Pa. 1993).
43. ETHICS COMMITTEE OF THE AMERICAN ACADEMY OF DERMATOLOGY, ETHICS IN MEDICAL PRACTICE, 1992, at 6.
44. 554 A.2d 954 (Pa. Super. Ct. 1989).
45. 640 So. 2d 476 (La. App. 3d Cir. 1994).
46. http://msnbc.msn.com/id/4505640/.
47. OKLA. STAT. ANN. 10, §§ 551–553.
48. OKLA. STAT. ANN. 10, §§ 551–553.
49. U.S. DEPT. OF HEALTH & HUMAN SERVICES, TASK FORCE ON ORGAN DONATION AND TRANSPLANTATION (1986).
50. 519 N.Y.S.2d 928 (N.Y. Sup. Ct. 1987).

51. http://humansubjects.stanford.edu/medical/VASampCons.html.

52. *Id.*

53. Blaz v. Michael Reese Hosp. Found., 74 F. Supp. 2d 803 (D.C. Ill. 1999).

54. 2 C.F.R. § 488.115 (1989).

55. *Id.*

56. Stokes, Mary Ellen and Bill, *Relentless Assault on a Research Hospital*, WALL ST. J., March 15, 2004, at A17.

57. 224 U.S. 200 (1927).

58. 337 F. Supp. 671 (E.D. Ohio 1971).

59. McKinney v. McKinney, 805 S.W.2d 66 (Ark. 1991).

60. 165 Cal. Rptr. 477 (Cal. Ct. App. 1980).

61. 730 A.2d 806 (N.J. 1999).

62. *Id.* at 18.

63. Smith v. Cote, 513 A.2d 344 (N.H. 1986).

64. *Id.* at 353.

65. 718 P.2d 635 (Kan. 1986).

66. 136 Md. App. 38 (2002).

67. Cowe v. Forum Group, Inc., 575 N.E.2d 630, 631 (Ind. 1991).

68. 707 F.2d 1544 (D.C. Cir. 1983).

69. *Id.* at 1557.

70. 805 P.2d 603 (N.M. 1991).

71. *Id.* at 612.

72. 582 A.2d 1384 (Pa. Super. Ct. 1990).

73. *Id.* at 1385.

74. 11 Pa. D. & C.2d 41, 46 (Lycoming Co. Ct. Com. Pl. 1957).

75. Chaffee v. Seslar, 786 N.E.2d 705 (2003).

chapter three

Health Care
Ethics Committee

LEARNING OBJECTIVES

The reader upon completion of this chapter will be able to:

- Understand the importance, development, structure, and goals of ethics committees

- Describe the functions of the ethics committee:

  ○ Policy and procedure development

  ○ Educational role

  ○ Consultation and conflict resolution

- Describe the expanding role of the ethics committee

- Describe the concept of reasoning and decision making

INTRODUCTION

Health care ethics committees are responsible for addressing ethical-legal issues that arise during the course of a patient's care and treatment. Ethics committees serve as a resource for patients, families, and staff. They offer objective counsel when dealing with difficult health care dilemmas. Ethics committees provide both educational and consultative services to patients, families, and caregivers. They enhance but do not replace important patient/family–physician relationships, yet they afford support for decisions made within those relationships.

The numerous ethical questions facing health professionals involve the entire life span, from the right to be born to the right to die. Ethics committees concern themselves with issues of morality, patient autonomy, legislation, and states' interests.

Although ethics committees first emerged in the 1960s in the United States, attention was focused on them in the 1976 landmark Quinlan case,[1] where parents of Karen Ann Quinlan were granted permission by the New Jersey Supreme Court to remove Karen from a ventilator after she had been in a coma for a year. She died 10 years later at the age of 31, having been in a persistent vegetative state the entire time. The Quinlan court looked to a prognosis committee to verify Karen's medical condition. It then factored in the committee's opinion with all other evidence to reach the decision to allow withdrawing her life-support equipment. To date, ethics committees do not have sole surrogate decision-making authority. However, they play an ever-expanding role in the development of policy and procedural guidelines to assist in resolving ethical dilemmas.

Most organizations describe the functioning of the ethics committee and how to access the committee at the time of admission in patient handbooks and informational brochures.

COMMITTEE STRUCTURE

To be successful, an ethics committee should be structured to include a wide range of community leaders in positions of political stature, respect, and diversity. The ethics committee should be comprised of a multidisciplinary group of people, whose membership should include an ethicist, educators, clinicians, legal advisors, and political leaders as well as members of the clergy, a quality improvement manager, and corporate leaders from the business community. Ethics committees all too often are comprised mostly of hospital employees and members of the medical staff with a token representation from the community.

GOALS OF THE ETHICS COMMITTEE

Ethics committees should:

- support and foster decision making by providing guidance to patients, families, and decision makers

- review cases, as requested, when there are conflicts in basic values and assist in clarifying situations that are ethical, legal, or religious in nature that extend beyond the scope of daily practice
- help clarify issues, discuss alternatives, and compromises
- provide institutional input and perspective
- determine what should trigger an ethics consultation
- facilitate knowledgeable reflection on ethical issues and concerns
- provide guidance, not decisions
- promote the rights of patients
- promote shared decision making between patients and their clinicians
- assist the patient and family, as appropriate, in coming to consensus with the options that best meet the patient's goal for care
- promote fair policies and procedures that maximize the likelihood of achieving good, patient-centered outcomes, and
- enhance the ethical tenor of both health care organizations and professionals.

COMMITTEE FUNCTIONS

The functions of ethics committees are multifaceted and include development of policy and procedure guidelines to assist in resolving ethical dilemmas; staff and community education; conflict resolution; case reviews, support, and consultation; and political advocacy. The degree to which an ethics committee serves each of these functions varies in different health care organizations.

Policy and Procedure Development

The ethics committee is a valuable resource for developing hospital policies and procedures to assist health care professionals in making difficult decisions.

Educational Role

The ethics committee typically provides education on current ethical concepts and issues to committee members, staff, and the community at large. Some community hospitals provide ethics education to the staff at ambulatory care facilities, home health agencies, long-term care facilities, and physicians' offices. Such education helps reduce the need for emergent end-of-life consultations in acute care settings.

The ethics committee helps to develop resources for educational purposes to help staff develop the appropriate competencies for addressing ethical, legal, and spiritual issues. Educational programs on ethical issues are developed for ethics committee members, staff, patients, and the community (e.g., how to prepare an advance directive).

Consultation and Conflict Resolution

Ethics committees often provide consultation services for patients, families, and caregivers struggling with difficult treatment decisions and end-of-life dilemmas. Always mindful of its basic orientation toward the patient's best interests, the committee provides options and suggestions for resolution of conflict in actual cases. Consultation with an ethics committee is not mandatory, but is conducted at the request of a physician, patient, family member, or other caregiver.

The ethics committee strives to provide viable alternatives that will lead to the optimal resolution of dilemmas confronting the continuing care of the patient. It is important to remember that an ethics committee functions in an advisory capacity and should not be considered a substitute proxy for the patient.

Requests for an ethics committee consultation often involve
• clarification of issues regarding decision-making capacity, informed consent, and advance directives,
• do not resuscitate orders,
• withdrawal of treatment, and
• assistance in conflict resolution.

Consultations must be conducted in a timely manner. The ethics committee member initially contacted should consider the following:

• Who requested the consultation?
• What are the issues?
• Is there is a problem that needs referral to another service?
• What specifically is being requested of the ethics committee (e.g., clarification of the problem or mediation)?

When conducting a consultation, all patient records must be reviewed and discussed with the attending physician, family members, and other caregivers involved in the patient's treatment. If an issue can be resolved easily, a designated member of the ethics committee should be able to consult on the case without the need for a full committee meeting. If the problem is unusual, problematic, delicate, or has important legal ramifications, a full committee meeting should be called. Others who can be invited to an ethics committee case review, as appropriate, include the patient, if competent; relatives, agent, or surrogate decision maker; and caregivers.

Evaluation of a case consultation should take the following into consideration:

• patient's current medical status, diagnosis, and prognosis
• benefits and burdens of recommended treatment, or alternative treatments

- effect(s) of no treatment
- life expectancy, treated and untreated
- views of caregivers and consultants
- pain and suffering
- quality-of-life issues
- financial burden on family (e.g., if the patient is in a comatose state with no hope of recovery, should the spouse deplete his or her finances to maintain the spouse on a respirator).

Decisions concerning patient care must take into consideration the patient's

- value system,
- personal assessment of the quality of life,
- current expressed choices,
- advance directives,
- competency to make decisions,
- ability to process information rationally to compare risks, benefits, and alternatives to treatment,
- ability to articulate major factors in decisions and reasons for them, and
- ability to communicate.

The patient must have all the information necessary to allow a reasonable person to make a prudent decision on his or her own behalf. The patient's choice must be voluntary and free from coercion by family, physicians, or others.

Family members must be identified and the following questions considered when making decisions:

- Do family members understand the patient's wishes?
- Is the family in agreement with what is believed to be the patient's wishes?
- Does the patient have an advance directive?
- Has the patient appointed an agent?
- Are there any religious proscriptions?
- Are there any financial concerns?
- Are there any legal factors (applicable state statutes and case law)?

When an ethics committee is engaged in the consulting process, its recommendations should be offered as suggestions, imposing no obligation for acceptance on the part of the patient, organization, its governing body, medical staff, attending physicians, or other persons. Exhibit 3–1 presents a suggested form for documenting an ethics committee consultation.

ETHICS CONSULTATION

Date: _____ Time: _____ Caller: _____

Reason for call: _____

Action taken: _____

Patient: _____ Age: _____ Record #: _____

Consultation requested by: _____ Relationship (e.g., caregiver, spouse) _____

Attending physician: _____ Other physicians: _____

Will the patient participate in the consultation? ❏ Yes ❏ No

Does the patient have decision-making capacity? ❏ Yes ❏ No Explain _____

Surrogate decision maker? ❏ Yes ❏ No If yes, name: _____

Phone #: _____ Advance directives (e.g., living will)? _____

Availability of advance directive _____

Consultation participants:

❏ Family/relationship _____

❏ Physicians _____

❏ Nurses _____

❏ Ethics committee members _____

_____

_____

Medical Treatment/Care Information

Diagnoses _____Prognosis _____

Course of illness _____

Treatment options appropriate _____

Treatment options medically beneficial: _____

Treatment options available: _____

Would the patient have wanted the treatment? _____

Ethical issues: _____

Legal issues: _____

Alternatives, risks, & benefits: _____

Other persons to contact for input, if any? _____

_____

Consultative guidance: _____

Guidance communicated? ❏ Yes ❏ No If yes, to whom? _____

Consultation noted on the medical record: ❏ Yes ❏ No

Disposition: _____

Form completed by: _____ Date/Time: _____

_____

Exhibit 3–1 Ethics Committee Consultation

When conducting a formal consultation, ethics committees should

1. Identify the ethical dilemma, i.e., reasons why the consult was requested.
   a. Be sure the appropriate "Consultation Request" form has been completed.
2. Identify relevant facts.
   a. diagnosis and prognosis
   b. patient goals and wishes
   c. regulatory and legal issues
   d. professional standards and codes of ethics
   e. institutional policies and values
3. Identify the stakeholders.
4. Identify moral issues.
   a. human dignity
   b. common good
   c. justice
   d. beneficence
   e. respect for autonomy
   f. informed consent
   g. medical futility, and so on
5. Identify legal issues.
6. Consider alternative options.
7. Conduct consultation.
   a. Review, discuss, and provide reasoning for recommendations made.
8. Review and follow up.
9. Committee discussion should include family members once the committee has had an opportunity to review the request for consultation.
10. Family members should be asked what their hopes and expectations are.
11. Each formal consultation should be documented and reviewed at subsequent ethics committee meetings for educational purposes.

CASE: ETHICS COMMITTEE SERVES AS GUARDIAN

The Kentucky Supreme Court ruled in *Woods v. Commonwealth,* 1999-SSC-0773 (August 24, 2004), that Kentucky's Living Will Directive, allowing a court-appointed guardian or other designated surrogate to remove a patient's life support systems, is constitutional. The patient in this case, Woods, had been placed on a ventilator after having a heart attack. It was generally agreed that he would never regain consciousness and would die in two to ten years. After a recommendation of the hospital ethics committee, Woods' guardian at the time asked for approval to remove Woods' life support. The Kentucky Supreme Court affirmed an appeals court decision, holding that,

- "if there is no guardian," but the family, physicians, and ethics committee all agree with the surrogate, there is no need to appoint a guardian.
- "if there is a guardian," and all parties agree, there is no need for judicial approval.
- "if there is disagreement," the parties may petition the courts.

Life support will be prohibited, absent clear and convincing evidence that: the patient is permanently unconscious, or is in a persistent vegetative state; and removal of life support is in the patient's best interest.

Ethical and Legal Issues

1. Discuss the ethical issues of this case.
2. Discuss under what circumstances an ethics committee should serve as a legal guardian.
3. Discuss the pros and cons of an ethics committee serving as a patient's guardian. ■

EXPANDING ROLE OF ETHICS COMMITTEES

The need recognized by the founders of ethics committees does exist. In fact, there have long been internal discussion forums where ethical problems and conflicts have been addressed case by case. However, the scale of current problems seems to have overwhelmed the capacity of this system. The benefits of having interdisciplinary committees, which facilitate medical treatment based on an informed debate of morally complex problems from a clear ethical standpoint, are clearly much greater. The only question is whether the scale of institutionalization envisioned by creating clinical ethics committees is really necessary. To that extent, it is unclear whether this kind of ethical guidance will last in hospitals. Its further development lies not least in the hands of hospitals themselves.[2]

Typically, hospital ethics committees concern themselves with biomedical issues as they relate to end-of-life issues; unfortunately, they often fail to address external decisions that affect internal operations. The role of an organization's ethics committee is evolving into more than a group of individuals who periodically gather together to meet regulatory requirements, and review and address advance directives and end-of-life issues. The function of an organizational ethics committee has an ever-expanding role. This expanded role involves addressing external issues that affect internal operations (e.g., managed care; malpractice insurance; and complicated Health Insurance Portability and Accountability Act regulations that increase legal and other financial costs, thus burdening hospitals and slowing the progress of medicine). Ethics committees need to periodically review their functions and redefine themselves.

The ethics committee is health care's sleeping giant. Because of its potential to bring about change, its mission must not be limited to end-of-life issues. Its vision must not be restricted to issues internal to the organization, but must include external matters that affect internal operations.

Failure to increase the good of others when one is knowingly in a position to do so is morally wrong. Preventative medicine and active public health interventions exemplify this conviction. After methods of treating yellow fever and smallpox were discovered, for example, it was universally agreed that positive steps ought to be taken to establish programs to protect public health.

The wide variety of ethical issues that an ethics committee can be involved in is somewhat formidable. Although an ethics committee cannot address every issue that one could conceivably imagine, the ethics committee should periodically re-evaluate its scope of activities and effectiveness in addressing ethical issues. Some of the internal and external issues facing an organization's ethics committee are presented below.

Internal Ethical Issues

1. Dilemma of blind trials: who gets the placebo when the investigational drug looks very promising?
2. Informed consent: are patients adequately informed as to the risks, benefits, and alternative procedures that may be equally effective, knowing that one procedure may be more risky or damaging than another (e.g., lumpectomy versus a radical mastectomy)?
3. What is the physician's responsibility for informing the patient of his or her education, training, qualifications, and skill in treating a medical condition or performing an invasive procedure?
4. What is the role of the ethics committee when the medical staff is reluctant or fails to take timely action, knowing that one of its members practices questionable medicine?
5. Should a hospital's medical staff practice evidence-based medicine or follow its own best judgment?
6. To what extent should the organization participate in and/or support genetic research?
7. How should the ethics committee address confidentiality issues?
8. To what extent should medical information be shared with the patient's family?
9. To what extent should the scope of issues that the ethics committee addresses be controlled by the organization's leadership?
10. What are the demarcation lines as to what information should or should not be provided to the patient when mistakes are made relative to his or her care?

External Ethical Issues

1. Does the ethics committee have a role in addressing questionable reimbursement schemes?

2. Should an ethics committee have its own letterhead? What value would this serve?

3. What role, if any, should an ethics committee play in the following scenario?

> Emergency services ambulance personnel regularly transport suspected stroke patients to Hospital A. This hospital has no neurologists or neurosurgeons on its medical staff but does provide coffee and donuts to transport personnel. Ambulance personnel have an option to take the suspected stroke victim to Hospital B, which is within five blocks of Hospital A. Hospital B has a well-trained stroke team with staff neurologists and neurosurgeons on staff and readily available.

Organizational politics may prevent an ethics committee from becoming involved in many of the issues just described. Although the committee's involvement is strictly advisory, its value to an organization has yet to be fully realized.

CONVENING THE ETHICS COMMITTEE

The ethics committee is not a decision maker but a resource that provides advice to help guide others in making wiser decisions when there is no clear best choice. A unanimous opinion is not always possible when an ethics committee convenes to consider the issues of an ethical dilemma. However, consultative advice as to a course of action to follow in resolving the dilemma is often the role of the ethics committee. Any recommendations for issue resolution reached by the ethics committee need to be communicated to those most closely involved with the patient's care. Sensitivity to each family member's values and assisting them in coping with whatever consensus decision is reached is a must. There are often unresolved issues that need to be addressed and a course of action followed. Each new consultation presents new opportunities for learning and teaching others how to cope with similar issues. Guidelines for resolving ethical issues will always be in a state of flux. Each new case presents new challenges and learning opportunities.

Making a decision, suggesting a course of action, recommending a path to follow, and making a choice require accepting the fact that there will be elements of right and wrong in the final decision. The idea is to cause the least pain and provide the greatest benefit.

CASE: BIOETHICS COMMITTEE NOT CONVENED

In this medical malpractice suit, the Stolles (appellants) sought damages from physicians and hospitals (appellees) for disregard of their instructions not to use "heroic efforts" or artificial means to prolong the life of their child, Mariel, who was born with brain damage. The Stolles argued that such negligence resulted in further brain damage to Mariel, prolonged her life, and caused them extraordinary costs that will continue as long as the child lives.

The Stolles had executed a written "Directive to Physicians" on behalf of Mariel in which they made known their desire that Mariel's life not be artificially prolonged under the circumstances provided in that directive.

Mariel suffered a medical episode after regurgitating her food. An unnamed, unidentified nurse-clinician administered chest compressions for 30 to 60 seconds and Mariel survived.

The Stolles sued alleging the following, among other things: Appropriate medical entries were not made in the medical record to reflect the Stolles' wishes that caregivers refrain from "heroic" life-sustaining measures; life-saving measures were initiated in violation of the physician's orders; the hospital did not follow the physician's orders, which were in Mariel's medical chart, when chest compressions and mechanically administered breathing to artificially prolong Mariel's life were applied; and *a bioethics committee meeting was not convened to consider the Stolles' wishes* and the necessity of a "do not resuscitate" order.

The central issue in this case is whether appellees are immune from liability under the Texas Natural Death Act. Section 672.016(b) of the Texas Natural Death Act provides: "A physician, or a health professional acting under the direction of a physician, is not civilly or criminally liable for failing to effectuate a qualified patient's directive" [TEX. HEALTH & SAFETY CODE ANN. § 672.016(b) (Vernon 1992)]. A "qualified patient" is a "patient with a terminal condition that has been diagnosed and certified in writing by the attending physician and one other physician who have personally examined the patient." A "terminal condition" is an "incurable condition caused by injury, disease, or illness that would produce death regardless of the application of life-sustaining procedures, according to reasonable medical judgment, and in which the application of life-sustaining procedures serves only to postpone the moment of the patient's death."

Mariel was not in a terminal condition, as appellees alleged. The Stolles failed to cite any authority that would have allowed the withdrawal of life-sustaining procedures in a lawful manner. The Texas Natural Death Act, therefore, provided immunity to the caregivers for their actions in the treatment and care of Mariel.[3]

Ethical and Legal Issues

1. Describe the ethical principles at conflict in this case.
2. Do you agree with the court's decision? Explain your answer. ■

REASONING AND DECISION MAKING

Reason guides our attempt to understand the world about us. Both reason and compassion guide our efforts to apply that knowledge ethically, to understand other people, and have ethical relationships with other people.

MOLLEEN MATSUMURA

The logical application of reasoning is important in the decision-making process. "Knowing" ethical theories, principles, values, and morals and "understanding" how to apply them must go hand in hand. Reason includes the capacity for logical inference; the ability to conduct inquiry, solve problems, evaluate, criticize, and deliberate about how we should act; and to reach an understanding of ourselves, other people, and the world.[4] *Partial reasoning* involves bias for or against a person based on one's relationship with that person. *Circular reasoning* describes a person who has already made up his or her mind on a particular issue and sees no need for deliberation (i.e., "Don't confuse me with the facts."). For example, consider the following: "Mr. Smith has lived a good life, it's time to pull the plug. He is over 65 and, therefore, should not have any rights to donated organs. Donated organs should be given to younger people." The rightness or wrongness of this statement is a moral issue and should be open for discussion, fact-finding, evaluation, reasoning, and consensus decision making.

Ethical decision making is the process of deciding the right thing to do when facing a moral dilemma. Decision making is not easy when there is more than one road, an alternative route, to take. Health care dilemmas often occur when there are alternative choices, limited resources, and differing values among patients, family members, and caregivers. Coming to an agreement may mean sacrificing one's personal wishes and following the road where there is consensus. Consensus building can happen only when the parties involved can sit and reason together. The process of identifying the various alternatives to an ethical dilemma, determining the pros and cons of each choice, and making informed decisions requires a clear unbiased willingness to listen, learn, and, in the end, make an informed decision.

Ethical dilemmas arise when ethical principles and values are in conflict. An ethical dilemma arises when, for example, the principles of *autonomy* and *beneficence* conflict with one another. The following case illustrates how one's right to make his or her decision can conflict with the principle of doing no harm.

CASE: PATIENT REFUSES BLOOD

Mrs. Jones has gangrene of her left leg. Her hemoglobin slipped to 6.4. She has a major infection and is diabetic. There is no spouse and no living will. The patient has decided that she does not want to be resuscitated if she should go into cardiopulmonary arrest. She may need surgery. She has agreed to surgery but refuses a blood transfusion, even though she is not a Jehovah's Witness. The surgeon will not perform the surgery, which is urgent, without Jones agreeing to a blood transfusion, if it becomes necessary. The attending physician questions the patient's capacity to make decisions. Her children have donated blood. She says she is not afraid to die.

Ethical and Legal Issues

1. Should the physician refuse to treat this patient? Explain your answer.
2. Should the family have a right to override the patient's decision to refuse blood? Explain your answer. ▪

CASE: A SON'S GUILT, A FATHER'S WISHES

Following a massive stroke, Mr. Smith was transported from the Rope Nursing Facility to a local hospital by ambulance on July 4, 2004. Smith, 94 years of age, had been a resident at the Rope nursing facility for the past 12 years. Prior to being placed in Rope, Smith had been living with Mr. Curry, a close friend, for the previous eight years. He had an advance directive indicating that he would never want to be placed on a respirator.

Smith's son and only child, Barry, who now lives in Los Angeles and had been estranged from his dad for more than 20 years, was notified by Curry that his dad had been admitted to the hospital in a terminal condition. Smith had mistakenly been placed on a respirator by hospital staff contrary to the directions in his advance directive, which had been placed on the front cover of Smith's medical chart. Curry, who was legally appointed by Smith to act as his health care surrogate decision maker, called Barry and explained that, according to his dad's wishes and advance directives, he was planning to ask hospital staff to have the respirator removed. Barry asked Curry to wait until he flew in from California to see his dad. Curry agreed to wait for Barry's arrival the following day, July 5. Upon arriving at the hospital, Barry told Curry that he would take responsibility for his dad's care and that Curry's services would no longer be needed. Barry told hospital staff that he objected to the hospital's plan to remove his father from the respirator. He said that he needed time to say goodbye to his dad, which he did by whispering his sorrows in his dad's ears. Smith, however, did not respond. Barry demanded that the hospital do everything that it could to save his dad's life, saying, "I don't know if dad heard me. We have to wait until he wakes up so that I can tell him how sorry I am for not having stayed in touch with him over the years." Smith's physicians explained to Barry that there was no chance Smith would ever awaken out of his coma. Barry threatened legal action if the hospital did not do everything it could to keep his dad alive. Smith's physician again spoke to Barry about the futility of maintaining his dad on a respirator. Barry remained uncooperative. The hospital chaplain was called to speak to Barry, but had little success. Finally, hospital staff requested an ethics consult.

Ethical and Legal Issues

1. Discuss the ethical dilemmas in this case.
2. Discuss the issues and the role of the ethics committee in this case. ▪

HELPFUL HINTS

The reason for studying ethical and legal issues is to understand and help guide others through the decision-making process as it relates to ethical dilemmas. The following are some helpful guidelines when faced with ethical dilemmas:

- Be aware of how everyday life is full of ethical decisions, and that numerous ethical issues can arise when caring for patients.
- Help guide others to make choices.
- Ask your patient how you might help him or her.
- Be aware of why you think the way you do. Do not impose your beliefs on others.
- Ask yourself whether you agree with the things you do. If the answer is no, ask yourself how you should change.
- When you are not sure what to do, the wise thing to do is to talk it over with another, someone whose opinion you trust.
- Do not sacrifice happiness for devotion to others.
- Do not lie to avoid hurting someone's feelings.

CHAPTER REVIEW

1. An ethics committee serves as a hospital resource to patients, families, and staff, offering an objective counsel when dealing with difficult health care issues and decisions.
2. To be successful, an ethics committee should be structured to include a wide range of community leaders in positions of political stature, respect, and diversity.
3. The goals of the ethics committee are to:
    a. promote the rights of patients;
    b. promote shared decision making between patients and their clinicians;
    c. assist the patient and family, as appropriate, in coming to consensus regarding the options that best meet the patient's goal for care;
    d. promote fair policies and procedures that maximize the likelihood of achieving good, patient-centered outcomes; and
    e. enhance the ethical tenor of both health care organizations and professionals.
4. The functions of ethics committees are multifaceted and include:
    a. development of policy and procedure guidelines to assist in resolving ethical dilemmas;
    b. staff and community education;
    c. conflict resolution;
    d. case reviews, support, and consultation; and
    e. political advocacy.

5. The role of the ethics committee should include addressing external issues that affect internal operations.

6. The ethics committee is not a decision maker but a resource that provides advice to help guide others toward making wiser decisions when there is no clear best choice.

7. Decision making is not easy when there are alternative choices, limited resources, a variety of value beliefs from patients, family members, and caregivers.

8. Patients and family should be encouraged to participate in patient care and decision-making processes.

9. One needs to know the *reasons* for his or her beliefs, and be able to state why decisions are made.
   a. *Partial reasoning* involves bias for or against a person based on one's relationship with that person.
   b. *Circular reasoning* describes a person who has already decided the correctness of something.

10. The process of identifying the various alternatives to an ethical dilemma, determining the pros and cons of each choice, and making informed decisions requires a clear unbiased willingness to listen, learn, and, in the end, make an informed decision.

TEST YOUR UNDERSTANDING

Terminology

ethics committee
ethics consultation
reasoning and decision making
circular reasoning
partial reasoning
conflict resolution

REVIEW QUESTIONS

1. Discuss how ethical dilemmas that arise during a patient's stay in a health care facility can be addressed.

2. Discuss the consultative role of the ethics committee.

3. Discuss the educational role of the ethics committee.

4. Discuss the ever-expanding role of ethics committees, including internal operational issues and external influences that affect internal operations.

HELPFUL WEB SITES

Advance Directives
www.mindspring.com/~scottr/will.html
Bioethics (comprehensive web site on bioethics)
www.bioethics.net
Biotech & Health Care Ethics
www.scu.edu/ethics/practicing/focusareas/medical
Centre for Bio-Ethics and Health Law
www.uu-cbg.nl/research-hce.htm
Happiness
http://www.cybernation.com/victory/quotations/subjects/quotes_
happiness.html
Living Wills/Advance Directives
www.mindspring.com/~scottr/will.html
Merriam-Webster On-Line Dictionary
http://www.m-w.com
National Advisory Board on Health Care Ethics
www.etene.org/e/index.shtml
National Center for Biotechnology Information
www.ncbi.nlm.nih.gov
Questia
www.questia.com/Index.jsp?CRID=medical_ethics&OFFID=se1
TransWeb
www.transweb.org

NOTES

1. In re Quinlan, 355 A.2d 647 (N.J. 1976).
2. http://www.hospital.be/2003Hospital/Hospital5I2003/CoverClinical.html.
3. Stolle v. Baylor College of Medicine, 981 S.W.2d 709 (1998).
4. George Lakoff & Mark Johnson, *Philosophy In The Flesh*, 3–4 (Basic Books, 1999).

chapter four

End-of-Life Dilemmas

. . . When we finally know we are dying,
And all other sentient beings are dying with us,
We start to have a burning, almost heartbreaking sense
of the fragility and preciousness of each moment and each being,
and from this can grow a deep, clear, limitless compassion for all beings.

SOGYAL RINPOCHE

LEARNING OBJECTIVES

The reader upon completion of this chapter will be able to:

- Understand and describe end-of-life dilemmas

- Present an historical overview of the right to self-determination

- Understand and describe the following topics:

  o Euthanasia

  o Physician-assisted suicide

  o Oregon's Death with Dignity Act

  o Patient Self-Determination Act of 1990

  o Advance directives

  o Appointed decision makers

  o Futility of treatment

  o Withdrawal of treatment

- "Men Don't Cry."

INTRODUCTION

One of the most tension-producing, thought-provoking issues facing health care providers focuses on end-of-life issues. Although it is established that competent terminally ill patients may refuse life-sustaining treatment, physician-assisted suicide continues to raise much debate.

The human struggle to survive and dreams of immortality have been instrumental in pushing humankind to develop means to prevent and cure illness. Advances in medicine and related technologies that have resulted from human creativity and ingenuity have given society the power to prolong life. However, the process of dying also can be prolonged. Those victims of long-term pain and suffering, as well as patients in vegetative states and irreversible comas, are the most directly affected. Rather than watching hopelessly as a disease destroys a person or as a body part malfunctions, causing death to a patient, physicians now can implant artificial body organs. Exotic machines and antibiotics are weapons in a physician's arsenal to help extend a patient's life. Such situations have generated vigorous debate. This section reviews many of those issues that inevitably come as one approaches the end of life.

SELF-DETERMINATION: SIGNIFICANT EVENTS

1976   The New Jersey Supreme Court granted the parents of Karen Ann Quinlan permission to remove her from a ventilator. In California, the first living will legislation was enacted, permitting a person to sign a declaration stating that if there is no hope of recovery, no heroic measures need to be taken to prolong life. This provision is now available in every state.

1980   The Hemlock Society is formed to advocate for physician-assisted dying for the terminally ill, mentally competent patient.

1983   California enacted the first durable power of attorney legislation permitting an advance directive to be made describing the kind of health care that one would desire when facing death by designating an agent to act on the patient's behalf.

1990   • The Supreme Court ruled that the parents of Nancy Cruzan, a 32-year-old woman who had been unconscious since a 1983 car accident, could have her feeding tube removed.[1]
        • Dr. Jack Kevorkian used a suicide machine to assist Janet Adkins, a 54-year-old woman with Alzheimer's disease, in ending her life at her request.
        • Congress passed the Patient Self-Determination Act (PSDA). The Act requires federally funded health care organizations to explain to patients that they have a right to complete an advance directive.
        • Timothy Quill, a primary care physician, published an article describing how he had prescribed a lethal dose of sedatives to end the life of a young woman whose suffering from leukemia had become unbearable.

- Derek Humphry's popular text, *Final Exit: The Practicalities of Self Deliverance and Assisted Suicide for the Dying*, is published.

1993   If the attending physician, the hospital, or nursing home ethics committee where a patient resides, and the legal guardian or next of kin, all agree and document the patient's wishes and the patient's condition, and if no one disputes their decision, no court order is required to proceed to carry out the patient's wishes. Future criminal sanctions or civil liability turn not on the existence or absence of a court order, but on the facts of the case. No liability attaches to a decision to refuse or withdraw treatment if the necessary facts are established and carefully documented by the parties involved. On the other hand, the court cannot absolve the parties from liability where the facts do not exist to support the action taken.[2]

1994   Oregon vote legalized physician-assisted dying. The law took three years to become effective.

1996   The Second and Ninth U.S. Circuit Courts of Appeals ruled that there is a constitutional right under the Fourteenth Amendment for a terminally ill person to receive help from a physician when dying.

1997   • Physician-assisted suicide, through referendum, became a legal medical option within narrowly prescribed circumstances for terminally ill Oregon residents.
   • Kevorkian was charged with murder in five cases of physician-assisted suicide and was acquitted.
   • Supreme Court overturns both 1996 circuit decisions, ruling that it is up to the states to enact laws regarding medically assisted death.

1998   • Oregon voters reaffirm their support for the Death with Dignity Act by a 60 percent majority.
   • Kevorkian administered a lethal injection to Thomas Youk, a 52-year-old man with Lou Gehrig's disease, on national television.
   • Michigan voters defeated a ballot measure that would legalize physician-assisted suicide.

1999   • Kevorkian was convicted of second-degree murder for Youk's death and sentenced to 10 to 20 years in prison.
   • Twenty-three terminally ill patients were reported as receiving lethal doses of medication since passage of Oregon's Death with Dignity Act.

2001   U.S. Attorney General John Ashcroft abrogated Janet Reno's mandate allowing physician-assisted suicide. Instead, he decided that physician-assisted suicide was a violation of the federal Controlled Substance Act. In *State of Oregon v. Aschcroft*, CV01-1647 (D. Oregon), the judge allowed Oregon's law to remain in effect.

2001   Since 1991, the total number of physician-assisted suicide cases totals 129. April 17: U.S. District Court Judge Robert Jones upheld the "Death with Dignity Act."

2002   Attorney General John Ashcroft filed an appeal, asking the 9th U.S. Circuit
            Court of Appeals to lift the District Court's ruling.

2003   Forty-two residents of the State of Oregon ingested medications under provi-
            sions of the Death with Dignity Act.

EUTHANASIA

When patients and their families perceive a deterioration of the quality of life
and no end to unbearable pain, conflict often arises between health care professionals, who are trained to save lives, and patients and their families, who
wish to end the suffering. This conflict centers on the concept of euthanasia
and its place in the modern world. There seems to be an absence of controversy only when a patient who is kept alive by modern technology is still able
to appreciate and maintain control over his or her life.

Any discussion of euthanasia obliges a person to confront humanity's
greatest fear—death. The courts and legislatures have faced it and have
made advances in setting forth some guidelines to assist decision makers in
this arena. However, much more must be accomplished. Society must be
protected from the risks associated with permitting the removal of life-support systems. Society cannot allow the complex issues associated with this
topic to be simplified to the point where it is accepted that life can be terminated based on subjective quality-of-life considerations. The legal system
must ensure that the constitutional rights of the patient are maintained,
while at the same time protect society's interests in preserving life, preventing suicide, and maintaining the integrity of the medical profession. For
example, can competent adult patients who ask that no extraordinary lifesaving measures be taken recover damages for finding themselves alive after
unwanted resuscitative measures? During a medical emergency, it seems
unrealistic to ask a caregiver to first look in a patient's medical record for an
advance directive before tending to the immediate needs of the patient. In
the final analysis, the boundaries of patient rights remain very uncertain.

From its inception, euthanasia has evolved into an issue with competing
legal, medical, and moral implications, which continue to generate debate,
confusion, and conflict. Currently, there is a strong movement advocating
death with dignity, which excludes machines, monitors, and tubes.

Even the connotation of the word euthanasia has changed with time
depending upon who is attempting to define it. Euthanasia originated from
the Greek word *euthanatos*, meaning "good death" or "easy death," and was
accepted in situations in which people had what were considered to be incurable diseases. Euthanasia is defined broadly as "the mercy killing of the
hopelessly ill, injured, or incapacitated."[3]

In the Confucian and Buddhist religions, suicide was an acceptable
answer to unendurable pain and incurable disease. The Celtics went a step
farther, believing that those who chose to die of disease or senility, rather
than committing suicide, would be condemned to Hell. Such acceptance

began to change during the 1800s when Western physicians refused to lessen suffering by shortening a dying patient's life. Napoleon's physician, for example, rejected Napoleon's plea to kill plague-stricken soldiers, insisting that his obligation was to cure rather than to kill people.

In the late 1870s, writings on euthanasia began to appear, mainly in England and the United States. Although such works were written, for the most part, by lay authors, the public and the medical community began to consider the issues raised by euthanasia. Then defined as "the act or practice of painlessly putting to death persons suffering from incurable conditions or diseases," it was considered to be a merciful release from incurable suffering. By the beginning of the 20th century, however, there were still no clear answers or guidelines regarding the use of euthanasia. Unlike in prior centuries when society as a whole supported or rejected euthanasia, different segments of today's society apply distinct connotations to the word, generating further confusion. Some believe euthanasia is meant to allow a painless death when one suffers from an incurable disease, yet is not dying. Others, who remain in the majority, perceive euthanasia as an instrument to aid only dying people in ending their lives with as little suffering as possible.

It has been estimated that of the two million Americans who die each year, 80 percent die in hospitals or nursing homes, and 70 percent of those die after a decision to forgo life-sustaining treatment has been made. Although such decisions are personal in nature and based on individual moral values, they must comply with the laws applicable to the prolonging of the dying process. Courts have outlined the ways in which the government is allowed to participate in the decision-making process. Yet the misconceptions and lack of clear direction regarding the policies and procedures have resulted in wide disparity among jurisdictions, both in legislation and in judicial decisions. As a result, the American Medical Association, the American Bar Association, legislators, and judges are actively attempting to formulate and legislate clear guidelines in this sensitive, profound, and not yet fully understood area. To ensure compliance with the law, while serving the needs of their patients, it is incumbent on health care providers to keep themselves informed of the legislation enacted in this ever-changing field.

To properly address the topic of euthanasia, it is necessary to understand the precise meaning of the recognized forms of it. Rhetorical phrases such as right to die, right to life, and death with dignity have obfuscated, rather than clarified, the understanding of euthanasia. The dividing of euthanasia into two categories, active or passive, is for many the most controversial aspect of this topic.

Active or Passive Euthanasia

Active euthanasia is commonly understood to be the intentional commission of an act, such as giving a patient a lethal drug that results in death. The act, if committed by the patient, is thought of as suicide. Moreover, because the patient cannot take his or her own life, any person who assists in the causing of the death could be subject to criminal sanction for aiding and abetting suicide.

Passive euthanasia occurs when lifesaving treatment (such as a respirator) is withdrawn or withheld, allowing the terminally ill patient to die a natural death. Passive euthanasia is generally accepted pursuant to legislative acts and judicial decisions. These decisions, however, generally are based on the facts of a particular case. Regardless of the definitional differences, the end result in both active and passive euthanasia is the same.

The distinctions are important when considering the duty and liability of a physician who must decide whether to continue or initiate treatment of a comatose or terminally ill patient. Physicians are obligated to use reasonable care to preserve health and to save lives, so unless fully protected by the law, they will be reluctant to abide by a patient's or family's wishes to terminate life-support devices.

Although there may be a duty to provide life-sustaining equipment in the immediate aftermath of cardiopulmonary arrest, there is no duty to continue its use after it has become futile and ineffective to do so in the opinion of qualified medical personnel. An example is a patient who suffered severe brain damage, placing him in a comatose and vegetative state, from which, according to tests and examinations by other specialists, he was unlikely to recover. The patient, on the written request of his family, was taken off life-support equipment. The patient's family (his wife and eight children) made the decision together after consultation with the physicians. Evidence had been presented that the patient, before his incapacitation, had expressed to his wife that he would not want to be kept alive by a machine. Decisions by family members are based upon love and concern for the dignity of their loved one. [*Barber v. Superior Court,* 147 Cal. App. 3d 1006 (Cal. Ct. App. 1983.]

Voluntary or Involuntary Euthanasia

Both active and passive euthanasia may be either voluntary or involuntary. Voluntary euthanasia occurs when a person suffering an incurable illness makes the decision to die. To be considered voluntary, the request or consent must be made by a legally competent adult and be based on material information concerning the possible ramifications and alternatives available.

Involuntary euthanasia, however, occurs when the decision to terminate the life of an incurable person (i.e., an incompetent or unconsenting competent) is made by someone other than that incurable person.

The patient's lack of consent could be due to mental impairment or a comatose state. Important value questions face courts grappling with making decisions regarding involuntary euthanasia:

- Who should decide to withhold or withdraw treatment?
- On what factors should the decision be based?

- Are there viable standards to guide the courts?
- Should criminal sanctions be imposed on a person assisting in ending a life?
- When does death occur?

Constitutional Considerations

To analyze the important questions regarding whether life-support treatment can be withheld or withdrawn from an incompetent patient, it is necessary to consider first what rights a competent patient possesses. Both statutory law and case law have presented a diversity of policies and points of view. Some courts point to common law and the early case of *Schloendorff v. Society of New York Hospital*[4] to support their belief in a patient's right to self-determination. The Schloendorff court stated:

> Every human being of adult years has a right to determine what shall be done with his own body; and the surgeon who performs an operation without his patient's consent commits an assault for which he is liable for damages.[5]

This right of self-determination was emphasized in *In re Storar*[6] when the court announced that every human being of adult years and sound mind has the right to determine what shall be done with his or her own body.

The Storar case was a departure from the New Jersey Supreme Court's rationale in the case of *In re Quinlan*.[7] The Quinlan case was the first to significantly address the issue of whether euthanasia should be permitted when a patient is terminally ill. The Quinlan court, relying on *Roe v. Wade*,[8] announced that the constitutional right to privacy protects a patient's right to self-determination. The court noted that the right to privacy "is broad enough to encompass a patient's decision to decline medical treatment under certain circumstances, in much the same way as it is broad enough to encompass a woman's decision to terminate pregnancy under certain conditions."[9]

The Quinlan court, in reaching its decision, applied a test balancing the state's interest in preserving and maintaining the sanctity of human life against Karen's privacy interest. It decided that, especially in light of the prognosis (physicians determined that Karen Quinlan was in an irreversible coma), the state's interest did not justify interference with her right to refuse treatment. Thus, Karen Quinlan's father was appointed her legal guardian, and the respirator was shut off.

In the same year as the Quinlan decision, the case of Superintendent of *Belchertown State School v. Saikewicz*[10] was decided. There, the court, using the balancing test enunciated in Quinlan, approved the recommendation of a court-appointed guardian ad litem that it would be in Saikewicz's best interests to end chemotherapy treatment. Saikewicz was a mentally retarded, 67-year-old patient suffering from leukemia. The court found from the evidence that the prognosis was dim, and even though a "normal person" would probably have chosen chemotherapy, it allowed Saikewicz to die without treatment to spare him the suffering.

Although the court also followed the reasoning of the Quinlan opinion in giving the right to an incompetent to refuse treatment, based on either the objective "best interests" test or the subjective "substituted judgment" test, which it favored because Saikewicz always had been incompetent, the court departed from Quinlan in a major way. It rejected the Quinlan approach of entrusting a decision concerning the continuance of artificial life support to the patient's guardian, family, attending physicians, and a hospital "ethics committee." The Saikewicz court asserted that even though a judge might find the opinions of physicians, medical experts, or hospital ethics committees helpful in reaching a decision, there should be no requirement to seek out the advice. The court decided that questions of life and death with regard to an incompetent should be the responsibility of the courts, which would conduct detached but passionate investigations. The court took a "dim view of any attempt to shift the ultimate decision-making responsibility away from duly established courts of proper jurisdiction to any committee, panel, or group, ad hoc or permanent."[11]

This main point of difference between the Saikewicz and Quinlan cases marked the emergence of two different policies on the incompetent's right to refuse treatment. One line of cases has followed Saikewicz and supports court approval before physicians are allowed to withhold or withdraw life support. Advocates of this view argue that it makes more sense to leave the decision to an objective tribunal than to extend the right of a patient's privacy to a number of interested parties, as was done in Quinlan. They also attack the Quinlan method as being a privacy decision effectuated by popular vote.[12]

Six months after Saikewicz, the Massachusetts Appeals Court narrowed the need for court intervention in *In re Dinnerstein*[13] by finding that "no code" orders are valid to prevent the use of artificial resuscitative measures on incompetent terminally ill patients. The court was faced with the case of a 67-year-old woman who was suffering from Alzheimer's disease. It was determined that she was permanently comatose at the time of trial. Further, the court decided that Saikewicz-type judicial proceedings should take place only when medical treatment could offer a reasonable expectation of effecting a permanent or temporary cure of or relief from the illness.

The Massachusetts Supreme Judicial Court attempted to clarify its Saikewicz opinion with regard to court orders in *In re Spring*.[14] It held that such different factors as the patient's mental impairment and his or her medical prognosis with or without treatment must be considered before judicial approval is necessary to withdraw or withhold treatment from an incompetent patient. The problem in all three cases is that there is still no clear guidance as to exactly when the court's approval of the removal of life-support systems would be necessary. Saikewicz seemed to demand judicial approval in every case. Spring, however, in partially retreating from that view, stated that it did not have to articulate what combination of the factors it discussed, thus making prior court approval necessary.

The inconsistencies presented by the Massachusetts cases have led most courts since 1977 to follow the parameters set by Quinlan, requiring judicial intervention. In cases where physicians have certified the irreversible nature of a patient's loss of consciousness, an ethics committee (actually a neurologic team) could certify the patient's hopeless neurologic condition. Then a guardian would be free to take the legal steps necessary to remove life-support systems. The main reason for the appointment of a guardian is to ensure that incompetents, like all other patients, maintain their right to refuse treatment. Most holdings indicate that because a patient has the constitutional right of self-determination, those acting on the patient's behalf can exercise that right when rendering their best judgment concerning how the patient would assert the right. This substituted judgment doctrine could be argued on standing grounds, whereby a second party has the right to assert the constitutional rights of another when that second party's intervention is necessary to protect the other's constitutional rights. The guardian's decision is more sound if based on the known desires of a patient who was competent immediately before becoming comatose.

An advance directive, such as a living will, is persuasive evidence of an incompetent's wishes. An incompetent patient can act as a guardian and in accordance with the terms of a living will. An agent can substitute his or her judgment for that of the patient.

A court may require the attending physician to certify that a patient is in a permanent vegetative state, with no reasonable chance for recovery, before a family member or guardian can request termination of extraordinary means of medical treatment.

The decision maker would attempt to ascertain the incompetent patient's actual interests and preferences. Court involvement would be mandated only to appoint a guardian in one of the following cases:

- family members disagree as to the incompetent's wishes
- physicians disagree on the prognosis
- the patient's wishes cannot be known because he or she always has been incompetent
- evidence exists of wrongful motives or malpractice
- no family member can serve as a guardian[15]

Defining Death

When is a patient considered to be legally dead, and what type of treatment can be withheld or withdrawn? Most cases dealing with euthanasia speak of the necessity for a physician to diagnose a patient as being either in a persistent vegetative state or terminally ill.

Traditionally the definition of death adopted by the courts has been according to Black's Law Dictionary: "cessation of respiration, heartbeat, and certain indications of central nervous system activity, such as respiration and pulsation."[16] At present, however, modern science has the capacity to sustain vegetative functions of those in irreversible comas. Machinery can sustain heartbeat and respiration even in the face of brain death. It is now generally accepted that the irreversible cessation of brain function constitutes death.

Ethicists who advocate the prohibition on taking action to shorten life agree that "where death is imminent and inevitable, it is permissible to forgo treatments that would only provide a precarious and painful prolongation of life, as long as the normal care due to the sick person in similar cases is not interrupted."[17]

Relying on the 1968 Harvard Criteria set forth by the Ad Hoc Committee of the Harvard Medical School To Examine the Definition of Brain Death, the American Medical Association in 1974 accepted that death occurs when there is "irreversible cessation of all brain functions including the brain stem."[18] Most states now recognize brain death by statute or judicial decision. New York, for example, in *People v. Eulo*,[19] in rejecting the traditional cardiopulmonary definition of death, announced that the determination of brain death can be made according to acceptable medical standards. The court also repeated its holding in *In re Storar*[20] that clear and convincing evidence of a person's desire to decline extraordinary medical care may be honored and that a third person may not exercise this judgment on behalf of a person who has not or cannot express the desire to decline treatment.

Some courts hold that artificial nutrition can be withheld from a patient who is unable to converse or feed himself or herself. Unequivocal proof of a patient's wishes will suffice when the decision to terminate life support is at issue. Factors for determining the existence of clear and convincing evidence of a patient's intention to reject the prolongation of life by artificial means include:

- the persistence of statements regarding an individual's beliefs
- the desirability of the commitment to those beliefs
- the seriousness with which such statements were made
- the inferences that may be drawn from the surrounding circumstances

The family of a patient who is in a persistent vegetative state cannot necessarily order physicians to remove artificial nutrition. In 1983, Nancy Cruzan sustained injuries in a car accident in which her car overturned, after which she was found face down in a ditch without respiratory or cardiac function. Although the patient was unconscious, her breathing and heartbeat were restored at the site of the accident. On examination at the hospital, a neurosurgeon diagnosed her as having suffered cerebral contusions and anoxia. It was estimated that she had been deprived of oxygen for 12 to 14 minutes. After remaining in a coma for three weeks, Cruzan went into an unconscious state. At first she was able to ingest some food orally. Thereafter, surgeons implanted a gastrostomy feeding and hydration tube, with the consent of her husband, to facilitate feeding her. She did not improve, and until December 1990 she lay in a Missouri state hospital in a persistent vegetative state that was determined to be irreversible, permanent, progressive, and ongoing. She was not dead, according to the accepted definition of death in Missouri, and physicians estimated that she could live in the vegetative state for an additional 30 years. Because of the prognosis, Cruzan's parents asked the hospital staff to cease all artificial nutrition and hydration procedures. The staff refused to comply with their wishes without court approval. The state trial court granted authorization for termination, finding that Cruzan had a fundamental right—grounded in both the state and federal constitutions—to refuse or direct the withdrawal of death-prolonging procedures. Testimony at trial from a former roommate of Cruzan indicated to the court that she had stated that if she were ever sick or injured, she would not want to live unless she could live halfway normally. The court interpreted that conversation, which had taken place when Cruzan was 25 years old, as meaning that she would not want to be forced to take nutrition and hydration while in a persistent vegetative state.

The case was appealed to the Missouri Supreme Court, which reversed the lower court decision. The court not only doubted that the doctrine of informed consent applied to the circumstances of the case, it moreover would not recognize a broad privacy right from the state constitution that would support the right of a person to refuse medical treatment in every circumstance. Because Missouri recognizes living wills, the court held that Cruzan's parents were not entitled to order the termination of her treatment, because "no person can assume that choice for an incompetent in the absence of the formalities required under Missouri's Living Will statutes or the clear and convincing, inherently reliable evidence absent here."[21] The court found that Cruzan's statements to her roommate did not rise to the level of clear and convincing evidence of her desire to end nutrition and hydration.

In June 1990, the U.S. Supreme Court heard oral arguments and held that:

- The U.S. Constitution does not forbid Missouri from requiring that there be clear and convincing evidence of an incompetent's wishes as to the withdrawal of life-sustaining treatment.
- The Missouri Supreme Court did not commit constitutional error in concluding that evidence adduced at trial did not amount to clear and convincing evidence of Cruzan's desire to cease hydration and nutrition.
- Due process did not require the state to accept the substituted judgment of close family members, absent substantial proof that their views reflected those of the patient.[22]

In delivering the opinion of the Court, Justice Rehnquist noted that although most state courts have applied the common-law right to informed consent or a combination of that right and a privacy right when allowing a right to refuse treatment, the Supreme Court analyzed the issues presented in the Cruzan case in terms of a Fourteenth Amendment liberty interest. They found that a competent person has a constitutionally protected right grounded in the due process clause to refuse lifesaving hydration and nutrition. Missouri provided for the incompetent by allowing a surrogate to act for the patient in choosing to withdraw hydration and treatment. Moreover, it put into place procedures to ensure that the surrogate's action conforms to the wishes expressed by the patient when he or she was competent. Although recognizing that Missouri had enacted a restrictive law, the Supreme Court held that right-to-die issues should be decided pursuant to state law, subject to a due process liberty interest, and in keeping with state constitutional law. After the Supreme Court rendered its decision, the Cruzans returned to Missouri probate court, where on November 14, 1990, Judge Charles Teel authorized physicians to remove the feeding tubes from Cruzan. The judge determined that testimony presented to him early in November demonstrated clear and convincing evidence that Nancy would not have wanted to live in a persistent vegetative state. Several of her co-workers had testified that she told them before her accident that she would not want to live "like a vegetable." On December 26, 1990, two weeks after her feeding tubes were removed, Nancy Cruzan died.

Legislative Response

After the Cruzan decision, states began to rethink existing legislation and draft new legislation in the areas of living wills, durable powers of attorney, health care proxies, and surrogate decision making. Pennsylvania and Florida were two of the first states to react to the Cruzan decision. The new Pennsylvania law is applied to terminally ill or permanently unconscious patients. The statute, the Advance Directive for Health Care Act,[23] deals mainly with individuals who have prepared living wills. It includes in its definition of life-sustaining treatment the administration of hydration and nutrition by any means if it is stated in the individual's living will. The statute mandates that a copy of the living will be given to the physician to be effective. Further, the patient must be incompetent or permanently unconscious. If there is no evidence of the presence of a living will, the Pennsylvania probate codes allow an attorney-in-fact who was designated in a properly executed durable-power-of-attorney document to give permission for "medical and surgical procedures to be utilized on an incompetent patient."[24]

The Supreme Court stated in Cruzan that only 15 percent of the population has signed any living wills or other types of medical directives. In the light of that, more states will have to address the problem of surrogate decision making for an incompetent. Legislation would not only have to include direction to consider evidence of an incompetent's wishes that had been expressed when he or she was competent, but it also would have to include provisions for consideration and protection of an incompetent who never stated what he or she would want done if in a terminally ill or persistent vegetative state.

Unless there is some national uniformity in the legislation, patients and their families will shop for states that will allow them to have medical treatment terminated or withdrawn with as few legal hassles as possible. For example, on January 18, 1991, a Missouri probate court judge authorized a father to take his 20-year-old brain-damaged daughter, Christine Busalacchi, from the Missouri Rehabilitation Center to Minnesota for testing by a pro-euthanasia physician, Dr. Cranford. Cranford, who practices at the Hennepin County Medical Center, has been at the center of controversy in Minnesota. In January 1991, Pro Life Action Ministries demanded Cranford's resignation, claiming that he "desires to make Minnesota the killing fields for the disabled."[25] He, however, views himself as an advocate of patients' rights. However the situation involving Cranford is resolved, it is clear that the main reason Busalacchi sought authorization to take his daughter to Minnesota is that he believed that he would have to deal with fewer legal impediments there to allow his daughter to die.

Because of the continuing litigation concerning the right-to-die issue, it is clear that the public must be educated about the necessity of expressing their wishes concerning medical treatment while they are competent. Uniformity with regard to the legal instruments available for demonstrating what a patient wants should be a common goal of legislators, courts, and the medical profession. If living wills, surrogates, and durable powers of attorney were to be enacted pursuant to national rather than individual state guidelines, the result should be a greater ease in resolving the myriad conflicting issues in this area. Some states have addressed the problem by statutorily providing for these instruments, thereby enabling individuals to have a say in the medical care they should receive if they become unable to speak for themselves.

Chief Justice Dore of the Washington Supreme Court voiced his opinion that a legislative response to right-to-die issues could be better addressed by the legislature.

> The United States Supreme Court, in Cruzan, questioned whether a federally protected right to forgo nutrition and hydration existed. The Cruzan Court confronted the same philosophical issues that we face today and wisely recognized and deferred to the Legislature's superior policy-making abilities. As was the case in Cruzan, our legislature is far better equipped to evaluate this complex issue and should not have its power usurped by the court.[26]

PHYSICIAN-ASSISTED SUICIDE

Dr. Jack Kevorkian of Michigan announced in October 1989 that he had developed a device that would end one's life quickly, painlessly, and

humanely. He assisted a 54-year-old Alzheimer's disease patient in committing suicide on June 4, 1990. In December 1990, he was charged with first-
degree murder, but the charge was later dismissed because Michigan had no
law against assisted suicide. He was ordered, however, not to help anyone
else commit suicide or to give advice about it. On February 6, 1991, he violated the court order by giving advice about the preparation of the drug to a
terminally ill cancer patient.[27] Additional murder charges were lodged
against Kevorkian in October 1991, when he instructed two Michigan
women in the use of his "suicide machine." In dismissing the charges against
him, the Circuit Court Judge stated that "some people with intractable pain
cannot benefit from treatment." While emphasizing that Michigan has no
law against assisting suicide, the judge also expressed his belief that physician-assisted suicide remains an alternative for patients experiencing
"unmanageable pain."[28]

The Michigan House approved legislation placing a temporary ban on
assisted suicide on November 24, 1992. The Senate approved the temporary
ban after Kevorkian helped a sixth terminally ill patient kill herself. On
December 15, 1992, Michigan Governor John Engler signed the law just
hours after two more women committed suicide with Kevorkian's aid.

The new law, which became effective on April 1, 1993, made assisting
suicide a felony punishable by up to four years in prison and a $2,000 fine.
Under the new law, assisted suicide was banned for 15 months. During this
time period a special commission studied assisted suicide and submitted its
recommendations to the Michigan legislature for review and action. The new
law apparently raised constitutional questions and was challenged by the
Civil Liberties Union of Michigan because of the claim that it fails to recognize that the terminally ill have the right to end their lives painlessly and with
dignity.

Kevorkian faced prosecution for murdering two people and for assisting
in the suicides of three others. As a result, he appealed a Michigan Supreme
Court ruling that found there is no right to assisted suicide.[29] The U.S.
Supreme Court rejected his argument that assisted suicide is a constitutional
right. The high court's decision allowed the State of Michigan to move forward and prosecute Kevorkian on the pending charges. At the time of the
high court's ruling, Kevorkian had attended his twenty-second suicide,
involving a retired clergyman, less than a month after he was left facing murder charges in Michigan.[30] As of March 1998, Kevorkian had aided in or witnessed 100 suicides. Kevorkian is currently serving a 10-year sentence for
physician-assisted suicide.

In March 1995, a federal appeals court upheld the State of Washington's
ban on assisted suicide. Then, in June 1997, the United States Supreme
Court, in two unanimous and separate decisions, ruled that the laws in
Washington and New York prohibiting assisted suicide are constitutional.
Yet the U.S. Supreme Court has also ruled that states can allow physicians to
assist in the suicide of their terminally ill patients.

Criminalizing Assisted Suicide

The Supreme Court in *Quill v. Vacco*[31] found that neither the assisted suicide ban nor the law permitting patients to refuse medical treatment treats anyone differently from anyone else or draws any distinctions between persons. There is a distinction between letting a patient die and making one die. Most legislatures have allowed the former, but have prohibited the latter. The Supreme Court disagreed with the respondents' claim that the distinction is arbitrary and irrational.

In its decision, the Supreme Court determined that New York had valid reasons for distinguishing between refusing treatment and assisting suicide. Those reasons included prohibiting intentional killing and preserving life; preventing suicide; maintaining the physician's role as his or her patient's healer; and protecting vulnerable people from indifference, prejudice, and psychological and financial pressure to end their lives. All of those reasons, the Court decided, constitute valid and important public interests fulfilling the constitutional requirement that a legislative classification bear a rational relation to a legitimate end.

In the Washington case, *Washington v. Glucksberg*,[32] the Court applied the same "rationally related to the state's interest in preserving life" test (which includes preventing suicide and studying, identifying, and treating its causes; protecting vulnerable groups; and preventing the state from allowing euthanasia). The Court held that assisted suicide is not a liberty protected by the Constitution's due process clause. A majority of states now ban assisted suicide. These rulings, however, do not affect the right of patients to refuse treatment. It is clear that this emotionally charged issue is not settled. Legislative, judicial, and public debates continue to rage.

A Florida court ruled that a man dying of acquired immune deficiency syndrome had a right to physician-assisted suicide under the privacy issues of the state's constitution. The court emphasized that the patient had to administer the lethal dose of medication, which was prescribed by his physician. Prosecutors were enjoined from bringing criminal charges against the physician.[33]

In the end, caregivers must improve the variety of pain management alternatives to those who are dying, so that physician-assisted suicide does not become the answer for those who suffer. Society must learn to deal effectively with end-of-life issues. Thus far, progress is slow and inadequate.

Assisted Suicide: A Profound Question

The issue of assisted suicide presents profound questions of medicine and medical ethics, theology and sociology, and numerous other far-reaching public policy issues. These are precisely the kinds of issues in which public input is vital, and courts are simply not equipped to conduct the type of comprehensive, broad-based hearings at which witnesses and experts on all sides of the question would testify about the broader policy ramifications of creating and regulating a right to assisted suicide. The Legislative and Executive branches in our system are uniquely well-equipped to pursue these issues. Courts have before them only the legal arguments of lawyers and, while questions of law are certainly part of the equation, the core issues presented are fundamentally grounded in questions of policy and how we view ourselves as a society. In a democracy, these questions are best answered by those who must answer to the people for their policy product, not by those who have no accountability to the people.[34]

OREGON'S DEATH WITH DIGNITY ACT—1994

On October 27, 1997 physician-assisted suicide became a legal medical option for the terminally ill residents of Oregon. The Oregon Death with Dignity Act allows a terminally ill Oregon resident to obtain a lethal dose of medication from his or her physician. The Act legalizes physician-assisted suicide, but specifically prohibits euthanasia, where a physician or other person directly administers a medication to end another's life. The following are excerpts from the Oregon Death with Dignity Act:

Or. Rev. Stat. Sects. 127.800-.897

Section 1.01. *Definitions . . .*
(12) "Terminal disease" means an incurable and irreversible disease that has been medically confirmed and will, within reasonable medical judgment, produce death within (6) months. . . .

Section 2.01. *Who may initiate a written request for medication?*
An adult who is capable, is a resident of Oregon, and has been determined by the attending physician and consulting physician to be suffering from a terminal disease, and who has voluntarily expressed his or her wish to die, may make a written request for medication for the purpose of ending his or her life in a humane and dignified manner.

Section 2.02. *Form of the Written Request.*
(1) A valid request for medication . . . shall be in substantially the form described in ORS 127.897, signed and dated by the patient and witnessed by at least two individuals who, in the presence of the patient, attest that to the best of their knowledge and belief the patient is capable, acting voluntarily, and is not being coerced to sign the request. . . .

Section 3.01. *Attending physician responsibilities.*
The attending physician shall:
(1) Make the initial determination of whether a patient has a terminal disease, is capable, and has made the request voluntarily;
(2) Inform the patient of:
    (a) His or her medical diagnosis;
    (b) His or her prognosis;

(c) The potential risks associated with taking the medication to be prescribed;

(d) The probable result of taking the medication to be prescribed;

(e) The feasible alternatives, including, but not limited to, comfort care, hospice care, and pain control.

(3) Refer the patient to a consulting physician for medical confirmation of the diagnosis, and for a determination that the patient is capable and acting voluntarily. . . .

Section 3.06. *Written and oral requests.*

In order to receive a prescription for medication to end his or her life in a humane and dignified manner, a qualified patient shall have made an oral request and a written request, and reiterate the oral request to his or her attending physician no less than (15) days after making the initial oral request. At the time the qualified patient makes his or her second oral request, the attending physician shall offer the patient an opportunity to rescind the request.

Section 3.07. *Right to rescind request.*

A patient may rescind his or her request at any time and in any manner without regard to his or her mental state . . . .

Section 3.08. *Waiting periods.*

No less than (15) days shall elapse between the patient's initial oral request and the writing of a prescription. . . . No less than 48 hours shall elapse between the patient's written request and the writing of a prescription . . . .

Section 6.01. *Form of the request.*

A request for a medication . . . shall be in substantially the following form (as shown on page 106).

PATIENT SELF-DETERMINATION ACT—1990

The Patient Self-Determination Act of 1990 (PSDA)[35] provides that patients have a right to formulate advance directives and to make decisions regarding their health care. Self-determination includes the right to accept or refuse medical treatment. Health care providers (including hospitals, nursing homes, home health agencies, health maintenance organizations, and hospices) receiving federal funds under Medicare are required to comply with the new regulations. Providers are not entitled to reimbursement under the Medicare program if they fail to meet PSDA requirements.

ADVANCE DIRECTIVES

Because of the advances in modern medical technology, each person should give serious consideration as to their health care wishes, to decide what they would want done should they become incapacitated, to execute

REQUEST FOR MEDICATION TO END MY LIFE IN A HUMANE AND DIGNIFIED MANNER

I, _____, am an adult of sound mind.

I am suffering from _____, which my attending physician has determined is a terminal disease and which has been medically confirmed by a consulting physician.

I have been fully informed of my diagnosis, prognosis, the nature of medication to be prescribed and potential associated risks, the expected result, and the feasible alternatives, including comfort care, hospice care, and pain control.

I request that my attending physician prescribe medication that will end my life in a humane and dignified manner.

Initial One:

_____ I have informed my family of my decision and taken their opinions into consideration.

_____ I have decided not to inform my family of my decision.

_____ I have no family to inform of my decision.

I understand that I have the right to rescind this request at any time.

I understand the full import of this request and I expect to die when I take the medication to be prescribed.

I make this request voluntarily and without reservation, and I accept full moral responsibility for my actions.

Signed: _____

Dated: _____

Declaration of Witnesses

We declare that the person signing this request:
(a) Is personally known to us or has provided proof of identity;
(b) Signed the request in our presence;
(c) Appears to be of sound mind and not under duress, fraud or undue influence;
(d) Is not a patient for whom either of us is attending physician. . . .

advance directives and make their wishes known so that family and health care providers can respect their decision.

Patients have a right to make decisions about their health care with their physician. They may agree to a proposed treatment, choose among offered treatments, or say no to a treatment. Patients have this right even if they become incapacitated and are unable to make decisions regarding their health care.

Advance directives, in the form of a "living will" or "durable power of attorney," allow the patient to state in advance the kinds of medical care that he or she considers acceptable or not acceptable. The patient can appoint an agent, a surrogate decision maker, to make those decisions on his or her behalf. A patient should be asked at the time of admission if he or she has an advance directive. If a patient does not have an advance directive, the organization should provide the patient with information about an advance directive and the opportunity to execute a directive. A patient should clearly understand that an advance directive is a guideline for caregivers describing his or her wishes for medical care—what he or she would and would not want—in the event of incapacitation and inability to make decisions. This interaction should be documented in the patient's medical record. If the patient has an advance directive, a copy should be requested for insertion into the patient's record. If the patient does not have a copy of the advance directive with him or her, the substance thereof should be documented and flagged in the patient's medical record. Documentation should include the location of the advance directive, the name and telephone number of the designated health care agent, and any information that might be helpful in the immediate care situation (e.g., patient's desire for food and hydration). The purpose of such documentation should not be considered to be a need to recreate a new directive, but should be considered a desire to adhere to a patient's wishes in the event some untoward event occurs while waiting for a copy of the directive.

The patient can execute a new directive at any time if desired. Patient and family education should be provided regarding the existence of the directive and its contents. The patient should be periodically queried as to whether he or she wishes to make any changes with regard to an advance directive.

Living Will

A *living will* is the instrument or legal document that describes those treatments an individual wishes or does not wish to receive should he or she become incapacitated and unable to communicate treatment decisions. Typically, a living will allows a person, when competent, to inform caregivers in writing of his or her wishes with regard to withholding and withdrawing life-supporting treatment, including nutrition and hydration. The living will is

MY LIVING WILL

To my Family, Doctors, and All Those Concerned with My Care:

I, _____, being of sound mind, make this statement as a directive to be followed if for any reason I become incapacitated and unable to participate in decisions regarding my medical care.

If I should be in an incurable or irreversible mental or physical condition with no reasonable expectation of recovery, I direct my attending physician to withhold or withdraw treatment that merely prolongs my dying. I direct that my treatment in this instance be limited to comfort care and the control of and relief from pain.

Care I want:

_____
_____
_____
_____

To live as long as possible regardless of the quality of life that I may experience:
- I direct that all appropriate medical/surgical measures be provided to sustain my life regardless of my mental or physical condition.
- Upon my death, I want to donate any parts of my body that may be of benefit to others.

Care I do not want:

_____
_____
_____
_____

- I am permanently unconscious with and permanently connected to a ventilator.
- I am permanently unconscious with a feeding tube and/or intravenous hydration.
- I am on a ventilator when there is little or no chance of recovery.
- I am conscious but unable to communicate, being fed with a feeding tube and/or hydrated.
- I am in the end stage of a fatal irreversible mental or physical illness, disease, or condition.
- I do not want: ___ Mechanical ventilation ___ CPR ___ Dialysis ___ Feeding tubes
- Other exceptions and/or comments:

_____
_____

Additional Comments or Exceptions: _____

MY LIVING WILL (continued)

This living will describes my express wishes and legal right to accept or refuse treatment. As I am of sound mind, I expect my family, physician/s, and all those concerned with my care to regard themselves as legally and morally bound to act in accord with my wishes.

Signed _____ Date_____

Witness (Cannot be designated health care agent). I declare that the person who signed the document, or asked another to sign this document on his/her behalf, did so in my presence and that he/she appears to be of sound mind and free of duress or undue influence.

Signed _____ Date_____

Signed _____ Date_____

Note: A copy of the executed living will should be provided to the patient's physician, and health care agent.

helpful to health care professionals because it provides guidance about a patient's wishes for treatment, provides legally valid instructions about treatment, and protects the patient's rights and the provider who honors them.

The living will should be signed and dated by two witnesses who are not blood relatives or beneficiaries of property. A living will should be discussed with the patient's physician, and a signed copy should be placed in the patient's medical record. A copy also should be given to the individual designated to make decisions in the event the patient is unable to do so. A person who executes a living will when healthy and mentally competent cannot predict how he or she will feel at the time of a terminal illness. Therefore, it should be updated regularly so that it accurately reflects a patient's wishes. The written instructions become effective when a patient is either in a terminal condition, permanently unconscious, or suffering irreversible brain damage.

Durable Power of Attorney

A *durable power of attorney* is a legal device that permits one individual, known as the "principal," to give to another person, called the "attorney-in-fact," the authority to act on his or her behalf. The attorney-in-fact is authorized to handle banking and real estate affairs, incur expenses, pay bills, and handle a wide variety of legal affairs for a specified period of time. The power of attorney may continue indefinitely during the lifetime of the principal so long as that person is competent and capable of granting power of attorney. If the principal becomes comatose or mentally incompetent, the power of attorney automatically expires, just as it would if the principal dies.

Because a power of attorney is limited by the competency of the principal, some states have authorized a special legal device for the principal to express intent concerning the durability of the power of attorney, to allow it to survive disability or incompetency. The durable power of attorney is more general in scope, and the patient does not have to be in imminent danger of death, as is necessary in a living will situation. Although it need not delineate desired medical treatment specifically, it must indicate the identity of the principal's attorney-in-fact and that the principal has communicated his or her health care wishes to the attorney-in-fact. Although the laws vary from state to state, all 50 states and the District of Columbia have durable power of attorney statutes. This legal device is an important alternative to guardianship, conservatorship, or trusteeship. Because a durable power of attorney places a considerable amount of power in the hands of the attorney-in-fact, the power of attorney should be drawn up by an attorney in the state where the client resides. In the health care setting, a *durable power of attorney for health care* is a legal instrument that designates and grants authority to an agent, for example, to make health care decisions for another.

APPOINTED DECISION MAKERS

Guardianship

Guardianship is a legal mechanism by which the court declares a person incompetent and appoints a guardian. The court transfers the responsibility for managing financial affairs, living arrangements, and medical care decisions to the guardian.

The right to refuse medical treatment on behalf of an incompetent person is not limited to legally appointed guardians but may be exercised by health care proxies or surrogates, such as close family members or friends. When a patient has not expressed instructions concerning his or her future health care in the event of later incapacity but has merely delegated full responsibility to a proxy, designation of a proxy must have been made in writing.

Substituted Judgment

Mrs. Martin, in *In re Martin*, 517 N.W.2d 749 (Mich. Ct. App. 1994), wanted to withdraw her husband's life support. Mr. Martin's mother and sister did not wish to have Mrs. Martin removed as the patient's guardian. There was, however, sufficient evidence to show that the patient had a medical preference to decline treatment under circumstances such as those that occurred and that the patient's spouse was a suitable guardian. Evidence was clear that Mr. Martin would never regain sufficient decision-making capacity

DURABLE POWER OF ATTORNEY FOR HEALTH CARE

I, _____,

Appoint:

1. Name_____ Phone _____
   Address _____

as my attorney-in-fact or agent to make my health and personal care decisions for me if I become unable to make my own decisions. If the person I have named above is unable to act as my agent, I hereby designate the following person to serve as my agent:

2. Name_____ Phone _____
   Address _____

This *durable power of attorney* shall become effective upon my incapacity to make health or personal care decisions. Please initial the statement/s below that best expresses your wishes.

_____ I authorize my admission to or discharge from any medical, nursing, residential, or similar facility and to enter into agreements for my care.

_____ I authorize my agent to refuse or withdraw consent to any and all types of treatment, including, but not limited to nutrition and hydration administered by artificial or invasive means.

I have discussed with my agent my wishes for health care. If my agent is not able to determine what I would want, I trust my agent to make his/her decision based on what he/she believes would be my wishes. This durable power of attorney is meant to replace all others.

Signed _____ Date_____

Witness (Cannot be the principal's designated health care agent). I declare that the person who signed this document or asked another to sign this document on his/her behalf did so in my presence and that he/she appears to be of sound mind and free of duress or undue influence.

Signed _____ Date_____

Signed _____ Date_____

Primary Agent

I, _____, have read the above durable power of attorney and am the person identified as the agent for _____.
My signature below indicates that I acknowledge and accept responsibility to act as the agent and will exercise the powers herein granted in the best interest of the principal.

Signature _____ Date_____

Substitute Agent

I, _____, have read the above durable power of attorney and am the person identified as the agent for _____.

DURABLE POWER OF ATTORNEY FOR HEALTH CARE (continued)

My signature below indicates that I acknowledge and accept responsibility to act as the agent and will exercise the powers herein granted in the best interest of the principal.

Signature _____ Date_____

State of _____

County of: _____

On this date, the _____ day of _____, 200___, before me, the undersigned officer, personally appeared _____, known to me (satisfactorily proven) to be the person whose name is subscribed to the foregoing instrument, and acknowledged that he/she executed it for the purposes therein contained.

Witness my hand and official seal the day and year aforesaid _____.

Notary Public

Note: A copy of the executed durable power of attorney should be provided to the patient's physician, and health care agent.

that would enable him to make such a decision and that his condition and cognitive level of functioning would not improve in the future.

Testimony from two of Mr. Martin's friends described statements made by him that he would never want to be maintained in a coma or in a vegetative state. In addition, Mrs. Martin described numerous statements made to her by her husband prior to the accident saying that he would not want to be maintained alive given the circumstances described earlier. The court of appeals found no reason to dispute the trial court's finding as to Mrs. Martin's credibility. There was no evidence that Mrs. Martin had anything but her husband's best interest at heart. There were allegations, but no evidence of, financial considerations or pressure from another individual that would show that Mrs. Martin's testimony was influenced by other individuals.

Health Care Proxy

A health care proxy allows a person to appoint a health care agent to make treatment decisions in the event he or she becomes incompetent and is unable to make decisions for himself or herself. The agent must be made aware of the patient's wishes regarding nutrition and hydration in order to be allowed to make a decision concerning withholding or withdrawing them. In contrast to a living will, a health care proxy does not require a person to know about and consider in advance all situations and decisions that could arise. Rather, the appointed agent would know about and interpret the expressed wishes of the patient and then make decisions about the medical care and treatment to be administered or refused. The Cruzan decision indicates that the Supreme Court views advance directives as clear and convincing evidence of a patient's wishes regarding life-sustaining treatment.

Although most statutes fail to cover incompetents, cases such as Quinlan and Saikewicz created a constitutionally protected obligation to terminate the incurable incompetent's life when guardians use the doctrine of substituted judgment. Further, some states provide for proxy consent in the form of durable power of attorney statutes. Generally, these involve designation of a proxy to speak on the incompetent incurable's behalf. They represent a combination of the intimate wishes of the patient and the medical recommendations of the physicians.

Oral declarations are accepted only after the patient has been declared terminally ill. Moreover, the declarant bears the responsibility of informing the physician to ensure that the document becomes a part of the medical record. The California statute provides that the document be re-executed after five years. Other statutes differ in the length of time of effectiveness. Most states allow the document to be effective until revoked by the individual. To revoke, the patient must sign and date a new writing, destroy the first document himself or herself, direct another to destroy the first document in his or her presence, or orally state to the physician an intent to revoke. The effect of the directive varies among jurisdictions. However, there is unanimity in the promulgation of regulations that specifically authorize health care personnel to honor the directives without fear of incurring liability. The highest court of New York in *In re Eichner*[36] complied with the request of a guardian to withdraw life-support systems from an 83-year-old brain-damaged priest. The court reached its result by finding the patient's previously expressed wishes to be determinative.

Before exercising an incompetent patient's right to forgo medical treatment, the surrogate decision maker must satisfy the following conditions:

- The surrogate must be satisfied that the patient executed a document (e.g., Durable Power of Attorney for Health Care and Health Care Proxy) knowingly, willingly, and without undue influence, and that the evidence of the patient's oral declaration is reliable.
- The patient must not have reasonable probability of recovering competency so that the patient could exercise the right.
- The surrogate must take care to ensure that any limitations or conditions expressed either orally or in written declarations have been considered carefully and satisfied.

Surrogate Decision Maker

A surrogate decision maker is an agent who acts on behalf of a patient who lacks the capacity to participate in a particular decision.

A health care agent's rights are no greater than those of a competent patient. However, the agent's rights are limited to any specific instructions included in the proxy document. An agent's decisions take priority over any other person except the patient. The agent has the right to consent or refuse to consent to any service or treatment, routine or otherwise; to refuse life-sustaining treatment; and to access "all" of the patient's medical information to make informed decisions. The agent must make decisions based on the patient's moral and religious beliefs. If a patient's wishes are not known, decisions must be based on a good-faith judgment of what the patient would have wanted.

FUTILITY OF TREATMENT

Futility of treatment, as it relates to medical care, occurs when the physician recognizes that the effect of treatment will be of no benefit to the patient. Morally, the physician has a duty to inform the patient when there is little likelihood of success. The determination as to futility of medical care is a scientific decision.

After a diagnosis has been made that a person is terminally ill with no hope of recovery and is in a chronic vegetative state with no possibility of attaining cognitive function, a state generally has no compelling interest in maintaining life. The decision to forgo or terminate life-support measures is, at this point, simply a decision that the dying process will not be artificially extended. Although the state has an interest in the prolongation of life, it has no interest in the prolongation of dying, and although there is a moral and ethical decision to be made to end the process, that decision can be made only by the surrogate. The decision whether to end the dying process is a personal decision for family members or those who bear a legal responsibility for the patient.

A determination as to the futility of medical care is a decision that must be made by a physician. Even if death is not imminent but a patient's coma is irreversible beyond doubt and there are adequate safeguards to confirm the accuracy of the diagnosis with the concurrence of those responsible for the patient's care, it is not unethical to discontinue all means of life-prolonging medical treatment.

Right to Die without a Living Will

In *San Juan-Torregosa v. Garcia*,[37] the evidence at trial established that Garcia suffered a cardiac arrest. Although she was later resuscitated, she suffered oxygen deprivation to her brain for more than ten minutes and was in a chronic vegetative state. Medical opinion established that she was breathing reflexively, but there was no evidence that she would be able to recover "cortical functions." Garcia also had metastatic breast cancer. Her treating physician, Dr. Parrish, testified at trial that within a reasonable degree of medical certainty Garcia would not recover and that he had never seen anyone in her condition recover. He stated that Garcia was functioning on a low brain level, whereby the brainstem kept her blood circulating, maintained blood pressure, and maintained respiration; and that she was in a persistent vegetative state with a zero chance of recovering any cortex activity. Parrish further stated that he discussed the discontinuation of artificial nutrition and hydration with the family, and that they had ultimately decided to continue the fluids but stop the nutrition, which he felt was reasonable.

When asked why Garcia had been given life support in the first place, Parrish explained that although Garcia's injury initially seemed very severe, he could not say from the beginning whether she would recover, and wanted to give her every chance to improve if she could.

The trial court ruled that because Garcia, who was in a chronic vegetative state, had not executed a living will, the court had no authority to authorize discontinuance of artificial nutrition.

On appeal, the appellants asserted that the trial court erred in refusing to allow Garcia's family to terminate the artificial nutrition and hydration that was keeping her body alive, thereby failing to honor her wishes and denying her constitutional right to bodily integrity.

[The United States Supreme Court in *Cruzan v. Director, Missouri Dept. of Health*, 497 U.S. 261, 110 S. Ct. 2841 (1990), recognized that a competent person had a constitutionally protected liberty interest in refusing unwanted medical treatment. The Court stopped short of finding that an incompetent person would have the same right. However, the court said: "An incompetent person is not able to make an informed and voluntary choice to exercise a hypothetical right to refuse treatment, or any other right. Such a "right" must be exercised for her, if at all, by some sort of surrogate."]

Tennessee's public policy on this issue is set forth in the Legislative intent section of the Tennessee Right to Natural Death Act, codified at Tenn. Code Ann. §32-11-102. This statute reads: "The general assembly declares it to be the law of the state of Tennessee that every person has the fundamental and inherent right to die naturally with as much dignity as circumstances permit and to accept, refuse, withdraw from, or otherwise control decisions relating to the rendering of the person's own medical care, specifically including palliative care and the use of extraordinary procedures and treatment."

This policy belongs to every person and does not distinguish between those who are competent and those who are not. An individual has a right to refuse treatment so long as that individual is competent. When an individual is incompetent to make such a decision, the state had a duty to become involved by trying to determine what "the desires of the patient would have been had he been conscious and competent," and that the initial assumption would be that the patient desired lifesaving treatment unless that assumption was contradicted by previous statements made when competent. It is clear that from state court decisions, artificial nutrition and hydration are to be included in the realm of medical treatment that a patient has a right to refuse. Kevorkian is presently serving a 10- to 25-year prison sentence for participating in physician-assisted suicide.

The appeals court concurred with the trial court's fact finding that evidence is clear and convincing that Garcia would not want to be kept alive by artificial means and that her wishes, expressed while she was competent, would be to have these services discontinued. Courts have the duty to protect and when necessary enable individuals to exercise their constitutional rights. The appeals court ordered that a conservator be appointed to carry out Garcia's wishes, including the refusal for medical care.

WITHDRAWAL OF TREATMENT

Withdrawal of treatment is a decision not to initiate treatment or medical interventions for the patient. When death is imminent and cannot be prevented by available treatment, it is morally permissible to withhold treatment that can yield only a precarious prolongation of life that may involve a great burden for the patient or family. Palliative care should be encouraged in end-of-life situations.

Withdrawal of treatment should be considered when: (1) the patient is in a terminal condition and there is a reasonable expectation of imminent death of the patient; (2) the patient is in a non-cognitive state with no reasonable possibility of regaining cognitive function, and/or restoration of cardiac function will last for a brief period.

Patient Not in a Persistent Vegetative State

A guardian may "only" direct the withdrawal of life-sustaining medical treatment, including nutrition and hydration, if the incompetent ward is in a persistent vegetative state and the decision to withdraw is in the best interests of the ward.

Edna's sister and court-appointed guardian, Spahn, sought permission to direct the withholding of Edna's nutrition, claiming that her sister would not want to live in this condition. However, the only testimony presented at trial regarding Edna's views on the use of life-sustaining medical treatment involves a statement made 30 years earlier. At that time, Spahn and Edna were having a conversation about their mother, who was recovering from depression, and Spahn's mother-in-law, who was dying of cancer. Spahn testified that during this conversation, Edna said to her that she would rather die of cancer than lose her mind. Spahn further testified that this was the only time that she and Edna discussed the subject and that Edna never said anything specifically about withholding or withdrawing life-sustaining medical treatment.

The "ethics committee" at the nursing facility where Edna lives met to discuss the issue of withholding artificial nutrition from Edna. The committee approved withholding nutrition if no family member objected. However, one of Edna's nieces refused to sign a statement approving the withdrawal of nutrition.

The record speaks very little to what Edna's desires would be, and there was no clear statement of what her desires would be today under the current conditions. Her friends and family never had any conversations with her discussing her feelings or opinions about withdrawing nutrition or hydration, and she did not execute any advance directives expressing her wishes while she was competent.

Consequently, the court held that a guardian may only direct the withdrawal of life-sustaining medical treatment, including nutrition and hydration, if the incompetent ward is in a persistent vegetative state and the decision to withdraw is in the best interests of the ward. In this case, where the only indication of Edna's desires was made at least 30 years ago and under different circumstances, there is not a clear statement of intent such that Edna's guardian may authorize the withholding of her nutrition.

The circuit judge concluded his own questioning of one member of the ethics committee: "The way I understand it, what you really have is a liability problem, and that's why you want everybody to consent, is that correct?" Dr. Erickson answered: "That is correct."[38]

Removal of Life-Support Equipment

Although there may be a duty to provide life-sustaining equipment in the immediate aftermath of cardiopulmonary arrest, there is no duty to continue its use once it has become futile and ineffective to do so in the opinion of qualified medical personnel. Two physicians in *Barber v. Superior Court*[39] were charged with the crimes of murder and conspiracy to commit murder. The charges were based on their acceding to requests of the patient's family to discontinue life-support equipment and intravenous tubes. The patient had suffered a cardiopulmonary arrest in the recovery room after surgery. A team of physicians and nurses revived the patient and placed him on life-support equipment. The patient had suffered severe brain damage, placing him in a comatose and vegetative state from which, according to tests and examinations by other specialists, he was unlikely to recover. On the written request of the family, the patient was taken off life-support equipment. The family, his wife and eight children, made the decision together after consultation with the physicians. Evidence had been presented that the patient, before his incapacitation, had expressed to his wife that he would not want to be kept alive by a machine. There was no evidence indicating that the family was motivated in their decision by anything other than love and concern for the dignity of their loved one. The patient continued to breathe on his own. Showing no signs of improvement, the physicians again discussed the patient's poor prognosis with the family. The intravenous lines were removed, and the patient died sometime thereafter.

A complaint then was filed against the two physicians. The magistrate who heard the evidence determined that the physicians did not kill the deceased because their conduct was not the proximate cause of the patient's death. On motion of the prosecution, the superior court determined as a matter of law that the evidence required the magistrate to hold the physicians to answer and ordered the complaint reinstated. The physicians then filed a writ of prohibition with the court of appeals. The court of appeals held that the physicians' omission to continue treatment, although intentional and with knowledge that the patient would die, was not an unlawful failure to perform a legal duty. The evidence amply supported the magistrate's decision. The superior court erred in determining that, as a matter of law, the evidence required the magistrate to hold the physicians to answer. The preemptory writ of prohibition to restrain the Superior Court of Los Angeles from taking any further action in this matter, other than to vacate its order reinstating the complaint and to enter a new and different order denying the People's motion, was granted.

Feeding Tubes

Theologians and ethicists have long recognized a distinction between ordinary and extraordinary medical care. The theological distinction is based on the belief that life is a gift from God that should not be destroyed deliberately by humans. Therefore, extraordinary therapies that extend life by imposing grave burdens on the patient and family are not required. A patient, however, has an ethical and moral obligation to accept ordinary or life-sustaining treatment. Although the courts have accepted decisions to withhold or withdraw extraordinary care, especially the respirator, from those who are comatose or in a persistent vegetative state with no possibility of emerging, they have been unwilling until now to discontinue feeding, which they have considered ordinary care.

However, in 1985, the New Jersey Supreme Court heard the case of *In re Claire C. Conroy*.[40] The case involved an 84-year-old nursing home patient whose nephew petitioned the court for authority to remove the nasogastric tube that was feeding her. The court overturned the appellate division decision and held that life-sustaining treatment, including nasogastric feeding, could be withheld or withdrawn from incompetent nursing home patients who will, according to physicians, die within one year, in three specific circumstances. These are

1. when it is clear that the particular patient would have refused the treatment under the circumstances involved (the subjective test),
2. when there is some indication of the patient's wishes (but he or she has not "unequivocally expressed" his or her desires before becoming incompetent) and the treatment "would only prolong suffering" (the limited objective test), and
3. when there is no evidence at all of the patient's wishes, but the treatment "clearly and markedly outweighs the benefits the patient derives from life" (the pure objective test based on pain).[41]

A procedure involving notification of the state Office of the Ombudsman is required before withdrawing or withholding treatment under any of the three tests. The ombudsman must make a separate recommendation.

The court also found tubal feeding to be a medical treatment, and, as such, it is as intrusive as other life-sustaining measures. The court in its analysis emphasized duty, rather than causation, with the result that medical personnel acting in good faith will be protected from liability. If physicians follow the Quinlan/Conroy standards and decide to end medical treatment of a patient, the duty to continue treatment ceases. Thus, the termination of treatment becomes a lawful act.

Although Conroy presents case-specific guidelines, there is concern that the opinion will have far-reaching repercussions. There is fear that decisions to discontinue treatment will not be based on the "balancing of interests" test, but rather that a "quality-of-life" test similar to that used by Hitler will be used to end the lives of severely senile, very old, decrepit, and burdensome people.

Those quality-of-life judgments would be most dangerous for nursing home patients in which age would be a factor in the decision-making process. "Advocates of 'the right to life' fear that the 'right to die' for the elderly and handicapped will become a 'duty to die.'"[42] In both the Saikewicz and Spring cases, age was a determining factor weighing against life-sustaining treatment. Further, in *In re Hier,*[43] the court found that Mrs. Hier's age of 92 years made the "proposed gastrostomy substantially more onerous or burdensome . . . than it would be for a younger, healthier person." Moreover, a New York Superior Court held that the burdens of an emergency amputation for an elderly patient outweighed the benefit of continued life.[44] Finding that prolonging her life would be cruel, the court stated that life had no meaning for her. Although some courts have recognized the difference, other courts must still address the difference between Quinlan-type patients and elderly, confined, and conscious patients who can interact but whose mental or physical functioning is impaired.

However, in a New Jersey case, the ombudsman denied a request to remove feeding tubes from a comatose nursing home patient.[45] In applying the Conroy tests, the ombudsman decided that Hilda Peterson might live more than one year, the period that Conroy used as a criterion for determining whether life support can be removed.

To further complicate this issue, on March 17, 1986, the American Medical Association changed its code of ethics on comas. Now physicians may ethically withhold food, water, and medical treatment from patients in irreversible comas or persistent vegetative states with no hope of recovery—even if death is not imminent.[46] Although physicians can consider the wishes of the patient and family or the legal representatives, they cannot cause death intentionally. The wording is permissive, so those physicians who feel uncomfortable withdrawing food and water may refrain from doing so. The American Medical Association's decision does not comfort those who fear abuse or mistake in euthanasia decisions, nor does it have any legal value as such. There are physicians, nurses, and families who are unscrupulous and have their own, and not the patient's, interests in mind.

Even with the Conroy decision and the American Medical Association's Code of Ethics change, the feeding tube issue is not settled.

On April 23, 1986, the New Jersey Superior Court ruled that the husband of severely brain-damaged Nancy Jobes could order the removal of her life-sustaining feeding tube, which would ultimately cause the 31-year-old comatose patient, who had been in a vegetative state in a hospice for the past six years, to starve to death.[47] Dr. Fred Plum created and defined the term *persistent vegetative state* as one in which:

> . . . the body functions entirely in terms of its internal controls. It maintains temperature. It maintains digestive activity. It maintains heart beat and pulmonary ventilation. It maintains reflex activity of muscles and nerves for low-level conditioned responses. But there is no behavioral evidence of either self-awareness or awareness of the surroundings in a learned manner.[48]

Medical experts testified that the patient could, under optimal conditions, live another 30 years. Relieving the nursing home officials from performing the act on one of its residents, the court ruled that the patient may be taken home to die (with the removal to be supervised by a physician and medical care to be provided to the patient at home).

The nursing home had petitioned the court for the appointment of a "life advocate" to fight for continuation of medical treatment for Jobes, which, it argued, would save her life. The court disallowed the appointment of a life advocate, holding that case law does not support requiring the continuation of life-support systems in all circumstances. Such a requirement, according to the court, would contradict the patient's right of privacy.

The court's decision applied "the principles enunciated in Quinlan and . . . Conroy" and the "ruling by the American Medical Association's Council on Judicial Affairs that the provision of food and water is, under certain circumstances, a medical treatment like any other and may be discontinued when the physician and family of the patient feel it is no longer benefiting the patient."[49]

An Illinois court found that the authorized guardian of a terminally ill patient in an irreversible coma or persistent vegetative state has a common-law right to refuse artificial nutrition and hydration. The court found that there must be clear and convincing evidence that the refusal is consistent with the patient's interest. The court also required the concurrence of the patient's attending physician and two other physicians. "Court intervention is also necessary to guard against the remote, yet real possibility that greed may taint the judgment of the surrogate decision maker."[50] Dissenting, Judge Ward said, "The right to refuse treatment is rooted in and dependent on the patient's capacity for informed decision, which an incompetent patient lacks."[51]

Also, Elizabeth Bouvia, a mentally competent cerebral palsy victim, won her struggle to have feeding tubes removed even though she was not terminally ill.[52] The California Court of Appeals announced on April 16, 1986, that she could go home to die. The court found that Bouvia's decision to "let nature take its course" did not amount to a choice to commit suicide with people aiding and abetting it. The court stated that it is not "illegal or immoral to prefer a natural, albeit sooner, death than a drugged life attached to a mechanical device."[53] The court's finding that it was a moral and philosophic question, not a legal or medical one, leaves one wondering whether the courts are opening the door to permitting "legal starvation" to be used by those who are not terminally ill but who do wish to commit suicide.

Do Not Resuscitate Orders

Do Not Resuscitate (DNR) orders are those given by a physician indicating that in the event of a cardiac or respiratory arrest, "no" resuscitative measures should be used to revive the patient. A DNR order is an extremely difficult decision to make for both the patient and family. It is generally made when one's quality of life has been so diminished that "heroic" rescue methods are no longer in the patient's best interests. The attending physician or his/her designee may initiate a DNR order at the request of or with the agreement of the patient or the legally appointed health care decision maker. A DNR order may be written if the patient has an executable advance directive with instructions regarding DNR status and/or if the transfer information from an extended care facility indicates the patient should have a DNR order.

If a patient lacks the ability to make a decision regarding a DNR order, the patient's legally appointed decision maker can make such decisions provided it can be demonstrated that the decision maker is following the patient's wishes. Advanced directives, such as living wills, are helpful in determining a patient's wishes.

DNR orders must be in writing, signed and dated by the physician. Appropriate consents must be obtained either from the patient or his or her health care agent. Many states have acknowledged the validity of DNR orders in cases involving terminally ill patients in which the patients' families make no objections to such orders.

DNR orders must comply with statutory requirements, be of short duration, and be reviewed periodically to determine whether the patient's condition or other circumstances (e.g., change of mind by the patient or family) surrounding the "no code" orders have changed. Presently, it is generally accepted that if a patient is competent, the DNR order is considered to be the same as other medical decisions in which a patient may choose to reject life-sustaining treatment. In the case of an incompetent, absent any advance written directives, the best interests of the patient would be considered.

Competent Patients Make Their Own Decisions

Should relatives of a patient agree to a no code order when the patient is competent to make his or her own decision?

In *Payne v. Marion General Hospital*,[54] the Indiana Court of Appeals overturned a lower court decision in favor of the physician. The physician had issued a no code status on Payne despite evidence given by a nurse that up to a few minutes before his death Payne could communicate. The physician had determined that Payne was incompetent, thereby rendering him unable to give informed consent to treatment. Because Payne left no written directives, the physician relied on one of Payne's relatives who asked for the DNR order. The court found that there was evidence that Payne was not incompetent and should have been consulted before a DNR order was given. Further, the court reviewed testimony that one year earlier Payne had suffered and recovered from the same type of symptoms, leading to the conclusion that there was a possibility that he could have survived if resuscitation had continued. There was no DNR policy in place at the hospital to assist the physician in making his decision. To avoid this type of problem, health care providers should adopt an appropriate process with respect to issuing no code orders.

CASE: SPOUSAL RIGHTS IN DECISION MAKING

Mr. Martin sustained debilitating injuries as the result of an automobile accident. He suffered severe subcortical brain damage, significantly impairing his physical and cognitive functioning.[55] His injuries left him totally paralyzed on the left side. He could not speak or eat and had no bladder or bowel control. Martin remained conscious and had some awareness of his surroundings. He could communicate to a very minimal degree through head nods.

The trial court determined that Martin did not have nor would he ever have the ability to have the requisite capacity to make decisions regarding the withdrawal of life-support equipment. The evidence demonstrated that Martin's preference would have been to decline life-support equipment given his medical condition and prognosis. The trial court's decision was based on the following four-part test for determining whether a person has the requisite capacity to make a decision:

1. Does the person have sufficient mind to reasonably understand the condition?
2. Is the person capable of understanding the nature and effect of the treatment choices?
3. Is the person aware of the consequences associated with those choices?

4. Is the person able to make an informed choice that is voluntary and not coerced?

The trial court also determined that Mrs. Martin, the patient's spouse, was a suitable guardian for him.

Mrs. Martin petitioned to withdraw her husband's life support. Martin's mother and sister counter-petitioned to have Mrs. Martin removed as the patient's guardian.

The Michigan Court of Appeals held that the evidence was sufficient to support a finding that the patient lacked capacity to make decisions regarding the withholding or withdrawal of life-sustaining treatment. As to the patient's desire not to be placed on life-support equipment, there was sufficient evidence to show that the patient had a medical preference to decline treatment under circumstances such as those that occurred. There was also sufficient evidence to show that the patient's spouse was a suitable guardian.

The test for determining whether Martin had the requisite capacity to make a decision regarding the withholding or withdrawal of life-supporting medical treatment was clear and convincing—he did not have sufficient decision-making capacity. The evidence was just as clear that he never would regain sufficient decision-making capacity that would enable him to make such a decision. It was the general consensus of all of the experts that Martin's condition and cognitive level of functioning would not improve in the future.

Testimony from two of Martin's friends described statements made by him that he would never want to be maintained in a coma or in a vegetative state. In addition, Mrs. Martin described numerous statements made to her by Martin prior to the accident that he would not want to be maintained alive given the circumstances described above. The trial court found that Mrs. Martin was credible. The court of appeals found no reason to dispute the trial court's finding as to Mrs. Martin's credibility.

Contrary to allegations made by the patient's mother and sister, the evidence was clear that Mrs. Martin's testimony was credible. There was no evidence that Mrs. Martin had anything but her husband's best interest at heart. There were allegations, but no evidence of, financial considerations or pressure from another individual that would show that Mrs. Martin's testimony was influenced by other individuals.

Ethical and Legal Issues

1. Knowing that the patient had some ability to interact with his environment, discuss the four-part test for determining the patient's ability to make a decision.
2. Do you agree with the court's decision? Explain.
3. Should the concern of the mother and sister have carried more weight in removing custody from Mrs. Martin?
4. What influence do you believe the mother and sister might have had on Mrs. Martin? ◼

CASE: MEN DON'T CRY

Some say, "Men don't cry." Not true! You may find yourself crying alone someday. For now, you have to be strong for Sunshine.

Sunshine was her name, as given to her by her grandmother. For purposes of this case, she remains Sunshine. Not Miss or Ms. or Mrs., for Sunshine is her name. If you were to ask Sunshine what she thought about her life, this is what she would tell you.

As a hard-charging former district attorney, Sunshine knows what it's like to be under the constant threat of death. In the notorious 1990 "Angel Gabriel" case, a key witness to a cult leader's rape spree was murdered. As a result, the district attorney ordered that a panic alarm be placed in Sunshine's home.

Still, one enemy has done more damage than all of her former enemies combined. Sunshine has been battling systemic sclerosis for more than six years and has beaten the long-shot odds for survival.

Early on she lost 20 pounds in three weeks. One by one, from her esophagus to her bottom, her internal organs came under painful attack. Her skin hardened in patches. Her fingers became discolored and swollen, fingernails fell off, calcification set in, and she nearly lost several digits.

At the moment, she has a mysterious edema throughout her body.

Maintaining a full-time work schedule, she bounced from physician to physician for three years, seeking to find a reason for sudden illness. The clues were finally put together and her illness was diagnosed as systemic sclerosis—a degenerative connective tissue disease.

Most people don't know she has an illness. She's always in good spirits. She hides it well. Sunshine admits to putting a mask on in the morning. "When I cannot hide the pain, I disappear—go away or go home. I don't want to be defined by my illness. You go through mourning and anger. You feel tethered by the disease. It's a sadness you have to cope with."

With her mask firmly in place, a smiling Sunshine says she is not bitter. "I had a great life. I had fun. If it ended, I had fun."

Sunshine's prayer: *Strength to Cope*

O God, you know my feelings. You know that I want to feel better. I want to be better. I want to have my health restored.

But the hours of testing, the days of diagnosis, and the question marks concerning my future seem nearly more than I can take!

Grant me, O God, the strength to face each hour of this and every day. In fact, when it seems that I cannot face even this hour, fill me with strength to face the next five minutes. Amen.

UNIVERSITY OF PENNSYLVANIA HEALTH SYSTEM

Wherever Sunshine goes, the sun always shines, for she, as always, recognizes the beauty of each day.

Ethical and Legal Issues

1. Remembering Annie in the summary case in Chapter 1, do you think Mark is capable of making end-of-life decisions for Sunshine? Explain your answer.
2. Should Sunshine appoint Mark as her health care surrogate decision maker? Explain your answer. ◼

CHAPTER REVIEW

1. Euthanasia is defined broadly as "the mercy killing of the hopelessly ill, injured, or incapacitated." The debate over euthanasia is complex, and the legal system must maintain a balance between ensuring that the patient's constitutional rights are protected and protecting society's interests in preserving life, preventing suicide, and maintaining the integrity of the medical profession.
2. When there exists an element of uncertainty regarding a patient's wishes in an emergency situation, the situation should be resolved in a way that favors the preservation of life. This protects the patient's right to freedom of religion and self-determination.
   - Active euthanasia is the intentional commission of an act that will result in death.
   - Passive euthanasia is when a potentially lifesaving treatment is withdrawn or withheld.
3. Voluntary euthanasia occurs when a competent adult patient with an incurable condition who has been informed of the possible ramifications and alternatives available gives consent. Involuntary euthanasia is when the decision to terminate the life of an incurable person (i.e., an incompetent or unconsenting competent) is made by someone other than that incurable person.
4. The Supreme Court has ruled that there exists no constitutional right to assisted suicide. This decision allowed the state of Michigan to prosecute Kevorkian for assisting patients in committing suicide.
5. According to the Patient Self-Determination Act of 1990, health care organizations have a responsibility to explain to patients, staff, and families that patients have legal rights to direct their medical and nursing care as it corresponds to existing state law.
6. Because of the debate surrounding right-to-die issues, patients should be counseled to make decisions regarding their wishes while they are competent. Living wills, designation of surrogates, health care proxies, and powers of attorney are legal steps that allow patients to express their wishes.

7. Advance directives, in the form of a "living will" or "durable power of attorney," allow the patient to state in advance the kinds of medical care that he or she considers acceptable or not acceptable. The patient can appoint an agent, a surrogate decision maker, to make those decisions on his or her behalf.

8. A living will is the instrument or legal document that describes those treatments an individual wishes or does not wish to receive should he or she become incapacitated and unable to communicate treatment decisions.

9. A durable power of attorney is a legal device that permits one individual, known as the "principal," to give to another person, called the "attorney-in-fact," the authority to act on his or her behalf.

10. Guardianship is a legal mechanism by which the court declares a person incompetent and appoints a guardian. The court transfers the responsibility for managing financial affairs, living arrangements, and medical care decisions to the guardian.

11. A health care proxy allows a person to appoint a health care agent to make treatment decisions in the event he or she becomes incompetent and is unable to make decisions for himself or herself.

12. A surrogate decision maker is an agent who acts on behalf of a patient who lacks the capacity to participate in a particular decision.

13. A primary difference between health care proxies and living wills is that proxies do not require that a person know about and consider in advance every situation and decision that could arise. Instead, the appointed agent would have to interpret the patient's wishes based on the information given at the time that the patient is incapacitated and unable to make decisions for himself or herself.

14. Do not resuscitate orders are given by physicians and indicate that in the event of a cardiac or respiratory arrest, no resuscitative measures should be used to revive the patient. These orders must be in writing and must be signed and dated by the physician.

15. Futility of treatment, as it relates to medical care, occurs when the physician recognizes that the effect of treatment will be of no benefit to the patient. Morally, the physician has a duty to inform the patient when there is little likelihood of success. The determination as to futility of a medical care is a scientific decision.

TEST YOUR UNDERSTANDING

Terminology

euthanasia	substituted judgment
physician-assisted suicide	health care proxy
Oregon's Death with Dignity Act	surrogate decision maker
Patient Self-Determination Act of 1990	futility of treatment

advance directives
living will
durable power of attorney
guardianship
appointed decision-makers
futility of treatment
withdrawal of treatment

withdrawal of treatment
Do Not Resuscitate (DNR) order

REVIEW QUESTIONS

1. What are the differences between allowing a patient to die and physician-assisted suicide?

2. Examine this statement: "The inherent risk is that society's faith in doctors as healers would become subverted if doctors participate in physician-assisted suicide."

3. Constitutionally, what gives patients the right to self-determination?

4. What is "standing" with regard to who can bring an action, and who has standing when litigating the right to die?

5. Describe how a living will differs from a durable power of attorney for health care.

NOTES

1. Cruzan v. Director of the Mo. Dep't of Health, 497 U.S. 261 (1990).
2. DeGrella v. Elston, 858 S.W.2d 698 (1993).
3. J. Podgers, *Matters of Life and Death*, A.B.A.J. May 1992, at 60.
4. 105 N.E. 92 (N.Y. 1914).
5. *Id.* at 93.
6. 438 N.Y.S.2d 266, 272 (N.Y. 1981).
7. In re Quinlan, 355 A.2d 647 (N.J. 1976).
8. 410 U.S. 113 (1973).
9. Quinlan, 355 A.2d at 663.
10. 370 N.E.2d 417 (Mass. 1977).
11. *Id.* at 434.
12. Gelford, *Euthanasia and the Terminally Ill Patient*, 63 Neb. L. Rev. 741, 747 (1984).
13. 380 N.E.2d 134 (Mass. 1978).
14. 405 N.E.2d 115 (Mass. 1980).
15. John F. Kennedy Mem'l Hosp. v. Bludworth, 452 So. 2d 921, 925 (Fla. 1984) (*citing* In re Welfare of Colyer, 660 P.2d 738 (Wash. 1983), in which the court found prior court approval to be "unresponsive and cumbersome").
16. Schmitt v. Pierce, 344 S.W.2d 120 (Mo. 1961).

17. Connery, *Prolonging Life: The Duty and Its Limits, Moral Responsibility in Prolonging Life's Decisions*, in To Treat or Not to Treat 25 (1984).
18. *Statement of Medical Opinion Re: "Brain Death,"* A.M.A. House of Delegates Res. (June 1974).
19. 482 N.Y.S.2d 436 (1984).
20. 438 N.Y.S.2d 266 (1981).
21. *Id.* at 425.
22. Cruzan v. Director of the Mo. Dep't of Health, 497 U.S. 261 (1990).
23. Pa. S.646, Amendment A3506, Printer's No. 689, Oct. 1, 1990.
24. 20 Pa. Cons. Stat. Ann. § 5602(a)(9) (1988).
25. *Hospital Wants To Let Wife Die*, Newsday, Jan. 11, 1991, at 13.
26. Farnam v. Crista Ministries, 807 P.2d 830, 849 (Wash. 1991).
27. *Dr. Death at Work*, Newsday, Feb. 7, 1991, at 12.
28. *Kevorkian Charges Dropped*, Newsday, July 22, 1992, at 4.
29. Hobbins v. Attorney Gen. of Mich., No. 94–1473 (Mich. 1994); Kevorkian v. Michigan, No. 94–1490 (Mich. 1994).
30. *22nd Death for "Dr. Death,"* USA Today, May 9, 1995, at 2A.
31. 117 S. Ct. 2293 (1997).
32. 117 S. Ct. 2258 (1997).
33. McIver v. Krischer, No. CL-96-1504-AF (Jan. 31, 1997) (stay issued February 11, 1997).
34. Kevorkian v. Thompson, 947 F. Supp. 1152 (1997).
35. 42 U.S.C. 1395cc(a)(1).
36. 420 N.E.2d 64 (N.Y. 1981).
37. No. E2001-02906-COA-R3-CV (2002).
38. Spahn v. Eisenberg, 563 N.W.2d 485 (1997).
39. 195 Cal. Rptr. 484 (Cal. Ct. App. 1983).
40. 486 A.2d 1209 (N.J. Sup. Ct. 1985).
41. *Id.*
42. U.S. Congress, Off. of Technology Assessment, Pub. No. OTA-BA-306, Life-Sustaining Technolgoies and the Elderly 48 (1987).
43. 464 N.E.2d 959 (Mass. 1984).
44. In re Beth Israel Med. Ctr., 519 N.Y.S.2d 511, 517 (N.Y. Sup. Ct. 1987).
45. Sullivan, *Ombudsman Bars Food Tube Removal*, N.Y. Times, Mar. 7, 1986, at 82.
46. *AMA Changes Code of Ethics on Comas*, Newsday, Mar. 17, 1986, at 2.
47. In re Jobes, 529 A.2d 434 (N.J. 1987).
48. *Id.* at 438.
49. *Man Wins Right To Let Wife Die*, Newsday, Apr. 24, 1986, at 3.
50. *Id.* at 790.
51. *Id.* at 793.
52. Bouvia v. Superior Court (Glenchur), 225 Cal. Rptr. 297 (Cal. Ct. App. 1986).
53. *Id.* at 306.
54. 549 N.E.2d 1043 (Ind. Ct. App. 1990).
55. In re Martin, 517 N.W.2d 749 (Mich. Ct. App. 1994).

Section II

Law

chapter five

Development of Law

Laws are the very bulwarks of liberty; they define every man's rights, and defend the individual liberties of all men.

J.G. HOLLAND (1819–1881)

LEARNING OBJECTIVES

The reader upon completion of this chapter will be able to:

- Understand the development of law
- Describe the functioning of our legal system
- Describe the sources of law:
  - ○ Common law
  - ○ Statutory law
  - ○ Administrative law
- Describe the functions of the three branches of government:
  - ○ Legislative
  - ○ Judicial
  - ○ Executive
- Understand the concept of "separation of powers"

INTRODUCTION

It is appropriate here to provide the reader with a background of the law, as it is the law that enables society to uphold what is right and punish those who transgress its intent—to protect the moral fiber upon which this nation was founded. This chapter introduces the reader to the development of American law, the functioning of our legal system, and the roles of the different branches of government in creating, administering, and enforcing the law in the United States. It is important to understand the foundation of our legal system before one can appreciate or comprehend the specific laws and principles relating to health care.

The law is rooted in tradition, culture, customs, and beliefs (e.g., religious influence—the mosaic law). Laws constantly grow and change to meet the needs of the American culture, a mixture of many. Familiarity with the vocabulary enables one to understand the ideas, concepts, and structure of the law. Laws continually evolve due to the ever-changing political, social, religious, and personal values of society, which is comprised of many cultures that become more intertwined with each new generation.

Supreme Court Justice Oliver Wendell Holmes said that the law "is a magic mirror, wherein we see reflected not only our own lives but also the lives of those who went before us."[1] "The government of the United States has been emphatically termed a government of laws, and not of men. It will certainly cease to deserve this high appellation, if the laws furnish no remedy for the violation of a vested right."[2]

Most definitions of law define it as a system of principles and processes by which people in a society deal with their disputes and problems, seeking to solve or settle them without resorting to force. Simply stated, laws are general rules of conduct that are enforced by government, which imposes penalties when prescribed laws are violated.

Laws govern the relationships between private individuals and organizations and between both of these parties and government. *Public law* deals with the relationships between individuals and government; *private law* deals with relationships among individuals. Laws regulate the activities and behaviors of individuals in international, federal, state, local, and municipal settings.

One important segment of public law is criminal law, which prohibits conduct deemed injurious to public order and provides for punishment of those proven to have engaged in such conduct. Public law also consists of countless regulations designed to advance societal objectives by requiring private individuals and organizations to adopt specified courses of action in their activities and undertakings. The thrust of most public law is to attain what society deems to be valid public goals.

Private law is concerned with the recognition and enforcement of the rights and duties of private individuals and organizations. Tort and contract actions are two basic types of private law. In a *tort action*, one party asserts that the wrongful conduct of another has caused harm, and the injured party seeks compensation for the harm suffered. Generally, a *contract action* involves a claim by one party that another party has breached an agreement by failing to fulfill an obligation. Either remuneration or specific performance of the obligation may be sought as a remedy. It is clear that without an organized, clear system of laws that regulate society, anarchy would be the result.

The goal of this chapter is to help caregivers better understand the law and how it affects the difficulties they face, while trying to do the right thing by making health care decisions that are both morally and legally acceptable.

SOURCES OF LAW

The basic sources of law are *common law,* which is derived from judicial decisions; *statutory law,* which emanates from the federal and state legislatures; and *administrative law,* prescribed by administrative agencies. In those instances in which written laws are either silent, vague, or contradictory to other laws, the judicial system often is called on to resolve those disputes until such time as appropriate legislative action can be taken to clear up a particular legal issue. In the following sections, the sources of law that formed the foundation of our legal system are discussed.

Common Law

The term *common law* refers to the body of principles that has evolved and expanded from judicial decisions that arise during the trial of court cases. Many of the legal principles and rules applied today by courts in the United States have their origins in English common law. Common law has its roots in "reason and justice" for all.

Because it is impossible to have a law that covers every potential human event that might occur in society, the judicial system is thus doubly necessary. It not only serves as a mechanism for reviewing legal disputes that arise in the written law, but it is also an effective review mechanism for those issues on which the written law is silent or, in instances of a mixture of issues, involving both written law and common-law decisions.

During the colonial period, English common law began to be applied in the colonies. According to John Dickinson in his *Letters from a Farmer in Pennsylvania* in 1768:

> The common law of England is generally received . . .; but our courts EXERCISE A SOVEREIGN AUTHORITY, in determining what parts of the common and statute law ought to be extended: For it must be admitted, that the difference of circumstances necessarily require us, in some cases to REJECT the determination of both. . . . Some of the English rules are adopted, others rejected.[3]

Joseph Story, in an 1829 U.S. Supreme Court decision, wrote, "The common law of England is not to be taken in all respects to be that of America. Our ancestors brought with them its general principles, and claimed it as their birthright but they brought with them and adopted only that portion which was applicable to their situation."[4]

The size of the country and the abundance of its natural resources made impossible the importation of the common law exactly as it had been developed in England. Measured by English standards, America had superabundant land, timber, and mineral wealth. American law had to serve the primary need of the new society to master the vast land areas of the American continent. The decisive facts upon which the law had to be based were the seemingly limitless expanses of land and the wealth and variety of natural resources.[5]

After the Revolution, each state, with the exception of Louisiana, adopted all or part of the existing English common law. Laws were added as needed. Louisiana civil law is based to a great extent on the French and Spanish laws and, especially, on the Code of Napoleon. As a result, there is no national system of common law in the United States, and common law on specific subjects may differ from state to state.

Case law court decisions did not easily pass from colony to colony. There were no printed reports to make transfer easy, though in the 18th century some manuscript materials did circulate among lawyers. These could hardly have been very influential. No doubt custom and case law slowly seeped from colony to colony. Travelers and word of mouth spread knowledge of living law. It is hard to say how much; thus it is hard to tell to what degree there was a common legal structure.[6]

Judicial review started to become part of the living law during the decade before the adoption of the federal Constitution. During that time American courts first began to assert the power to rule on the constitutionality of legislative acts and to hold unconstitutional statutes void.[7]

Cases are tried applying common-law principles unless a statute governs. Even though statutory law has affirmed many of the legal rules and principles initially established by the courts, new issues continue to arise, especially in private-law disputes, which require decision making according to common-law principles. Common-law actions are initiated mainly to recover money damages and/or possession of real or personal property.

When a higher state court has enunciated a common-law principle, the lower courts within the state where the decision was rendered must follow that principle. A decision in a case that sets forth a new legal principle establishes a precedent. Trial courts or those on equal footing are not bound by the decisions of other trial courts. Also, a principle established in one state does not set precedent for another state. Rather, the rulings in one jurisdiction may be used by the courts of other jurisdictions as guides to the legal analysis of a particular legal problem. Decisions found to be reasonable will be followed.

The position of a court or agency, relative to other courts and agencies, determines the place assigned to its decision in the hierarchy of decisional law. The decisions of the United States Supreme Court are highest in the hierarchy of decisional law with respect to federal legal questions. Because of the parties or the legal question involved, most legal controversies do not fall within the scope of the Supreme Court's decision-making responsibilities. On questions of purely state concern—such as the interpretation of a state statute that raises no issues under the U.S. Constitution or federal law—the highest court in the state has the final word on proper interpretation. The following are explanations of some of the more important common-law principles:

- *Res Judicata.* In common law, the term *res judicata,* which means "the thing is decided," refers to that which has been previously acted on or decided by the courts. According to *Black's Law Dictionary,* it is a rule where "a final judgment rendered by a court of competent jurisdiction on the merits is conclusive as to the rights of the parties and their privies, and, as to them, constitutes an absolute bar to subsequent action involving the same claim, demand, or cause of action."[8]
- *Stare Decisis.* The common-law principle of *stare decisis* ("let the decision stand") provides that when a decision is rendered in a lawsuit involving a particular set of facts, another lawsuit involving an identical or substantially similar situation is to be resolved in the same manner as the first lawsuit. The resolution of future lawsuits is arrived at by applying rules and principles of preceding cases. In this manner, courts arrive at comparable rulings. Sometimes slight factual differences may provide a basis for recognizing distinctions between the precedent and the current case. In some cases, even when such differences are absent, a court may conclude that a particular common-law rule is no longer in accord with the needs of society and may depart from precedent. It should be understood that principles of law are subject to change, whether they originate in statutory or in common law. Common-law principles may be modified, overturned, abrogated, or created by new court decisions in a continuing process of growth and development to reflect changes in social attitudes, public needs, judicial prejudices, or contemporary political thinking.

Statutory Law

Statutory law is written law emanating from federal and state legislative bodies. Although a statute can abolish any rule of common law, it can do so only by stating it in express words. States and local jurisdictions can only enact and enforce laws that do not conflict with federal law. Statutory laws may be declared void by a court; for example, a statute may be found unconstitutional because it does not comply with a state or federal constitution, because it is vague or ambiguous, or, in the case of a state law, because it is in conflict with a federal law.

In many cases involving statutory law, the court is called on to interpret how a statute applies to a given set of facts. For example, a statute may state merely that no person may discriminate against another person because of race, creed, color, or sex. A court may then be called on to decide whether certain actions by a person are discriminatory and therefore violate the law.

Constitution of the United States

The principles and rules of statutory law are set in hierarchical order. The *Constitution of the United States* adopted at the Constitutional Convention in Philadelphia in 1787 is highest in the hierarchy of enacted law. Article VI of the Constitution declares:

> This Constitution, and the Laws of the United States which shall be made in Pursuance thereof; and all Treaties made, or which shall be made, under the Authority of the United States, shall be the supreme Law of the Land; and the Judges in every State shall be bound thereby, any Thing in the Constitution or Laws of any State to the Contrary notwithstanding.[9]

The clear import of these words is that the U.S. Constitution, federal law, and federal treaties take precedence over the constitutions and laws of specific states and local jurisdictions. Statutory law may be amended, repealed, or expanded by action of the legislature.

Bill of Rights

The Conventions of a number of the States, at the time of adopting the U.S. Constitution, expressed a desire to prevent the abuse of its powers. As a result of this concern, Congress ratified amendments to the Constitution of the United States. The *Bill of Rights*, the first ten amendments to the constitution, was added to protect the rights of citizens. The amendments included the right to privacy, equal protection, and freedom of speech and religion.

Administrative Law

Administrative law is the extensive body of public law issued by administrative agencies to direct the enacted laws of the federal and state governments. It is the branch of law that controls the administrative operations of government. Congress and state legislative bodies realistically cannot oversee their many laws; therefore, they delegate implementation and administration of the law to an appropriate administrative agency. Health care organizations in particular are inundated with a proliferation of administrative rules and regulations affecting every aspect of their operations.

The *Administrative Procedures Act*[10] describes the different procedures under which federal administrative agencies must operate.[11] The Act prescribes the procedural responsibilities and authority of administrative agencies and provides for legal remedies for those wronged by agency actions. The regulatory power exercised by administrative agencies includes power to license, power of rate setting (e.g., Centers for Medicare and Medicaid Services [CMS]), and power over business practices (e.g., National Labor Relations Board).

The rules and regulations established by an agency must be administered within the scope of the authority delegated to the agency by Congress. Agency regulations and decisions can be subject to judicial review.

GOVERNMENT ORGANIZATION

The three branches of the federal government are the legislative, executive, and judicial branches. A vital concept in the constitutional framework of government on both federal and state levels is the separation of powers. Essentially, this principle provides that no one branch of government is clearly dominant over the other two; however, in the exercise of its functions, each may affect and limit the activities, functions, and powers of the others.

Legislative Branch

On the federal level, legislative powers are vested in the Congress of the United States, which consists of a Senate and a House of Representatives. The function of the legislative branch is to enact laws that may amend or repeal existing legislation and to create new legislation. It is the legislature's responsibility to determine the nature and extent of the need for new laws and for changes in existing laws. The work of preparing federal legislation is the responsibility of the various committees of both houses of Congress. There are 16 standing committees in the Senate and 19 in the House of Representatives. "The membership of the standing committees of each house is chosen by a vote of the entire body; members of other committees are appointed under the provisions of the measure establishing them."[12]

Legislative proposals are assigned or referred to an appropriate committee for study. The committees conduct investigations and hold hearings where interested persons may present their views regarding proposed legislation. These proceedings provide additional information to assist committee members in their consideration of proposed bills. A bill may be reported out of a committee in its original form or it may be reported out with recommended amendments; or the bill might be allowed to lie in the committee without action. Some bills eventually reach the full legislative body, where, after consideration and debate, they may be approved or rejected.

The U.S. Congress and all state legislatures are bicameral (consisting of two houses), except for the Nebraska legislature, which is unicameral. Both houses in a bicameral legislature must pass identical versions of a legislative proposal before the legislation can be brought to the chief executive.

Judicial Branch

As I have said in the past, when government bureaus and agencies go awry, which are adjuncts of the legislative or executive branches, the people flee to the third branch, their courts, for solace and justice.[13]

JUSTICE J. HENDERSON,
SUPREME COURT OF SOUTH DAKOTA

The function of the judicial branch of government is adjudication—resolving disputes in accordance with law. As a practical matter, most disputes or controversies that are covered by legal principles or rules are resolved without resort to the courts.

Alexis de Tocqueville, a foreign observer commenting on the primordial place of the law and the legal profession, stated, "Scarcely any political question arises in the United States that is not resolved, sooner or later, into a judicial question."[14]

It is emphatically the province and duty of the judicial branch to say what the law is. Those who apply the rule to particular cases must of necessity expound and interpret that rule. If two laws conflict with each other, the courts must decide on the operation of each.

So if a law be in opposition to the constitution; if both the law and the constitution apply to a particular case, so that the court must either decide that case conformably to the law, disregarding the constitution; or conformably to the constitution, disregarding the law; the court must determine which of these conflicting rules govern the case. This is the very essence of judicial duty.

• • • •

. . ., it is apparent, that the framers of the constitution contemplated that instrument, as a rule for the government of courts, as well as of the legislature.

Why otherwise does it direct the judges to take such an oath to support it?[15]

Each state in the United States provides its own court system, which is created by the state's constitution and/or statutes. The oldest court in the United States, established in 1692, is the Supreme Judicial Court of Massachusetts.[16] Most of the nation's judicial business is reviewed and acted on in state courts. Each state maintains a level of trial courts that have original jurisdiction. This jurisdiction may exclude cases involving claims with damages less than a specified minimum, probate matters (i.e., wills and estates), and workers' compensation. Different states have designated different names for trial courts (e.g., superior, district, circuit, or supreme courts). Also on the trial court level are minor courts such as city, small claims, and justice of the peace courts. States such as Massachusetts have consolidated their minor courts into a statewide court system.

There is at least one appellate court in each state. Many states have an intermediate appellate court between the trial courts and the court of last resort. Where this intermediate court is present, there is a provision for appeal to it, with further review in all but select cases. Because of this format, the highest appellate tribunal is seen as the final arbiter in cases that possess importance in themselves or for the particular state's system of jurisprudence.

The trial court of the federal system is the U.S. District Court. There are 89 district courts in the 50 states (the larger states having more than one district court) and one in the District of Columbia. The Commonwealth of Puerto Rico also has a district court with jurisdiction corresponding to that of district courts in the different states. Generally, only one judge is required to sit and decide a case, although certain cases require up to three judges. The federal district courts hear civil, criminal, admiralty, and bankruptcy cases. The Bankruptcy Amendments and Federal Judgeship Act of 1984[17] provided that the bankruptcy judges for each judicial district shall constitute a unit of the district court to be known as the bankruptcy court.

The U.S. Courts of Appeals (formerly called Circuit Courts of Appeals) are appellate courts for the 11 judicial circuits. Their main purpose is to review cases tried in federal district courts within their respective circuits, but they also possess jurisdiction to review orders of designated administrative agencies and to issue original writs in appropriate cases. These intermediate appellate courts were created to relieve the U.S. Supreme Court of deciding all cases appealed from the federal trial courts.

The Supreme Court, the nation's highest court, is the only federal court created directly by the Constitution.

> The Judicial Power of the United States, shall be vested in one supreme Court, and in such inferior Courts as the Congress may from time to time ordain and establish. The Judges, both of the supreme and inferior Courts, shall hold their offices during good Behaviour, and shall, at stated Times, receive for their Services, a Compensation, which shall not be diminished during their Continuance in Office.[18]

Eight associate justices and one chief justice sit on the Supreme Court. The Court has limited original jurisdiction over the lower federal courts and the highest state courts. In a few situations, an appeal will go directly from a federal or state court to the Supreme Court, but in most cases today, review must be sought through the discretionary writ of certiorari, an appeal petition. In addition to the aforementioned courts, there are special federal courts that have jurisdiction over particular subject matters. The U.S. Court of Claims has jurisdiction over certain claims against the government. The U.S. Court of Appeals for the Federal Circuit has appellate jurisdiction over certain customs and patent matters. The U.S. Customs Court reviews certain administrative decisions by customs officials. Also, there is a U.S. Tax Court and a U.S. Court of Military Appeals.

Executive Branch

The primary function of the executive branch of government on the federal and state level is to administer and enforce the law. The chief executive, either the President of the United States or the governor of a state, also has a role in the creation of law through the power to approve or veto legislative proposals.

The U.S. Constitution provides that "the executive Power shall be vested in a President of the United States of America. He shall hold his Office during the Term of four Years, . . . together with the Vice President, chosen for the same Term."[19] The President serves as the administrative head of the executive branch of the federal government, which includes 14 executive departments, as well as a variety of agencies, both temporary and permanent.

The Cabinet, a creation of custom and tradition dating back to George Washington's administration, functions at the pleasure of the President. Its purpose is to advise the President upon any subject on which he requests information (pursuant to Article II, section 2, of the Constitution).

The Cabinet is composed of the 15 executive departments.[20] Each department is responsible for a different area of public affairs, and each enforces the law within its area of responsibility. For example, the Department of Health and Human Services (HHS) administers much of the federal health law enacted by Congress. Most state executive branches also are organized on a departmental basis. These departments administer and enforce state law concerning public affairs.

On a state level, the governor serves as the chief executive officer. The responsibilities of a state governor are provided for in the state's constitution. The Massachusetts State Constitution, for example, describes the responsibilities of the governor as

- presenting an annual budget to the state legislature
- recommending new legislation
- vetoing legislation
- appointing and removing department heads
- appointing judicial officers
- acting as Commander-in-Chief of the state's military forces (the Massachusetts National Guard)[21]

Separation of Powers

The concept of *separation of powers*—in effect, a system of checks and balances—is illustrated in the relationships among the branches of government with regard to legislation. On the federal level, when a bill creating a statute is enacted by Congress and signed by the President, it becomes law. If the President vetoes a bill, it takes a two-thirds vote of each house of Congress to override the veto. The President also can prevent a bill from becoming law by avoiding any action while Congress is in session. This procedure, known as a pocket veto, can temporarily stop a bill from becoming law and may permanently prevent it from becoming law if later sessions of Congress do not act on it favorably.

A bill that has become law may be declared invalid by the Supreme Court if the law violates the Constitution. "It is not entirely unworthy of observation, that in declaring what shall be the Supreme law of the land, the Constitution itself is first mentioned; and not the laws of the United States generally, but those only made in pursuance to the Constitution, have that rank."[22]

Even though a Supreme Court decision is final regarding a specific controversy, Congress and the President may generate new, constitutionally sound legislation to replace a law that has been declared unconstitutional. The procedures for amending the Constitution are complex and often time consuming, but they can serve as a way to offset or override a Supreme Court decision.

ADMINISTRATIVE DEPARTMENTS AND AGENCIES

There are a variety of federal departments and administrative agencies that affect the health care industry. Besides the federal-level departments and agencies, many departments and agencies on the state and local levels address many matters also considered on the federal level (e.g., public health, finance, education, welfare, labor, housing, and other needs and concerns of state residents).

The HHS is a cabinet-level department of the executive branch of the federal government, is concerned with people, and is most involved with the nation's human concerns. HHS is responsible for developing and implementing appropriate administrative regulations for carrying out national health and human services policy objectives. It is also the main source of regulations affecting the health care industry. The Secretary of HHS, serving as the Department's administrative head, advises the President with regard to health, welfare, and income security plans, policies, and programs. The following are operating divisions within the HHS operating divisions: (1) the Social Security Administration, (2) CMS, (3) the Office of Human Development Services, (4) the Public Health Service (PHS), and (5) the Family Support Administration. Within each division of HHS, there are a variety of "operating" divisions, for example, the Agency for Healthcare Research and Quality. The Agency for Toxic Substances and Disease Registry, Centers for

Disease Control and Prevention, Food and Drug Administration, Health Resources and Services Administration, Indian Health Services, National Institutes of Health, and the Substance Abuse and Mental Health Services Administration are operating divisions of the Public Health Service.

HHS also is responsible for many of the programs designed to meet the needs of senior citizens, including Social Security benefits (e.g., retirement, survivors, and disability), Supplemental Security Income (which ensures a minimum monthly income to needy persons and is administered by local Social Security offices), Medicare, Medicaid, and programs under the Older Americans Act (e.g., in-home services such as home health and home-delivered meals, and community services such as adult day care, transportation, and ombudsman services in long-term care facilities).[23]

CHAPTER REVIEW

1. A law is a general rule of conduct that is enforced by the government. When a law is violated, the government imposes a penalty.
   - Public laws deal with the relationships between individuals and the government. Criminal law is a segment of public law.
   - Private laws deal with relationships among individuals. Two types of private law are tort and contract actions.
2. Common law is derived from judicial decisions. U.S. common law has as its roots the English common-law system. The first English royal court was established in A.D. 1178. There were few written laws at the time, and a collection of principles evolved from the decisions of the court. These principles, known as "common law," were used to decide subsequent cases. During the colonial period, the United States based its law on English common law, but states had the authority to modify their legal systems.
3. A common-law principle established in a higher state court must be followed by the lower courts in that state. However, trial courts or those otherwise on equal footing are not bound by the decisions of other trial courts, and a principle established in one state does not set precedent within another state. Common-law principles can be modified, overturned, abrogated, or created by new court decisions.
4. Statutory law is a written law that emanates from a legislative body. Using express words, a statute can abolish any rule of common law. The Constitution is the highest level of enacted law; it takes precedence over the constitutions and laws of specific states and local jurisdictions.
5. Statutory law can be amended, repealed, or expanded by the legislature. States and local jurisdictions can only enact and enforce laws that do no conflict with federal laws.

6. Administrative law is public law issued by administrative agencies to administer the enacted laws of the federal and state governments. This branch of law controls the administrative operations of the government.

7. Administrative agencies implement and administer the administrative law. The rules and regulations established by an agency must be administered within the scope of the authority delegated to the agency by Congress.

8. The concept of separation of powers provides that no one branch of the government—legislative, executive, or judicial—will be clearly dominant over the other two. The legislative branch, composed of the House of Representatives and the Senate, both enacts laws that can amend or repeal existing legislation and creates new legislation. The judicial branch resolves disputes in accordance with the law. The executive branch administers and enforces the law.

9. The HHS develops and implements administrative regulations for carrying out national health and human services policy objectives. It is the main source of regulations that affect the health care industry.

TEST YOUR UNDERSTANDING

Terminology

law	statutory law
public law	Constitution of the United States
private law	Bill of Rights
common law	administrative law
res judicata	separation of power
stare decisis	

REVIEW QUESTIONS

1. Define the term *law* and describe the sources from which law is derived.

2. Describe and contrast the legal terms *res judicata* and *stare decisis*.

3. Describe the function of each branch of government.

4. What is the meaning of separation of powers?

5. What is the function of an administrative agency?

WEB SITES

American Bar Association
www.abanet.org

American Health Lawyers Association
www.healthlawyers.org

American Society of Law, Medicine and Ethic
www.aslme.org

Answers to Your Legal Questions
www.legalscholar.com

Court Reporters
www.courtreporters.com

Court Room Sciences
www.courtroomsciences.com

Experts
Hgexperts.com

Federal Law
www.thecre.com/fedlaw/default.htm

FindLaw
www.findlaw.com

Healthcare Law Net
www.healthcarelawnet.com

Health Law Resource
www.netreach.net/~wmanning

Law.com
www.law.com

Lawyers
www.lawyers.com

Legal Information Institute
www.law.cornell.edu/topical.html

Legal Research
http://bender.lexisnexis.com/bender/us/catalog?action=home

National Court Reporters Association
www.verbatimreporters.com

NoLo
www.nolo.com

Quackwatch
www.quackwatch.com

Resources for Attorneys
www.resourcesforattorneys.com

Specialty Law
www.specialtylaw.com

Versus Law
www.versuslaw.com

WashLaw
www.washlaw.edu

Westlaw (subscription service)
    http://web2.westlaw.com/signon/default.wl
United States Supreme Court Opinions
    www.usscplus.com
Supreme Court Collection
    http://supct.law.cornell.edu/supct
U.S. Courts/Links
    http://www.uscourts.gov/allinks.html#7th
State legal links
    http://www.alllaw.com/state_resources

NOTES

1. B. Schwartz, The Law in America 1 (1974).
2. Marbury v. Madison, 5 U.S. (Cranch) 137, 163 (1803).
3. Schwartz, *supra* note 1, at 29.
4. *Id.*
5. *Id.* at 30–31.
6. L. Friedman, A History of American Law 92 (1985).
7. Schwartz, *supra* note 1, at 51.
8. Black's Law Dictionary 1305 (6th. ed. 1990).
9. U.S. Const. art. VI, § 1, cl. 2. http://www.archives.gov/national_archives_experience/constitution_transcript.html.
10. 5 U.S.C.S. §§ 500–576 (Law. Co-op. 1989).
11. An "agency means each authority of the Government of the United States, . . . but does not include (A) the Congress; the Courts of the United States; . . ." 5 U.S.C.S. § 551(1) (Law. Co-op. 1989).
12. Office of the Federal Register, National Archives and Records Administration, The United States Government Manual 2000/2001 29 (2000) [hereinafter Manual].
13. Heritage of Yankton, Inc. v. South Dakota Dep't of Health, 432 N.W.2d 68, 77 (S.D. 1988).
14. Schwartz, *supra* note 1, at 15.
15. Marbury v. Madison, 5 U.S. (Cranch) 137, 177–180 (1803).
16. Levitan, *supra* note 46, at 32.
17. 28 U.S.C. § 151.
18. U.S. Const. art. III, § 1.
19. U.S. Const. art. II, §1, cl. 1.
20. http://dir.yahoo.com/Government/U_S_Government/Executive_Branch/Departments_and_Agencies/
21. D. Levitan, Your Massachusetts Government 14 (10th ed. 1984).
22. Marbury v. Madison, 5 U.S. (Cranch) 137, 180 (1803).
23. http://www.os.dhhs.gov/about/index.html.

chapter six

Introduction to Law

*Every instance of a man's suffering the penalty of the law, is an
instance of the failure of that penalty in effecting its purpose, which
is to deter from transgression.*

WHATELY

LEARNING OBJECTIVES

The reader upon completion of this chapter will be able to:

- Identify and explain the elements of negligence and how
  they apply to health professionals

- Identify and describe intentional torts and how they apply
  to health professionals:

  ○ Assault and battery

  ○ False imprisonment

  ○ Defamation of character

  ○ Invasion of privacy

  ○ Infliction of mental distress

- Identify and describe criminal law and how it applies to
  health professionals:

  ○ Criminal trial

  ○ Criminal negligence

- Manslaughter
- Murder
- Fraud
- Identify and describe contract law and how it applies to health professionals:
  - Elements of a contract
  - Employment contracts
  - Exclusive contracts
  - Commercial ethics and noncompetitive agreements
- Understand the pre-trial and trial process and how it applies to health professionals.

INTRODUCTION

This chapter introduces the health care professional to tort law, criminal law, contract law, and trial procedures.

TORT LAW

A *tort* is a civil wrong, other than a breach of contract, committed against a person or property (real or personal) for which a court provides a remedy in the form of an action for damages. Tort actions touch an individual both on a personal and a professional level, which is why those involved in the health care field should be armed with the knowledge necessary to make them aware of their rights and responsibilities.

The basic objectives of tort law are: preservation of peace—between individuals by providing a substitute for retaliation; culpability—to find fault for wrongdoing; deterrence—to discourage the wrongdoer (tort-feasor) from committing future torts; and compensation—to indemnify the injured person(s) of wrongdoing.

NEGLIGENCE

Negligence is a tort, a civil or personal wrong. It is the unintentional commission or omission of an act that a reasonably prudent person would or would not do under given circumstances.

Commission of an act would include: (1) administering the wrong medication; (2) administering the wrong dosage of a medication; (3) administering medication to the wrong patient; and (4) performing a surgical procedure without patient consent; performing a surgical procedure on the wrong patient; surgically removing the wrong body part; failing to assess and reassess a patient's nutritional needs.

Omission of an act would include: (1) failing to administer medications; (2) failing to order diagnostic tests; and (3) failing to follow up on abnormal test results.

Negligence is a form of conduct caused by heedlessness or carelessness that constitutes a departure from the standard of care generally imposed on reasonable members of society. It can occur where (1) one has considered the consequences of an act and has exercised his or her best possible judgment; (2) one fails to guard against a risk that should be appreciated; and (3) one engages in certain behavior expected to involve unreasonable danger to others.

Malpractice is the negligence or carelessness of a professional person (e.g., a nurse, pharmacist, physician, accountant). Criminal negligence is the reckless disregard for the safety of another (e.g., willful indifference to an injury that could follow an act).

Negligence generally involves one of the following acts: (1) *malfeasance*—execution of an unlawful or improper act (e.g., performing an abortion in the third trimester when such is prohibited by state law); (2) *misfeasance*—improper performance of an act, resulting in injury to another (e.g., wrong-sided surgery); and (3) *nonfeasance*—failure to act, when there is a duty to act as a reasonably prudent person would in similar circumstances (e.g., failing to order diagnostic tests or prescribe medications that should have been ordered or prescribed under the circumstances).

Elements of Negligence

The four elements that must be present for a plaintiff to recover damages caused by negligence are (1) *duty to care*, (2) *breach of duty, (3) injury*, and (4) *causation*. All four elements must be present in order for a plaintiff to recover for damages suffered as a result of a negligent act.

Duty to Care

The first requirement in establishing negligence is that the plaintiff prove the existence of a legal relationship between himself or herself and the defendant. *Duty* is defined as a legal obligation of care, performance, or observance imposed on one to safeguard the rights of others. This duty may arise from a special relationship such as that between a physician and a patient. The existence of this relationship implies that a physician–patient relationship was in effect at the time an alleged injury occurred. The duty to care can arise from a simple telephone conversation or out of a physician's voluntary act of assuming the care of a patient. Duty also can be established by statute or contract between the plaintiff and the defendant.

Standard of Care Expected

A duty of care carries with it a corresponding responsibility not only to provide care, but also to provide it in an acceptable manner. Because of this obligation to conform to a recognized standard of care, the plaintiff must show that the defendant failed to meet this standard. Just because an injury is suffered is not sufficient for imposing liability without proof that the defendant deviated from the practice of competent members of his or her profession.

The standard of care describes what conduct is expected of an individual in a given situation. The general standard of care that must be exercised is that which a reasonably prudent person would do acting under the same or similar circumstances.

The "reasonably prudent person" concept describes a nonexistent, hypothetical person who is put forward as the community ideal of what would be considered reasonable behavior. It is a measuring stick representing the conduct of the average person in the community under the circumstances facing the defendant at the time of the alleged negligence. The reasonableness of conduct is judged in light of the circumstances apparent at the time of injury and by reference to different characteristics of the actor (e.g., age, sex, physical condition, education, knowledge, training, mental capacity).

The actual performance of an individual in a given situation will be measured against what a reasonably prudent person would or would not have done. Deviation from the standard of care will constitute negligence if there are resulting damages.

Ethicists and the Standard of Care

Some medical standards of care are influenced by medical ethics. For example, a decision concerning termination of resuscitation efforts is an area in which the standard of care includes an ethical component. Under these circumstances, it occasionally may be appropriate for a medical expert to testify about the ethical aspects underlying the professional standard of care. In *Neade v. Portes*, 710 N.E.2d 418 (Ill. App. Ct. 1999), a physician expert was allowed to base an opinion on breach of standard of care upon violation of an ethical standard established by the American Medical Association.

Duty Created by Statute

Some duties are created by statute, which occurs when a statute specifies a particular standard that must be met. Many such standards are created by administrative agencies under the provisions of a statute. For liability to be established, based on a defendant's failure to follow the standard of care outlined by statute, the following elements must be present: (1) the defendant must have been within the specified class of persons outlined in the statute; (2) the plaintiff must have been injured in a way that the statute was designed to prevent; and (3) the plaintiff must show that the injury would not have occurred if the statute had not been violated.

Duty to Provide Timely Care

The surviving parents in *Hastings v. Baton Rouge Hospital*[1] brought a medical malpractice action for the wrongful death of their 19-year-old son. The action was brought against the hospital; the emergency department physician, Dr. Gerdes; and the thoracic surgeon on call, Dr. McCool. The patient had been brought to the emergency department at 11:56 PM because of two stab wounds and weak vital signs. Gerdes decided that a thoracotomy had to be performed. He was not qualified to perform the surgery and called McCool, who was on call that evening for thoracic surgery. Gerdes described the patient's condition, indicating he had been stabbed in a major blood vessel. At trial, McCool claimed that he did not recall Gerdes saying that a major blood vessel could be involved. McCool asked Gerdes to transfer the patient to the Earl K. Long Hospital. Gerdes said, "I can't transfer this patient." McCool replied, "No. Transfer him." Kelly, an emergency department nurse on duty, was not comfortable with the decision to transfer the patient and offered to accompany him in the ambulance. Gerdes reexamined the patient, who exhibited marginal vital signs, was restless, and was draining blood from his chest. The ambulance service was called at 1:03 AM, and by 1:30 AM the patient had been placed in the ambulance for transfer. The patient began to fight wildly, the chest tube came out, and the bleeding increased. An attempt to revive him from a cardiac arrest was futile, and the patient died after having been moved back to the emergency department. The patient virtually bled to death.

The duty to care in this case cannot be reasonably disputed. Louisiana, by statute, imposes a duty on hospitals licensed in Louisiana to make emergency services available to all persons residing in the state regardless of insurance coverage or economic status. The hospital's own bylaws provided that no patient should be transferred without due consideration for his or her condition and the facilities existing for his or her care.

Duty to Hire Competent Staff

Texas courts recognize that an employer has a duty to hire competent employees, especially if they are engaged in an occupation that could be hazardous to life and limb and requires skilled or experienced persons. For example, the appellant in *Deerings West Nursing Center v. Scott*[2] was found to have negligently hired an incompetent employee that it knew or should have known was incompetent, thereby causing unreasonable risk of harm to others.

Hopper testified that he was hired sight unseen over the telephone by the Deerings' Director of Nursing. Even though the following day he went to the nursing facility to complete an application, he still maintained that he was hired over the phone. In his application he falsely stated that he was a Texas-licensed vocational nurse (LVN). Additionally, he claimed that he had never been convicted of a crime. In reality, he had been previously employed by a bar, was not a LVN, had committed more than 56 criminal offenses of theft, and was on probation at the time of his testimony.

The duty of care in this case is clear. The appellant violated the very purpose of Texas licensing statutes by failing to validate whether or not Hopper had a current LVN license. The appellant then placed him in a position of authority and not only allowed him to dispense drugs, but also made him a shift supervisor. This negligence eventually resulted in the inexcusable assault on an elderly woman.

Breach of Duty

After a duty to care has been established, the plaintiff must demonstrate that the defendant breached that duty by failing to comply with the accepted standard of care required. Breach of duty, the second element that must be present for a plaintiff to establish negligence, is the failure to conform to or the departure from a required obligation owed to a person. The obligation to perform according to a standard of care may encompass either doing or refraining from doing a particular act.

The court in *Hastings v. Baton Rouge Hospital*,[3] discussed earlier, found a severe breach of duty when hospital regulations provide that when a physician cannot be reached or refuses a call, the chief of service is to be notified so that another physician can be obtained. This was not done. It is not necessary to prove that a patient would have survived if proper treatment had been administered, but only that the patient would have had a chance of survival. As a result of Dr. Gerdes' failure to make arrangements for another physician and Dr. McCool's failure to perform the necessary surgery, the patient had no chance of survival. The duty to provide for appropriate care under the circumstances was breached.

Injury/Actual Damages

A defendant may be negligent and still not incur liability if no *injury* or actual damages, the third element necessary to establish negligence, result to the plaintiff. The term *injury* includes more than physical harm. Without harm or injury, there is no liability. Injury is not limited to physical harm but includes loss of income or reputation and compensation for pain and suffering.

The mere occurrence of an injury "does not establish negligence for which the law imposes liability, since the injury may be the result of an unavoidable accident, or an act of God, or some cause so remote to the person sought to be held liable for negligence that he cannot be charged with responsibility for the injury."[4] In *Hastings*, the patient's death was a direct result of the breach of duty.

Proximate Cause/Causation

The fourth element necessary to establish negligence requires that there be a reasonable, close, and causal connection or relationship between the defendant's negligent conduct and the resulting damages suffered by the plaintiff.

In other words, the defendant's negligence must be a substantial factor causing the injury. *Proximate cause* is a term referring to the relationship between a breached duty and the injury. The breach of duty must be the proximate cause of the resulting injury.

Causation in the *Hastings*[5] case was well established. In the ordinary course of events, a person does not bleed to death in a hospital emergency department over a two-hour period without some surgical intervention to save the patient's life.

Foreseeability and Anticipation of Harm

Foreseeability is the reasonable anticipation that harm or injury is likely to result from an act or an omission of an act. The test for foreseeability is whether one of ordinary prudence and intelligence should have anticipated the danger to others caused by his or her negligent act. "The test is not what the wrongdoer believed would occur; it is whether he or she ought reasonably to have foreseen that the event in question, or some similar event, would occur."[6]

There is no expectation that a person can guard against events that cannot reasonably be foreseen. Foreseeability involves guarding against that which is probable and likely to happen, not against that which is only remotely and slightly possible. In *Hastings*, it was highly probable that the patient would die if the bleeding was not stopped. "The broad test of negligence is what a reasonably prudent person would foresee and would do in the light of this foresight under the circumstances."[7]

CASE: COMEDY OF ERRORS

All the elements necessary to establish negligence were well established in *Niles v. City of San Rafael.*[8] On June 26, 1973, at approximately 3:30 PM, Kelly Niles, a young boy, got into an argument with another boy on the ball field. He was hit on the right side of his head. He rode home on his bicycle and waited for his father, who was to pick him up for the weekend. At approximately 5:00 PM, his father arrived. By the time they arrived in San Francisco, Kelly appeared to be in a great deal of pain. His father then decided to take him to Mount Zion Hospital, which was a short distance away. He arrived at the hospital emergency department at approximately 5:45 PM. On admission to the emergency department, Kelly was taken to a treatment room by a registered nurse. The nurse obtained a history of the injury and took Kelly's pulse and blood pressure. During his stay in the emergency department, he was irritable, vomited several times, and complained that his head hurt. An intern who had seen Kelly wrote "pale, diaphoretic, and groggy" on the patient's chart. Skull X-rays were ordered and found to be negative except for soft tissue swelling that was not noted until later. The intern then decided to admit the patient. A second-year resident was called, and he agreed with the intern's decision. An admitting clerk called the intern and indicated that the patient had to be admitted by an attending physician. The resident went as far as to write "admit" on the chart and later crossed it out. A pediatrician who was in the emergency department at the time was asked to look at Kelly. The pediatrician was also the paid director of the Mount Zion Pediatric Out-Patient Clinic. The pediatrician asked Kelly a few questions and then decided to send him home. The physician could not recall what instructions he gave the patient's father, but he did give the father his business card.

The pediatrician could not recall giving the father a copy of the emergency department's "Head Injury Instructions," an information sheet that had been prepared for distribution to patients with head injuries. The sheet explained that an individual should be returned to the emergency department should any of the following signs appear: a large, soft lump on the head; unusual drowsiness (cannot be awakened); forceful or repeated vomiting; a fit or convulsion (jerking or spells); clumsy walking; bad headache; and/or one pupil larger than the other.

Kelly was taken back to his father's apartment at about 7:00 PM. A psychiatrist friend stopped by at approximately 8:45 PM. He examined Kelly and noted that one pupil was larger than the other. Because the pediatrician could not be reached, the patient was taken back to the emergency department. A physician on duty noted an epidural hematoma during his examination and ordered that a neurosurgeon be called.

Today, the patient can move only his eyes and neck. A lawsuit against Mount Zion and the pediatrician for $5 million was instituted. The city of San Rafael and the public school district also were included in the lawsuit as defendants. Expert testimony by two neurosurgeons during the trial indicated that the patient's chances of recovery would have been very good if he had been admitted promptly. This testimony placed the proximate cause of the injury with the hospital. The final judgment was $4 million against the medical defendants, $2.5 million for compensatory damages, and another $1.5 million for pain and suffering.

Case Lessons

Each case presented in this textbook illustrates actual experiences of plaintiffs and defendants. It is anticipated that the reader will learn from these experiences and apply them to real-life situations. The many lessons in *Niles v. City of San Rafael* include:

- An organization can improve the quality of patient care rendered in the facility by establishing and adhering to policies, procedures, and protocols that facilitate the delivery of quality care across all disciplines.
- The provision of quality health care requires collaboration across disciplines.
- A physician must conduct a thorough and responsible examination and order the appropriate tests for each patient, evaluating the results of those tests prior to discharging the patient.

- A patient's vital signs must be monitored closely and documented in the medical record.
- Corrective measures must be taken when a patient's medical condition signals a medical problem.
- A complete review of a patient's medical record must be accomplished before discharging a patient.
- Review of the record must include review of test results, nurses' notes, residents' and interns' notes, and the notes of any other physician or consultant who may have attended the patient.
- An erroneous diagnosis leading to the premature dismissal of a case can result in liability for both the organization and physician.

Ethics and Negligent Acts: The Real Lesson Here

Duty to care involves a responsibility to do the "right thing." The right thing is based on an acceptable standard of care. If breaching the standard causes harm to the patient, there is not only a legal issue but there are ethical principles that have been violated. *Nonmaleficence*, for example, requires caregivers to avoid causing harm to patients.

The real lesson in *Niles v. City of San Rafael* is that if the "ethical theories, principles and values" discussed in Chapter 1 had been adopted, put in place, understood, and practiced, Kelly Niles would be leading a normal life today.

INTENTIONAL TORTS

An intentional tort is one that is committed deliberately. Proof of intent is based on the premise that the defendant intended the harmful consequences of his or her behavior. An individual's reason to cause harm is irrelevant and does not protect him or her from responsibility for the damages suffered as the result of an intentional act.

Assault and Battery

It has long been recognized by law that a person possesses a right to be free from aggression and the threat of actual aggression against one's person. The right to expect others to respect the integrity of one's body has roots in both common and statutory law. The distinguishing feature between assault and battery is that "assault" effectuates an infringement on the mental security or tranquility of another whereas "battery" constitutes a violation of another's physical integrity.

An *assault* is defined as the deliberate threat, coupled with the apparent present ability to do physical harm to another. No actual contact is necessary. It is the deliberate threat or attempt to injure another or the attempt by one to make bodily contact with another without his or her consent. To commit the tort of assault, two conditions must exist. First, the person attempting to touch another unlawfully must possess the apparent present ability to commit the battery. Second, the person threatened must be aware of or have actual knowledge of an immediate threat of a battery and must fear it.

A *battery* is the intentional touching of another's person, in a socially impermissible manner, without that person's consent. It is intentional conduct that violates the physical security of another. An act that otherwise would be considered to be an assault may be permissible if proper consent has been given or if it is in defense of oneself or of a third party. The receiver of the battery does not have to be aware that a battery has been committed (e.g., a patient who is unconscious and has surgery performed on him or her without consent, either expressed or implied, is the object of a battery). The unwanted touching may give rise to a cause of action for any injuries brought about by the touching. No actual damages need be shown to impose liability.

False Imprisonment

False imprisonment is the unlawful restraint of an individual's personal liberty or the unlawful restraining or confining of an individual. The personal right to move freely and without hindrance is basic to our legal system. Any intentional infringement on this right may constitute false imprisonment. Actual physical force is not necessary to constitute false imprisonment. All that is necessary is that an individual who is physically confined to a given area experience a reasonable fear that force, which may be implied by words, threats, or gestures, will be used to detain the individual or to intimidate him or her without legal justification. Excessive force used to restrain a patient may produce liability for both false imprisonment and battery.

Defamation of Character

Defamation of character involves communications to someone other than the person defamed that tends to hold that person's reputation up to scorn and ridicule.

Slander is the oral form of defamation. For example, the nurse's aide, in *Eli v. Griggs County Hospital & Nursing Home*,[9] was terminated as the result of an incident in the hospital dining room, where the aide in the presence of patients and visitors cursed at her supervisor and complained that personnel were working short staffed. Given the nature of her employment, such behavior justified her termination on a charge of reported breach of patient-specific and facility-specific information. No defamation resulted from the entry of such charges in the aide's personnel file because the record established that the charges were "true."

Libel is the written form of defamation. Libel can be presented in signs, photographs, letters, cartoons, and various other forms of written communication. To be an actionable wrong, defamation must be communicated to a third person. Defamatory statements communicated only to the injured party are not grounds for an action. Truth of a statement is a complete defense.

Defamation on its face is actionable without proof of special damages. In certain cases, a court will presume that the words caused injury to the person's reputation. There are four generally recognized exceptions whereby no proof of actual harm to reputation is required to recover damages: (1) accusing someone of a crime, (2) accusing someone of having a loathsome disease, (3) using words that affect a person's profession or business, and (4) calling a woman unchaste.

Invasion of Privacy

Invasion of privacy is a wrong that invades the right of a person to personal privacy. Absolute privacy has to be tempered with reality in the care of any patient, and the courts recognize this fact. Disregard for a patient's right to privacy is legally actionable, particularly when patients are unable to protect themselves adequately because of unconsciousness or immobility.

The right to privacy is implied in the Constitution. It is recognized by the law as the right to be left alone—the right to be free from unwarranted publicity and exposure to public view, as well as the right to live one's life without having one's name, picture, or private affairs made public against one's will. Health care organizations and professionals may become liable for invasion of privacy if, for example, they divulge information from a patient's medical record to improper sources or if they commit unwarranted intrusions into a patient's personal affairs.

Patients have a right to personal privacy and a right to the confidentiality of their personal and clinical records. The information in a patient's medical record is confidential and should not be disclosed without the patient's permission. Those who come into possession of the most intimate personal information about patients have both a legal and an ethical duty not to reveal confidential communications. The legal duty arises because the law recognizes a right to privacy. To protect this right, there is a corresponding duty to obey. The ethical duty is broader and applies at all times. There are, however, occasions when there is a legal obligation or duty to disclose information. The reporting of communicable diseases, gunshot wounds, child abuse, and other matters is required by law.

Infliction of Mental Distress

The *intentional or reckless infliction of mental distress* is characterized by conduct that is so outrageous that it goes beyond the bounds tolerated by a decent society. It is a civil wrong for which a tort-feasor can be held liable for damages. Mental distress includes mental suffering resulting from painful emotions such as grief, public humiliation, despair, shame, and wounded pride. Liability for the wrongful infliction of mental distress may be based on either intentional or negligent misconduct. A plaintiff may recover damages if he or she can show that the defendant intended to inflict mental distress, and knew or should have known that his or her actions would give rise to it. Recovery generally is permitted even in the absence of physical harm.

Ethical Issues Abound: Access to Care Delayed

The plaintiff, while in the custody of the defendant-penal institution, alleged that because the defendant's employees failed to timely diagnose her breast cancer, her right breast had to be removed. The defendant contended that even if its employees were negligent, the plaintiff's cancer was so far developed when discovered that it would nevertheless have required removal of her breast.[10]

The day following her examination, the plaintiff examined her own breasts. At that time she discovered a lump in her right breast, which she characterized as being about the size of a pea. The plaintiff then sought an additional medical evaluation at the defendant's medical clinic. Testimony indicated that fewer than half of the inmates who sign the clinic list are actually seen by medical personnel the next day. Also, those not examined on the day for which the list is signed are given no preference in being examined on the following day. In fact, their names are simply deleted from the daily list and their only recourse is to continually sign the list until they are examined. The evidence indicated that after May 27, the plaintiff constantly signed the clinic list and provided the reason she was requesting medical care.

A nurse finally examined the plaintiff on June 21. The nurse noted in her nursing notes that the plaintiff had a "moderate large mass in right breast." The nurse recognized that the proper procedure was to measure such a mass but she testified that this was impossible because no measuring device was available. The missing measuring device to which she alluded was a simple ruler. The nurse concluded that Evans should again examine the plaintiff.

On June 28, Evans again examined the plaintiff. He recorded in the progress notes that the plaintiff had "a mass on her right wrist. Will send her to hospital and give her Benadryl for allergy she has."[11] Evans meant to write "breast" not "wrist." He again failed to measure the size of the mass on the plaintiff's breast.

The plaintiff was transferred to the Franklin County Prerelease Center (FCPR) on September 28. On September 30, a nurse at FCPR examined the plaintiff; the nurse recorded that the plaintiff had a "golf ball-sized" lump in her right breast. The plaintiff was transported to the hospital on October 27, where Dr. Walker treated her. The plaintiff received a mammogram examination, which indicated that the tumor was probably malignant. This diagnosis was confirmed by a biopsy performed on November 9. The plaintiff was released from confinement on November 13.

On November 16, Dr. Lidsky, a surgeon, examined the plaintiff. Lidsky noted the existence of the lump in the plaintiff's breast and determined that the size of the mass was approximately four to five centimeters and somewhat fixed. He performed a modified radical mastectomy upon the plaintiff's right breast, by which nearly the plaintiff's entire right breast was removed.

The plaintiff, while in the custody of the defendant-penal institution, alleged that because the defendant's employees failed to timely diagnose her breast cancer, her right breast had to be removed. The defendant contended that even if its employees were negligent, the plaintiff's cancer was so far developed when discovered that it would nevertheless have required removal of her breast.[12]

Pursuant to the defendant's policy of medically evaluating all new inmates, on May 26, 1989, Dr. Evans gave the plaintiff a medical examination. He testified that his physical evaluation included an examination of the plaintiff's breasts. However, he stated that his examination was very cursory.

The Ohio Court of Appeals held that the delay in providing the plaintiff treatment fell below the medically acceptable standard of care. The court was "appalled" that the physician had characterized his evaluation as a medical examination or to imply that what he described as a "cursory breast examination" should be considered a medically sufficient breast examination. It seemed incredible to the court that a physician would deliberately choose not to take the additional few minutes or seconds to thoroughly palpitate the sides of the breasts, which is a standard minimally intrusive cancer detection technique.

CRIMINAL LAW

Laws are made to restrain and punish the wicked; the wise and good do not need them as a guide, but only as a shield against rapine and oppression; they can live civilly and orderly, though there were no law in the world.

JOHN MILTON (1608–1674)

Criminal law is society's expression of the limits of acceptable human and institutional behavior. A *crime* is any social harm defined and made punishable by law. The *objectives of criminal law* are to maintain public order and safety, to protect the individual, to use punishment as a deterrent to crime, and to rehabilitate the criminal for return to society.

Crimes are generally classified as misdemeanors or felonies. The difference between a misdemeanor and a felony revolves around the severity of the crime. A *misdemeanor* is an offense punishable by less than one year in jail and/or a fine (e.g., petty larceny). A *felony* is a much more serious crime (e.g., rape, murder) and is generally punishable by imprisonment in a state or federal penitentiary for more than one year.

Peculiar to health care organizations is the fact that patients are often helpless and at the mercy of others. Health care facilities are far too often places where the morally weak and mentally deficient prey on the physically and sometimes mentally helpless. The very institutions designed to make the public well and feel safe can sometimes provide the setting for criminal conduct.

The U.S. Department of Justice and state and local prosecutors are vigorously pursuing and prosecuting health care organizations and individuals for criminal conduct. Health care fraud, patient abuse, and other such crimes have caused law enforcement agencies to assume a *zero-tolerance level* for such acts. This reality requires health care professionals to be observant in their environments and to report suspicious conduct, as appropriate.

The Criminal Prosecution Procedure

Arrest

Prosecutions for crimes generally begin with the arrest of a defendant by a police officer or with the filing of a formal action in a court of law and the issuance of an arrest warrant or summons. On arrest, the defendant is taken to the appropriate law enforcement agency for processing, which includes paperwork and fingerprinting. The police also prepare accusatory statements, such as misdemeanor complaints and felony complaints. Detectives are assigned to cases when necessary to gather evidence, interview persons suspected of committing a crime and witnesses to a crime, and assist in preparing a case for possible trial. After processing has been completed, a person is either detained or released on bond.

A felony complaint or an indictment commences a criminal proceeding; however, an individual may be tried for a felony after indictment by a grand jury unless the defendant waives presentment to the grand jury and pleads guilty by way of a superior court. Felony cases are presented to a grand jury by a district attorney or an assistant district attorney. The grand jury is presented with the prosecution's evidence and then charged that they may indict the target if they find reasonable cause to believe from the evidence presented to them that all the elements of a particular crime are present. The grand jury may request that witnesses be subpoenaed to testify. A defendant may choose to testify and offer information if he or she wishes. Actions of a grand jury are handed up to a judge, after which the defendant will be notified to appear to be arraigned for the crimes charged in the indictment.

Arraignment

The arraignment is a formal reading of the accusatory instrument and includes the setting of bail. The accused should appear with counsel or have counsel appointed by the court if he or she cannot afford his or her own. After the charges are read, the defendant pleads guilty or not guilty. A not guilty plea is normally offered on a felony. On a plea of not guilty, the defense attorney and prosecutor make arguments regarding bail. After arraignment of the defendant, the judge sets a date for the defendant to return to court. Between the time of arraignment and the next court date, the defense attorney and the prosecutor confer about the charges and evidence in the possession of the prosecutor. At that time, the defense will offer any mitigating circumstances that it believes will convince the prosecutor to lessen or drop the charges.

Conference

If the defendant does not plead guilty, both felony and misdemeanor cases are taken to conference, and plea bargaining commences with the goal of an agreed-upon disposition. If no disposition can be reached, the case is adjourned, motions are made, and further plea bargaining takes place. Generally after several adjournments, a case is assigned to a trial court.

Prosecutor

The role of the prosecutor in the criminal justice system is well defined in *Berger v. United States*:

> The United States Attorney is the representative not of an ordinary party to a controversy, but of a sovereignty whose obligation to govern impartially is as compelling as its obligation to govern at all; and whose interest, therefore, in a criminal prosecution is not that it shall win a case, but that justice will be done. As such, he is in a peculiar and very definite sense the servant of the law, the twofold aim of which is that guilt shall not escape or innocence suffer.[13]

The potential of the prosecutor's office is not always fully realized in many jurisdictions. In many cities the combination of the prosecutor's staggering caseload and small staff of assistants prevents sufficient attention being given to each case.[14]

Defense Attorney

The defense attorney generally sits in the proverbial hot seat, being perceived as the bad guy. Although everyone seems to understand the attorney's function in protecting the rights of those represented, the defense attorney often is not very popular.

> There is a substantial difference in the problem of representing the "run-of-the-mill" criminal defendant and one whose alleged crimes have aroused great public outcry. The difficulties in providing representation for the ordinary criminal defendant are simple compared with the difficulties of obtaining counsel for one who is charged with a crime which by its nature or circumstances incites strong public condemnation.[15]

Criminal Trial

Most of the processes of a criminal trial are similar to that of a civil trial. They include jury selection, opening statements, presentation of witnesses and other evidence, summations, instructions to the jury by the judge, jury deliberations, verdict, and opportunity for appeal to a higher court. In a criminal trial, the jury verdict must be unanimous, and the standard of proof must be beyond a reasonable doubt.

Manslaughter: An Angry Surgeon, A Patient's Death

It was alleged that a surgeon unlawfully killed a teenage cancer patient when he lost his temper as she lay on an operating table. The physician is said to have become angry because the operation at the hospital was making him late for his next appointment. The physician denied manslaughter at the opening of the trial.

Part of the patient's heart was punctured and she died from massive internal bleeding. A staff nurse, who was assisting in the operating room, told the court that she was aghast at the physician's behavior and language during the operation. She told the jury that the physician was unable to insert a needle and guide wire into the patient, and that the physician pushed and shoved quite aggressively, using such force that the patient's whole body shook.

The nurse was asked by the prosecutor if she had ever seen that sort of behavior or anything like it, and she replied that she had not. The physician accepted that something had gone wrong but that it was a rare and recognized complication.[16]

Murder

The tragedy of murder in institutions that are dedicated to the healing of the sick has been a frequent occurrence. Cullen, a former nurse, for example, pleaded guilty to 13 murders and attempting to kill two others in New Jersey and Pennsylvania.[17] Cullen had refused to cooperate with prosecutors unless they promised not to seek the death penalty. Cullen had claimed responsibility for the deaths of 30 to 40 patients over a 16-year nursing career. "The case raises concerns about hospital oversight of medical errors, narcotics security, and background checks on prospective employees. Cullen was fired from five hospitals and resigned from two amid questions about his job performance."[18]

Cullen was found violating nursing standards from the beginning of his career. He had problems in every one of the ten institutions that he worked for in New Jersey and Pennsylvania. Apparently not one of the institutions in which Cullen worked gave him a bad reference. "It amounted to a policy of 'see no evil, speak no evil'—one that gave Cullen, in effect, a license to kill."[19]

In a case involving Angelo, a registered nurse on the cardiac/intensive care unit at a Long Island hospital, the defendant was found guilty of second-degree murder for injecting two patients with the drug Pavulon. He was found guilty of the lesser charges of manslaughter and criminally negligent homicide in the deaths of two other patients. Angelo had committed the murders in a bizarre scheme to revive the patients and be thought of as a hero. The attorney for the estate of one of the alleged victims had filed a wrongful death suit against Angelo and the hospital a day before the verdict was rendered by the jury.[20]

Home Care Fraud

Today, more Americans are living longer into older age than ever before. As medicine has advanced, the average life expectancy has increased by 50 percent. There is an ever-escalating number of elderly persons receiving in-home care, dependent upon family and health care providers to attend to their physical, financial, emotional, and health care needs. Medicare home health benefits allow individuals with restricted mobility to remain home outside an institutional setting by providing home care benefits. Home care services and supplies are generally provided by nurses, home nursing aides, speech therapists, and physical therapists under a physician-certified plan of care.

Home care is rapidly being recognized as a breeding ground for abuse. The numerous scams in home care fraud are caused by the difficulty in supervising services provided in the home, Medicare's failure to monitor the number of visits per patient, beneficiaries paying no co-payments except for medical equipment, and the lack of accountability to the patient by failing to explain services provided.

Home care fraud generally is not easy to detect. It involves charging insurers for more services than patients received, billing for more hours of care than were provided, falsifying records, and charging higher nurses' rates for care given by aides. The trend toward shorter hospital stays has created a multibillion dollar market in home care services. This new market is attracting opportunities for fraud.

CONTRACTS

A *contract* is a special kind of agreement, either written or oral, that involves legally binding obligations between two or more parties. The major purpose of a contract is to specify, limit, and define the agreements that are legally enforceable.

Elements of a Contract

Whether contracts are executed in writing or agreed to orally, they must contain the following elements to be enforceable: (1) offer/communication, (2) consideration, and (3) acceptance.

Offer/Communication

An offer must be communicated to the other party so that it can be accepted or rejected. Unless the offeror specifically requires that the acceptance be received before a contract is formed, communication of the acceptance to the offeror is not necessary.

Consideration

An *offer* is a promise by one party to do (or not to do) something if the other party agrees to do (or not do) something. Not all statements or promises are offers. Generally, advertisements of goods for sale are not offers but are invitations to the public to come to the place of business, view the merchandise, and be made an offer. An opinion is not an offer. Preliminary negotiations are not offers.

Acceptance

Upon proper acceptance of an offer, a contract is formed. It involves:

- *Meeting of the Minds.* Acceptance requires a "meeting of the minds" (mutual assent). The parties must understand and then agree on the terms of the contract.
- *Definite and Complete.* Acceptance requires mutual assent to be found between the parties. The terms must be so complete that both parties understand and agree to what has been proposed.
- *Duration.* Generally, the other party may revoke an offer at any time prior to a valid acceptance. When the offeror does revoke the proposal, the revocation is not effective until the offeree (the person to whom the offer is made) receives it. After the offeree has accepted the offer, any attempt to revoke the agreement is too late and is invalid.
- *Complete and Conforming.* The traditional rule is that the acceptance must be the mirror image of the offer. In other words, the acceptance must comply with all the terms of the offer and not change or add any terms.

Employment Contracts

An employer's right to terminate an employee can be limited by express agreement with the employee or through a collective bargaining agreement to which the employee is a beneficiary. No such agreement was found to exist in *O'Connor v. Eastman Kodak Co.*,[21] in which the court held that an employer had a right to terminate an employee at will at any time, and for any reason or no reason. The plaintiff did not rely on any specific representation made to him during the course of his employment interviews, nor did he rely on any documentation in the employee handbook, which would have limited the defendant's common-law right to discharge at will. The employee had relied on a popular perception of Kodak as a "womb-to-tomb" employer.

Exclusive Contracts

An organization often enters into an exclusive contract with physicians and/or medical groups for the purpose of providing a specific service to the organization. Exclusive contracts generally occur within the organization's ancillary service departments (e.g., radiology, anesthesiology, and pathology). Physicians who seek to practice at organizations in these ancillary areas but who are not part of the exclusive group have attempted to invoke the federal antitrust laws to challenge these exclusive contracts. These challenges generally have been unsuccessful.

A hospital and its governing body were immune from liability under the Federal Health Care Quality Improvement Act of 1986, in *Taylor v. Kennestone Hosp.*,[22] for claims arising out of their decision to deny a physician's application to renew his medical staff privileges. A peer review board found that reasonable investigation had adduced evidence demonstrating that the physician had a history of sexual misconduct toward both nurses and patients. He admitted that he had sexual harassment problems, that he stopped seeing patients at the hospital, and sought psychiatric treatment. He admitted that he failed to fully comply with his own psychiatrist's plan of care before he could resume seeing patients in the hospital. The evidence established that the peer reviewers could reasonably believe that their actions were warranted and that those actions furthered the quality of health care.

Tennessee Code permitted the hospital authority to enter into an exclusive contract with a radiology group. The governing body's decision to close the staff of the Imaging Department did not violate medical staff bylaws, and the defendant radiologists were not legally or constitutionally entitled to a hearing if their privileges were terminated upon entry of the hospital authority into an exclusive provider contract.[23]

Commercial Ethics and Noncompetition Agreements

The purpose in allowing noncompetition agreements is to foster "commercial ethics" and to protect the employer's legitimate interests by preventing unfair competition, not ordinary competition.

The respondent-hospital in *Washington County Memorial Hospital v. Sidebottom*[24] employed the appellant-nurse practitioner from October 1993 through April 1998. Prior to beginning her employment, the nurse entered into an employment agreement with the hospital. The agreement included a noncompetition clause providing in part that the nurse ". . . during the term of [the] Agreement and for a period of one (1) year after the termination of her employment with . . . will not, anywhere within a fifty (50) mile radius . . . directly or indirectly engage in the practice of nursing . . . without the express direction or consent . . ." of the hospital. In February 1994, the nurse requested the hospital's permission to work for the Washington County Health Department doing prenatal nursing care. Because the hospital was not then doing prenatal care, the hospital gave her permission to accept that employment, but reserved the ability to withdraw the permission if the services the nurse was providing later came to be provided by the hospital. In January 1996, the nurse and the hospital entered into a second employment agreement that continued the parties' employment relationship through January 9, 1998. This agreement included a noncompetition clause identical to the 1993 employment agreement. It also provided for automatic renewal for an additional two years unless either party gave written termination notice no less than 90 days prior to the expiration of the agreement.

The hospital's interest lies in protecting its patient base as a primary source of revenue. The specific enforcement of the nurse's noncompetition clause is reasonably necessary to protect the hospital's interest. Actual damage need not be proven to enforce a covenant not to compete. Rather, the employee's opportunity to influence customers justifies enforcement of the covenant. Thus, the quality, frequency, and duration of an employee's exposure to an employer's customers are crucial in determining the covenant's reasonableness. The nurse had opportunity to influence the hospital's patients. Prior to her employment with the hospital, the nurse had never worked in Washington County nor did she have a patient base there. The nurse helped to establish two rural health care clinics for the hospital, one of which she managed during her first year of employment. During her almost five years of employment with the hospital, the nurse saw more than 3,000 patients. Pursuant to a collaborative practice agreement with a physician, the nurse treated patients, diagnosed illnesses and injuries, prescribed and dispensed medications, and ordered and interpreted laboratory tests. The nurse got to know the patients and families to whom she provided these services. At the clinic, she had her own telephone number, receptionist, appointment book, medical assistant, patient charts, laboratory, and examination rooms. Her offices were physically separated from the other medical practitioner at the clinic. Further, during her employment, the hospital promoted the nurse as a nurse practitioner in the community by paying for advertisements with her picture and telephone number in the newspaper. In general, the nurse had a good rapport with her patients, and she had patients who requested her for medical services.

TRIAL PROCEDURES AND THE COURTROOM

This next section presents the reader with a brief review of the law as applied in the courtroom. Although many of the procedures leading up to and followed during a trial are discussed in this chapter, civil procedure and trial practice are governed by each state's statutory requirements. Cases on a federal level are governed by federal statutes.

Pleadings

The pleadings of a case (e.g., summons and complaint), which include all the allegations of each party to a lawsuit, are filed with a court. The pleadings may raise questions of both law and fact. If only questions of law are at issue, the judge will decide the case based on the pleadings alone. If questions of fact are involved, the purpose of a trial is to determine those facts.

Summons and Complaint

The *parties* to a controversy are the plaintiff and the defendant. The *plaintiff* is the person who initiates an action by filing a complaint; the *defendant* is the person against whom a suit is brought. Many cases have multiple plaintiffs and defendants. Filing an order with a court clerk to issue a writ or summons commences an action.

Although the procedures for beginning an action vary according to jurisdiction, there are procedural common denominators. All jurisdictions require service of process on the defendant (usually through a summons) and a return to the court of that process by the person who served it. Where a summons is not required to be issued directly by a court, an attorney, as an officer of the court, may prepare and cause a summons to be served without direct notice to or approval of a court. Notice to a court occurs when an attorney files a summons and complaint in a court, thereby indicating to the court that an action has been commenced.

The first pleading filed with the court in a negligence action is the *complaint*. The complaint identifies the parties to a suit, states a cause of action, and includes a demand for damages. It is filed by the plaintiff and is the first statement of a case by the plaintiff against the defendant. In some jurisdictions, a complaint must accompany a summons (an announcement to the defendant that a case has been commenced).

Answer

After service of a complaint, a response is required from the defendant in a document called the *answer*. In the answer, the defendant responds to each of the allegations contained in the complaint by stating his or her defense and by admitting to or denying each of the plaintiff's allegations. If the defendant fails to answer the complaint within the prescribed time, the plaintiff can seek judgment by default against the defendant.

Bill of Particulars

Because a complaint may provide very little information regarding the claim, the defense attorney may request a *bill of particulars*. This document requests more specific and detailed information than is provided in the complaint. If a counterclaim has been filed, the plaintiff's attorney may request a bill of particulars from the defense attorney.

Discovery of Evidence

Discovery is the process of investigating the facts of a case before trial. The objectives of discovery are to: (1) obtain evidence that might not be obtainable at the time of trial; (2) isolate and narrow the issues for trial; (3) gather knowledge of the existence of additional evidence that may be admissible at trial; and (4) obtain leads to enable the discovering party to gather further evidence.

The parties to a lawsuit have the right to discovery and to examine witnesses before trial. Examination before trial (EBT) is one of several discovery techniques used to enable the parties of a lawsuit to learn more regarding the nature and substance of each other's case. An EBT consists of oral testimony under oath and includes cross-examination. A deposition, taken at an EBT, is the testimony of a witness that has been recorded in a written format. Testimony given at a deposition becomes part of the permanent record of the case. Each question and answer is transcribed by a court stenographer and may be used at the subsequent trial. Truthfulness and consistency are important because answers that differ from those given at trial will be used to attack the credibility of the witness.

Preparation of Witnesses

The manner in which a witness handles questioning at a deposition or trial is often as important as the facts of the case. Each witness should be well prepared before testifying. Preparation should include a review of all pertinent records. Helpful guidelines for witnesses undergoing examination in a trial or a court hearing include the following:

- Review the records (e.g., medical records and other business records) on which you might be questioned.
- Do not be antagonistic when answering the questions. The jury may already be somewhat sympathetic toward a particular party to the lawsuit; antagonism may only serve to reinforce such an impression.
- Be organized in your thinking and recollection of the facts regarding the incident.
- Answer only the questions asked.
- Explain your testimony in simple, succinct terminology.
- Do not overdramatize the facts you are relating.
- Do not allow yourself to become overpowered by the cross-examiner.
- Be polite, sincere, and courteous at all times.
- Dress appropriately, and be neatly groomed.
- Pay close attention to any objections your attorney may have as to the line of questioning being conducted by the opposing counsel.
- Be sure to have reviewed any oral deposition in which you may have participated during EBT.
- Be straightforward with the examiner. Any answers designed to cover up or cloud an issue or fact will, if discovered, serve only to discredit any previous testimony that you may have given. Do not show any visible signs of displeasure regarding any testimony with which you are in disagreement.
- Be sure to have questions that you did not hear repeated and questions that you did not understand rephrased.
- If you are not sure of an answer, indicate that you are not sure or that you just do not know the answer.

The Court

A case is heard in the court that has jurisdiction over the subject of controversy. The judge decides questions of law and is responsible for ensuring that a trial is conducted properly in an impartial atmosphere and that it is fair to both parties of a lawsuit. He or she determines what constitutes the general standard of conduct required for the exercise of due care. The judge informs the jury of what the defendant's conduct should have been, thereby making a determination of the existence of a legal duty.

The judge decides whether evidence is admissible, charges the jury (defines the jurors' responsibility in relation to existing law), and may take a case away from the jury (by directed verdict or judgment notwithstanding the verdict) if he or she believes that there are no issues for the jury to consider or that the jury has erred in its decision. This right on the part of the judge with respect to the role of the jury narrows the jury's responsibility with regard to the facts of the case. The judge maintains order throughout the suit, determines issues of procedure, and is generally responsible for the conduct of the trial.

The Jury

The right to a trial by jury is a constitutional right in certain cases. Not all cases entitle the parties to a jury trial as a matter of right. For example, in many jurisdictions, a case in equity (a case seeking a specific course of conduct rather than monetary damages) may not entitle the parties to a trial by a jury. An example of an equity case is one that seeks a declaration as to the title to real property.

An individual may waive the right to a jury trial. If this right is waived, the judge acts as judge and jury, becomes the trier of facts, and decides issues of law.

Members of the jury are selected from a jury list. They are summoned to court by a paper known as the jury process. Impartiality is a prerequisite of all jurors. The number of jurors who sit at trial is 12 in common law. If there are fewer than 12, the number must be established by statute.

Counsel for both parties of a lawsuit question each prospective jury member for impartiality, bias, and prejudicial thinking. This process is referred to as the *voir dire*, the examination of jurors. Once members of the jury are selected, they are sworn in to try the case.

The jury makes a determination of the facts that have occurred, evaluating whether the plaintiff's damages were caused by the defendant's negligence and whether the defendant exercised due care. The jury makes a determination of the particular standard of conduct required in all cases in which the judgment of reasonable people might differ. The jury must pay close attention to the evidence presented by both sides of a suit in order to render a fair and impartial verdict.

The jury also determines the extent of damages, if any, and the degree to which the plaintiff's conduct may have contributed to any injuries suffered.

Subpoenas

A *subpoena* is a legal order requiring the appearance of a person and/or the presentation of documents to a court or administrative body. Attorneys, judges, and certain law enforcement and administrative officials, depending on the jurisdiction, may issue subpoenas.

A *subpoena ad testificandum* orders the appearance of a person at a trial or other investigative proceeding to give testimony. Witnesses have a duty to appear and may suffer a penalty for contempt of court should they fail to appear.

A subpoena for records, known as a *subpoena duces tecum*, is a written command to bring records, documents, or other evidence described in the subpoena to a trial or other investigative proceeding. The subpoena is served on a person able to produce such records.

Opening Statements

During the opening statement, the plaintiff's attorney attempts to prove the wrongdoing of the defendant by presenting credible evidence favorable to his or her client. The opening statement by the plaintiff's attorney provides in capsule form the facts of the case, what he or she intends to prove by means of a summary of the evidence to be presented, and a description of the damages to his or her client.

The defense attorney makes his or her opening statement indicating the position of the defendant and the points of the plaintiff's case he or she intends to refute. The defense attorney explains the facts as they apply to the case for the defendant.

Burden of Proof

The burden of proof requires that the plaintiff's attorney show that the defendant violated a legal duty by not following an acceptable standard of care and that the plaintiff suffered injury because of the defendant's breach. If the evidence presented does not support the allegations made, the case is dismissed.

Evidence

Evidence consists of the facts proved or disproved during a lawsuit. The law of evidence is a body of rules under which facts are proved. Evidence must be competent, relevant, and material to be admitted at trial.

Direct Evidence

Direct evidence is proof offered through direct testimony. It is the jury's function to receive testimony presented by witnesses and to draw conclusions in the determination of facts.

Demonstrative Evidence

Demonstrative (real) *evidence* is evidence furnished by things themselves. It is considered the most trustworthy and preferred type of evidence. It consists of tangible objects to which testimony refers (e.g., medical instruments and broken infusion needles) that can be requested by a jury. Demonstrative evidence is admissible in court if it is relevant, has probative value, and serves the interest of justice. It is not admissible if it will prejudice, mislead, confuse, offend, inflame, or arouse the sympathy or passion of the jury. Other forms of demonstrative evidence include photographs, motion pictures, X-ray films, drawings, human bodies as exhibits, pathology slides, fetal monitoring strips, safety committee minutes, infection committee reports, medical staff bylaws, rules and regulations, nursing policy and procedure manuals, census data, and staffing patterns.

The plaintiff's injuries are admissible as an exhibit if the physical condition of the body is material to the complaint. The human body is considered the best evidence as to the nature and extent of the alleged injury/injuries. If there is no controversy about either the nature or the extent of an injury, presenting such evidence could be considered prejudicial and an objection can be made as to its presentation to a jury.

Documentary Evidence

Documentary evidence is written evidence capable of making a truthful statement (e.g., drug manufacturer inserts, autopsy reports, birth certificates, and medical records). Documentary evidence must satisfy the jury as to authenticity. Proof of authenticity is not necessary if the opposing party accepts its genuineness. In some instances, concerning wills, for example, witnesses are necessary. In the case of documentation, the original of a document must be produced unless it can be demonstrated that the original has been lost or destroyed, in which case a properly authenticated copy may be substituted.

Examination of Witnesses

After conclusion of the opening statements, the judge calls for the plaintiff's witnesses. An officer of the court administers an oath to each witness, and direct examination begins. On cross-examination by the defense, an attempt is made to challenge or discredit the plaintiff's witness. The plaintiff's attorney may ask the same witness more questions in an effort to overcome the effect of the cross-examination. Re–cross-examination may also take place if necessary for the defense of the defendant.

Expert Witness Necessary

Laymen are quite able to render opinions about a great variety of general subjects, but for technical questions, the opinion of an expert is necessary. At the time of testifying, each expert's training, experience, and special qualifications will be explained to the jury. The experts will be asked to give an opinion concerning hypothetical questions based on the facts of the case. Should the testimony of two experts conflict, the jury will determine which expert opinion to accept. Expert witnesses may be used to assist a plaintiff in proving the wrongful act of a defendant or to assist a defendant in refuting such evidence. In addition, expert testimony may be used to show the extent of the plaintiff's damages or to show the lack of such damages.

Defense of One's Actions

The defendant's case is presented to discredit the plaintiff's cause of action and prevent recovery of damages. Principles of law that may relieve a defendant from liability include assumption of a risk, comparative negligence, contributory negligence, Good Samaritan laws, ignorance of fact and unintentional wrongs, the statute of limitations, and sovereign immunity. These are discussed next.

Assumption of a Risk

Assumption of a risk is knowing that a danger exists and voluntarily accepting the risk by exposing oneself to it, knowing that harm might occur. Assumption of a risk may be implicitly assumed, as in alcohol consumption, or expressly assumed, as in relation to warnings found on cigarette packaging.

This defense provides that the plaintiff expressly has given consent in advance, relieving the defendant of an obligation of conduct toward the plaintiff and taking the chances of injury from a known risk arising from the defendant's conduct. For example, one who agrees to care for a patient with a communicable disease and then contracts the disease would not be entitled to recover from the patient for damages suffered. In taking the job, the individual agreed to assume the risk of infection, thereby releasing the patient from all legal obligations.

The following two requirements must be established in order for a defendant to be successful in an assumption of a risk defense: (1) the plaintiff must know and understand the risk that is being incurred, and (2) the choice to incur the risk must be free and voluntary.

Comparative Negligence

A defense of comparative negligence provides that the degree of negligence or carelessness of each party to a lawsuit must be established by the finder of fact and that each party then is responsible for his or her proportional share of any damages awarded. For example, if a plaintiff suffers injuries of $10,000 from an accident and is found to be 20 percent negligent, and the defendant is found to be 80 percent negligent, the defendant would be required to pay $8,000 to the plaintiff. Thus, with comparative negligence, the plaintiff can collect for 80 percent of the injuries, whereas an application of contributory negligence would deprive the plaintiff of any monetary judgment. This doctrine relieves the plaintiff from the hardship of losing an entire claim when a defendant has been successful in establishing that the plaintiff has contributed to his or her own injuries.

Contributory Negligence

Contributory negligence can be defined as any lack of ordinary care on the part of the person injured that, combined with the negligent act of another, caused the injury and without which the injury would not have occurred. A person is contributorily negligent when that person does not exercise reasonable care for his or her own safety. As a general proposition, if a person has knowledge of a dangerous situation and disregards the danger, then that person is contributorily negligent.

Good Samaritan Laws

The various states have enacted Good Samaritan laws that relieve health care professionals and, in some instances, laypersons, from liability in certain emergency situations. Good Samaritan legislation encourages health care professionals to render assistance at the scene of emergencies. Good Samaritan statutes provide a standard of care that delineates the scope of immunity for those persons eligible under the law.

Ignorance of Fact and Unintentional Wrongs

Ignorance of the law excuses no man; not that all men know the law, but because it is an excuse every man will plead, and no man can tell how to confute him.

JOHN SELDEN (1584–1654)

Ignorance of the law is not a defense, otherwise an individual would be rewarded by pleading ignorance. Arguing that a negligent act is unintentional is no defense. If such a defense were acceptable, all defendants would use it.

Statute of Limitations

The *statute of limitations* refers to legislatively imposed time constraints that restrict the period of time after an injury occurs during which a legal action must be commenced. Should a cause of action be initiated later than the period of time prescribed, the case cannot proceed. The statutory period begins when an injury occurs, although in some cases (usually involving foreign objects left in the body during surgery) the statutory period commences when the injured person discovers or should have discovered the injury.

Many technical rules are associated with statutes of limitations. Computation of the period when the statute begins to run in a particular state may be based on any of the following factors:

- the date that the physician terminated treatment
- the time of the wrongful act
- the time when the patient should have reasonably discovered the injury
- the date that the injury is discovered
- the date when the contract between the patient and the physician ended

Sovereign Immunity

Sovereign immunity refers to the common-law doctrine by which federal and state governments historically have been immune from liability for harm suffered from the tortious conduct of employees. For the most part, both federal and state governments have abolished sovereign immunity.

Closing Statements

Closing statements give attorneys an opportunity to summarize for the jury and the court what they have proven. They may point out faults in their opponent's case and emphasize points they want the jury to remember.

Judge's Charge to the Jury

After the attorneys' summations, the court charges the jury before the jurors recess to deliberate. Because the jury determines issues of fact, it is necessary for the court to instruct the jury with regard to applicable law. This is done by means of a charge. The charge defines the responsibility of the jury, describes the applicable law, and advises the jury of the alternatives available to it.

Jury Deliberation

After the judge's charge, the jury retires to the jury room and deliberates as to whether or not the defendant is liable. The jury returns to the courtroom upon reaching a verdict, and its determinations are presented to the court.

If a verdict is against the weight of the evidence, a judge may dismiss the case, order a new trial, or set his or her own verdict. At the time judgment is rendered, the losing party has an opportunity to motion for a new trial. If the new trial is granted, the entire process is repeated; if not, the judgment becomes final, subject to a review of the trial record by an appellate court.

Damages

Damages are often awarded to a plaintiff in a civil case in order to compensate the injured party as a result of the wrongful actions of the defendant(s).

Plaintiffs seek recovery for a great variety of damages. Damages are generally sought for emotional distress, physical pain and suffering, and economic loss. Punitive damages are sometimes awarded over and above that which is intended to compensate the plaintiff for economic losses resulting from the injury. Punitive damages cover such items as physical disability, mental anguish, loss of a spouse's services, physical suffering, injury to one's reputation, and loss of companionship. Punitive damages are referred to as "that mighty engine of deterrence" in *Johnson v. Terry*.[25] In *Estes Health Care Centers v. Bonnerman*, it was found that,

> While human life is incapable of translation into a compensatory measurement, the amount of an award of punitive damages may be measured by the gravity of the wrong done, the punishment called for by the act of the wrongdoer, and the need to deter similar wrongs in order to preserve human life.[26]

Appeals

An appellate court reviews a case on the basis of the trial record as well as written briefs and, if requested, concise oral arguments by the attorneys. A brief summarizes the facts of a case, testimony of the witnesses, laws affecting the case, and arguments of counsel. The party making the appeal is the appellant. The party answering the appeal is the appellee. After hearing the oral arguments, the court takes the case under advisement until such time as the judges consider it and agree on a decision. An opinion then is prepared, explaining the reasons for a decision. The appellate court may modify, affirm, or reverse the judgment, or may reorder a new trial on an appeal.

CHAPTER REVIEW

1. A tort is a civil wrong, not including breach of contract, that is committed against a person or property for which a court provides a correction in the form of an action for damages.

2. Negligence is a tort, a civil or personal wrong. It is the unintentional commission or omission of an act that a reasonably prudent person would or would not do under given circumstances. Intentional wrongdoing involves an act that violates another person's interests.

3. Negligence has three basic forms:
   - Malfeasance is the execution of an unlawful or improper act.
   - Misfeasance is the improper performance of an act that results in injury to another.
   - Nonfeasance is a failure to act when there is a duty to do so.

   To recover damages caused by negligence, four elements must be present: duty to care, breach of duty, injury, and causation.

- Duty to care exists when there is a legal obligation of care, performance, or observance imposed on one party to guard the rights of others.
- Breach of duty is the failure to meet a prevailing standard of care.
- Injury. Without proof of harm or injury, a defendant cannot be found liable.
- Causation refers to the idea that the defendant's negligence must be a substantial factor in having caused an injury.

4. Foreseeability is the reasonable anticipation that harm or injury will result from an act or a failure to act. The test for foreseeability is whether or not one should have reasonably anticipated that the event in question or a similar event would occur.

5. Assault is the infringement on the mental security or tranquility of another person; battery is the violation of another person's physical integrity.

6. False imprisonment is the unlawful restraint of an individual's personal liberty or the unlawful restraint or confinement of an individual.

7. Defamation of character is a false oral or written communication to someone other than the individual defamed subjecting that individual's reputation to scorn and ridicule. Two aspects of defamation of character are libel, which results from the written word, and slander, which results from the spoken word.

8. Fraud is a willful and intentional misrepresentation that could cause harm or loss to an individual or property.

9. The objectives of criminal law are to maintain public order and safety, protect individuals, use punishment as a deterrent to crime, and rehabilitate criminals for return to society.

10. A crime—a social harm defined and made punishable by law—is generally either a misdemeanor or a felony. A misdemeanor is an offense punishable by less than one year in jail and/or a fine. A felony, however, is generally punishable by imprisonment in a state or federal prison for a period of more than one year.

11. Criminal negligence is the reckless disregard for the safety of others and is the willful indifference to an injury that could result from an act. It differs from tort liability in that it provides for a more specific lack of care commonly characterized as "gross negligence" and "recklessness."

12. A contract is a written or oral agreement that involves legally binding obligations between two or more parties.

13. To be enforceable, contracts must contain an offer or communication, consideration, and acceptance.

14. Exclusive contracts allow organizations to contract with physicians and/or medical groups to provide specific services to the organization.

15. Before the trial, facts are investigated in a process called discovery. The discovery process helps to prevent surprises during trial. Examination before trial is part of the discovery process and allows for witnesses to be examined before the trial.

16. The jury determines the facts in a case and makes a determination of the particular standards of conduct required in all cases in which the judgment of reasonable people might differ.

17. A subpoena is a legal order requiring that a person appear in court or that documents be presented to a court or administrative body.

18. Facts proved or disproved during a lawsuit constitute evidence. Direct evidence is proof that is offered via direct testimony. Demonstrative evidence is offered by objects themselves. Written evidence capable of making a truthful statement is considered documentary evidence.

19. When the issues to be resolved in a case are outside the understanding or experience of the average juror, an expert witness is allowed to offer testimony to assist in explaining technical matters.

20. Principles of law that may relieve a defendant from liability include, among others:
    - Assumption of a risk
    - Borrowed servant doctrine
    - Contributory negligence
    - Good Samaritan laws
    - Statute of limitations

21. Damages can include nominal damages, compensatory damages, and punitive damages

TEST YOUR UNDERSTANDING

Terminology

tort	slander	demonstrative evidence
negligence	libel	documentary evidence
malpractice	invasion of privacy	assumption of a risk
standard of care	misdemeanor	contributory negligence
proximate cause	manslaughter	comparative negligence
foreseeability	contract	Good Samaritan law
assault	exclusive contract	statute of limitations
battery	subpoena	damages
false imprisonment	evidence	punitive damages
defamation	direct evidence	

REVIEW QUESTIONS

1. Describe the objectives of tort law.

2. Discuss the distinctions among negligent torts, intentional torts, and strict liability.

3. What forms of negligence are described in this chapter?

4. How does one distinguish between negligence and malpractice?

5. What are the elements that must be proven in order to be successful in a negligence suit? Illustrate your answer with a case. (The facts of the case can be hypothetical.)

6. Describe the categories of intentional torts.

7. How does slander differ from libel? Give an example of each.

8. What are the objectives of criminal law?

9. Describe the difference between a misdemeanor and a felony. Give an example of each.

10. Discuss why physicians have been so reluctant to remove a patient's life support systems.

11. What is a contract?

12. What are the elements of a contract?

13. Describe why exclusive contracts are so controversial.

14. Describe the trial process, including pre-trial motions and the functions of the judge, jury, and attorneys.

15. Describe the kinds of evidence that a plaintiff can present in order to establish a negligent act.

16. What defenses can a defendant present in order to refute a plaintiff's evidence?

17. Describe how statutes of limitations favor defendants in a lawsuit.

18. Describe the differences between nominal, compensatory, hedonic, and punitive damages.

NOTES

1. 498 So. 2d 713 (La. Ct. App. 1986).
2. 787 S.W.2d 494 (Tex. Ct. App. 1990).
3. 498 So. 2d 713 (La. Ct. App. 1986).
4. 57A Am. Jur. 2d *Torts* § 78 (1989).
5. 498 So. 2d 713 (La. Ct. App. 1986).
6. Clark v. Wagoner, 452 S.W.2d 437, 440 (Tex. 1970).
7. 57A Am. Jur. 2d *Torts* § 134 (1989).
8. 116 Cal. Rptr. 733 (Cal. Ct. App. 1974).
9. 385 N.W.2d 99 (N.D. 1986).
10. Tomcik v. Ohio Dep't of Rehabilitation & Correction, 598 N.E.2d 900 (Ohio Ct. App. 1991).
11. *Id.* at 904.
12. Tomcik v. Ohio Dep't of Rehabilitation & Correction, 598 N.E.2d 900 (Ohio Ct. App. 1991).
13. 295 U.S. 78, 88 (1935).
14. J. Kaplan, Criminal Justice Introductory Cases and Materials 228 (1973).
15. *Id.* at 259.
16. http://news.bbc.co.uk/1/hi/england/1695580.stm.
17. USA Today, November 30, 2004, at 3A.
18. USA Today, November 29, 2004, at 3A.
19. http:www.cbsnews.com/stories/2004/04/02/60minutes/printable610047.shtml.
20. Collwell, *The Verdict of Angelo*, 50(103) Newsday 1989, at 3.
21. 492 N.Y.S.2d 9 (N.Y. 1985).
22. No. A03A2308 (Ga. App. 2004).
23. City of Cookeville, No. M2001-00695-SC-R11-CV (Tenn. 2004).
24. 7 S.W.3d 542 (Mo. App. 1999).
25. No. 537-907 (Wis. Cir. Ct. Mar. 18, 1983).
26. 411 So. 2d 109, 113 (Ala. 1982).

seven

chapter seven

Government, Ethics, and the Law

Nothing is politically right which is morally wrong.

DANIEL O'CONNELL (1755–1847)[1]

LEARNING OBJECTIVES

The reader upon completion of this chapter will be able to:

- Describe the meaning and sources of public policy.
- Describe important laws designed to protect each individual's rights:
  - XIV Amendment to the U.S. Constitution
  - Sherman Antitrust Act
  - Civil Rights Act
  - Privacy Act
  - Emergency Medical Treatment and Active Labor Act
  - Health Care Quality Improvement Act
  - Agency for Healthcare Research and Quality
  - Ethics in Patient Referral Act
  - Patient Self-Determination Act

- ○ Uniform Controlled Substances Act
- ○ Federal Food, Drug and Cosmetic Act
- • Understand the concept of political malpractice.

INTRODUCTION

Public outcry over ever-increasing antisocial behavior, declining civility, and rampant unethical conduct have heightened discussions over the nation's moral decline and decaying value systems. The numerous instances of questionable political decisions, numbers-cooking, money-grabbing executives (including health care executives working for nonprofit organizations being paid high six-figure salaries plus all of the perks, bonuses, etc.), cheating at work and in school, and the proliferation of x-rated Web sites have led to this decline. Legislators, investigators, prosecutors, and the courts are finally stepping up to the plate and are taking action. The question, however, remains: Can this boat be turned around, or are we just plugging the holes with new laws and creating more leaks in a misdirected sinking boat? The answer is more likely to be a return to practicing the values upon which this nation was founded.

The continuing trend of consumer awareness about declining value systems, coupled with increased governmental regulations, mandates that caregivers understand ethics and the law and their interrelationships. Ethics and the law are not mutually exclusive—they are intertwined. Without the two, we would become a lawless land. The following pages present an overview of laws, influenced by ethical principles, designed to protect each individual's rights (e.g., the right to privacy and self-determination).

XIV AMENDMENT TO THE U.S. CONSTITUTION—1868

According to the Fourteenth Amendment to the Constitution, a state cannot act to deny any person equal protection of the laws. If a state or a political subdivision of a state, whether through its executive, judicial, or legislative branch, acts in such a way as to deny unfairly to any person the rights accorded to another, the amendment has been violated.

XIV Amendment

Section 1. All persons born or naturalized in the United States, and subject to the jurisdiction thereof, are citizens of the United States and of the state wherein they reside. No state shall make or enforce any law which shall abridge the privileges or immunities of citizens of the United States; nor shall any state deprive any person of life, liberty, or property, without due process of law; nor deny to any person within its jurisdiction the equal protection of the laws.

• • •

Section 5. The Congress shall have power to enforce, by appropriate legislation, the provisions of this article.

PUBLIC POLICY AS A PRINCIPLE OF LAW

Public policy is the principle of law that holds that no one can lawfully do that which tends to be injurious to the public or against the public good. The sources of public policy "include legislation; administrative rules, regulations, or decisions; and judicial decisions. In certain instances, a professional code of ethics may contain an expression of public policy."[2]

CIVIL RIGHTS ACT—1964

Civil rights are rights ensured by the U.S. Constitution and by the acts of Congress and the state legislatures. Generally, the term includes all the rights of each individual in a free society. Congress and the federal courts have dealt with discriminatory practices in health care organizations. Discrimination in the admission of patients and segregation of patients on racial grounds are prohibited in any organization receiving federal financial assistance. Pursuant to Title VI of the Civil Rights Act of 1964, the guidelines of the Department of Health and Human Services (HHS) prohibit the practice of racial discrimination by any organization or agency receiving money under any program supported by HHS. This includes all "providers of service" receiving federal funds under Medicare legislation.

SHERMAN ANTITRUST ACT—1890

The Sherman Antitrust Act, named for its author Senator John Sherman of Ohio, proscribes that every contract, combination in the form of trust or otherwise, or conspiracy, in restraint of trade or commerce among the several states is declared to be illegal. Those who monopolize, attempt to monopolize, or combine or conspire with any other person or persons to monopolize any part of the trade or commerce can be deemed guilty of a felony.[3] Areas of concern for health care organizations include reduced market competition, price fixing, actions that bar or limit new entrants to the field, preferred provider arrangements, and exclusive contracts.

A health care organization must be cognizant of the potential problems that may exist when limiting the number of physicians that it will admit to its medical staff. Because closed staff determinations can effectively limit competition from other physicians, the governing body must ensure that the decision-making process in granting privileges is based on legislative, objective criteria and is not dominated by those who have the most to gain competitively by denying privileges. Physicians have attempted to use state and federal antitrust laws to challenge determinations denying or limiting medical staff privileges. Generally, these actions claim that the organization conspired with other physicians to ensure that the complaining physician would not obtain privileges so that competition among physicians would be reduced.

PRIVACY ACT—1974

The Privacy Act of 1974, Title 5 United States Code (U.S.C.) 552, was enacted to safeguard individual privacy from the misuse of federal records, to give individuals access to records concerning themselves that are maintained by federal agencies, and to establish a Privacy Protection Safety Commission. Section 2 of the Privacy Act reads as follows:

> [a]The Congress finds that (1) the privacy of an individual is directly affected by the collection, maintenance, use, and dissemination of personal information by Federal agencies; (2) the increasing use of computers and sophisticated information technology, while essential to the efficient operations of the Government, has greatly magnified the harm to individual privacy that can occur from any collection, maintenance, use, or dissemination of personal information; (3) the opportunities for an individual to secure employment, insurance, and credit, and his right to due process, and other legal protections are endangered by the misuse of certain information systems; (4) the right to privacy is a personal and fundamental right protected by the Constitution of the United States; and (5) in order to protect the privacy of individuals identified in information systems maintained by Federal agencies, it is necessary and proper for the Congress to regulate the collection, maintenance, use, and dissemination of information by such agencies. [b] The purpose of this Act is to provide certain safeguards for an individual against an invasion of personal privacy by requiring Federal agencies, except as otherwise provided by law, to (1) permit an individual to determine what records pertaining to him are collected, maintained, used, or disseminated by such agencies; (2) permit an individual to prevent records pertaining to him obtained by such agencies for a particular purpose from being used or made available for another purpose without his consent; (3) permit an individual to gain access to information pertaining to him in Federal agency records, to have a copy made of all or any portion thereof, and to correct or amend such records; (4) collect, maintain, use, or disseminate any record of identifiable personal information in a manner that assures that such action is for a necessary and lawful purpose, that the information is current and accurate for its intended use, and that adequate safeguards are provided to prevent misuse of such information. . . .

EMERGENCY MEDICAL TREATMENT AND ACTIVE LABOR ACT—1986

In 1986, Congress passed the Emergency Medical Treatment and Active Labor Act (EMTALA), which forbids Medicare-participating hospitals from "dumping" patients out of emergency departments. The Act provides that:

> [i]n the case of a hospital that has a hospital emergency department, if any individual (whether or not eligible for benefits under this subchapter) comes to the emergency department and a request is made on the individual's behalf for examination or treatment for a medical condition, the hospital must provide for an appropriate medical screening examination within the capability of the hospital emergency department, including ancillary services routinely available to the emergency department, to determine whether or not an emergency medical condition . . . exists.[4]

CASE: EMTALA VIOLATED

In *Burditt v. U.S. Department of Health and Human Services*,[5] EMTALA was violated by a physician when he ordered a woman with dangerously high blood pressure (210/130) and in active labor with ruptured membranes transferred from the emergency department of one hospital to another hospital 170 miles away. The physician was assessed a penalty of $20,000. Dr. Louis Sullivan, Secretary of HHS at that time, issued a statement: "This decision sends a message to physicians everywhere that they need to provide quality care to everyone in need of emergency treatment who comes to a hospital. This is a significant opinion and we are pleased with the result."[6] The American Public Health Association, in filing an *amicus curiae*, advised the appeals court that "if Burditt wants to ensure that he will never be asked to treat a patient not of his choosing, then he ought to vote with his feet by affiliating only with hospitals that do not accept Medicare funds or do not have an emergency department."[7]

Ethical and Legal Issues

1. What are the main issues in this case?
2. What ethical theories, principles, and values are of concern? Describe them.
3. What action can be taken to prevent similar occurrences in the future?
4. What could have been done to prevent the ethical and legal issues from occurring in the first place?
5. If you were the judge in this case, what would you do in light of the American Public Health Association's comments?
6. Describe both the hospital and physician's ethical and legal responsibilities. ■

HEALTH CARE QUALITY IMPROVEMENT ACT—1986

The Health Care Quality Improvement Act of 1986 (HCQIA) was enacted in part to provide those persons giving information to professional review bodies and those assisting in review activities limited immunity from damages that may arise as a result of adverse decisions that affect a physician's medical staff privileges. Prior to enacting the HCQIA, Congress found that "[t]he increasing occurrence of medical malpractice and the need to improve the quality of medical care . . . [had] become nationwide problems," especially in light of "the ability of incompetent physicians to move from State to State without disclosure or discovery of the physician's previous damaging or incompetent performance" (42 U.S.C. § 11101). The problem, however, could be remedied through effective professional peer review combined with a national reporting system that made information about adverse professional actions against physicians more widely available. HCQIA was enacted by Congress to "facilitate the frank exchange of information among professionals conducting peer review inquiries without the fear of reprisals in civil lawsuits. The statute attempts to balance the chilling effect of litigation on peer review with concerns for protecting physicians improperly subjected to disciplinary action."

CASE: FAILURE TO MEET ETHICAL STANDARDS

Meyers applied for medical staff privileges at a hospital. Shortly thereafter, the Credentials Committee and the Medical Executive Committee (MEC) and the board of the hospital approved Meyers for appointment to the medical staff. All initial appointments to the medical staff were provisional for one year. At the end of that year the physician would once again be evaluated for advancement from associate to active staff.

The Credentials Committee began to evaluate Meyers for advancement to active staff privileges. The committee was concerned about Meyers' history: moving from hospital to hospital following disputes with hospital staff, his failure to timely and fully disclose disciplinary and corrective action taken against him in another state, and the quality of his patient care. The MEC voted to accept a Credentials Committee decision to revoke Meyers' staff privileges. The MEC was to consider the recommendation from the Credentials Committee and make a recommendation to the Board, which had the ultimate authority to grant, deny, or terminate Meyers' privileges.

The Board informed Meyers that it was assuming responsibility for determining his reappointment and advancement to active staff because of concerns with the manner in which the peer review process was being handled. Three members of the Board, acting as a Credentials Committee, conducted an independent review. This committee discussed concerns about Meyers' behavior and his inability to get along with others, in addition to questions about his surgical technique. The committee questioned Meyers about several incident reports concerning disruptive behavior, his history of problems at other hospitals, his failure to timely complete medical records, his hostility toward the operation room staff, reports of breaking the sterile field, and his failure to provide appropriate coverage for patients while he was out of town. Meyers acknowledged that he had a personality problem.

The three member committee of the Board voted to deny Meyers' appointment to active staff. The reasons cited for the committee's decision were Meyers' failure to satisfy requirements that he "abide by the ethics of the profession," work cooperatively with others, timely complete medical records, and abide by hospital standards. The committee outlined Meyers' pattern of rude, abusive, and disruptive behavior that included, but was not limited to, temper tantrums, attempted interference with the right of an attending physician to refer a patient to the surgeon of his choice or to transfer the patient, condescending remarks toward women, refusal to speak to a member of his surgical team during surgical procedures, and several instances of throwing a scalpel during surgery. The committee informed Meyers that this behavior could have an adverse effect on the quality of patient care. As for his failure to timely complete medical records, the committee stated that "delinquent medical records can put patients at risk by being inaccurate or incomplete if needed to assist in later diagnosis and treatment of a patient."

A Fair Hearing Committee issued its recommendation that Meyers not be reappointed to the hospital's staff because of his failure to meet "ethical standards" and his inability to work cooperatively with others. In May, the Board adopted and affirmed the Fair Hearing Committee's recommendation. Ultimately, following further appeals the Board revoked Meyers' privileges.

Meyers brought suit in seeking a permanent injunction to require the hospital to reinstate him to staff. The court denied the motion for an injunction that would require the hospital to reinstate Meyers' privileges.

The Court agreed with hospital defendants that the behavior of Meyers had the potential of affecting the health and welfare of patients, despite the fact that no patients were actually injured. Quality patient care demands that doctors possess at least a reasonable ability to work with others. Clearly, the hospital defendants were acting with a reasonable belief that the professional review action was in the furtherance of quality health care. They were concerned that Meyers' behavior would continue until a patient was injured as a result of his actions.[8]

Ethical and Legal Issues

1. Describe where Meyers failed to satisfy requirements that he abide by the ethics of his profession. (See the code of ethics adopted by the American Medical Association presented in the chapter on physician ethics and legal issues.)
2. Describe the ethical theories, principles, and values of concern in this case.
3. Describe what steps the organization can take to prevent similar occurrences in the future. ▪

AGENCY FOR HEALTHCARE RESEARCH AND QUALITY

It is well publicized that tens of thousands of patients die annually because hospitals fail to ensure safety, quality, and public accountability, this according to a report released on January 7, 2002, by the National Academy of Sciences.

The Agency for Healthcare Research and Quality (AHRQ), established in 1989, is charged with research designed to improve the quality of health care, reduce its costs, and broaden access to essential services. AHRQ was created as a result of the mistakes that have occurred and continue to occur in the delivery of care. The pain, misery, and financial drain on the injured, their families, and society has taken its toll. The numerous ethical and legal issues that have evolved spawned the need for the AHRQ.

ETHICS IN PATIENT REFERRAL ACT—1989

In 1989, the Ethics in Patient Referral Act was enacted, prohibiting physicians who have ownership interest or compensation arrangements with a clinical laboratory from referring Medicare patients to that laboratory. The law also requires all Medicare providers to report the names and provider numbers of all physicians or their immediate relatives with ownership interests in the provider entity prior to October 1, 1991.

PATIENT SELF-DETERMINATION ACT—1990

The Patient Self-Determination Act of 1990 (PSDA)[9] was enacted to ensure that patients are informed of their rights to execute advance directives and accept or refuse medical care. On December 1, 1991, the PSDA[10] took effect in hospitals, skilled nursing facilities, home health agencies, hospice organizations, and health maintenance organizations serving Medicare and Medicaid patients. As a result of implementation of the PSDA,[11] health care organizations participating in the Medicare and Medicaid reimbursement programs must address patient rights regarding life-sustaining decisions and other advance directives. Health care organizations have a responsibility to explain to patients, staff, and families that patients have a legal right to direct their own medical and nursing care as it corresponds to existing state law, including right-to-die directives. A person's right to refuse medical treatment is not lost when his or her mental or physical status changes. When a person is no longer competent to exercise his or her right of self-determination, the right still exists but the decision must be delegated to a surrogate decision maker. Those organizations that do not comply with a patient's medical directives or those of a legally authorized decision maker are exposing themselves to the risk of a lawsuit.

Each state is required under PSDA to provide a description of the law in the state regarding advance directives to providers, whether such directives are based on state statutes or judicial decisions. Providers must ensure that written policies and procedures with respect to all adult individuals regarding advance directives are established as follows:

(A) to provide written information to each such individual concerning
  (i) an individual's rights under State law (whether statutory or as recognized by the courts of the State) to make decisions concerning such medical care, including the right to accept or refuse medical or surgical treatment and the right to formulate advance directives . . ., and
  (ii) written policies of the provider organization respecting the implementation of such rights;
(B) to document in the individual's medical record whether or not the individual has executed an advance directive;
(C) not to condition the provision of care or otherwise discriminate against an individual based on whether or not the individual has executed an advance directive;
(D) to ensure compliance with requirements of State law (whether statutory or recognized by the courts of the State) respecting advance directives at the facilities of the provider or organization; and
(E) to provide (individually or with others) for education for staff and the community on issues concerning advance directives.[12]

Although the PSDA is being cheered as a major advancement in clarifying and nationally regulating this often obscure area of law and medicine, there are continuing problems and new issues that must be addressed.

HEALTH INSURANCE PORTABILITY AND ACCOUNTABILITY ACT—1996

The "Health Insurance Portability and Accountability Act" (HIPAA) of 1996 (Public Law 104-191) was designed to protect the privacy, confidentiality, and security of patient information. HIPAA standards are applicable to all health information in all its formats (e.g., electronic, paper, verbal). It applies to both electronically maintained and transmitted information. HIPAA privacy standards include restrictions on access to individually identifiable health information, and the use and disclosure of that information, as well as requirements for administrative activities such as training, compliance, and enforcement of HIPAA requirements.

SARBANES-OXLEY ACT—2002

The Sarbanes-Oxley Act was signed by President Bush on July 30, 2002, in response to the Enron debacle and high-profile cases of corporate mismanagement. The Act requires top executives of public corporations to vouch for the financial reports of their companies. The Act encourages self-regulation and the need to: promote due diligence; select a leader with morals and core values; examine incentives; constantly monitor the organization's culture;

build a strong, knowledgeable governing body; continuously search for conflicts of interest; focus attention on the right things; and have the courage to speak out.

"The tragedy of society is not the noisiness of the so-called bad people, but the appalling silence of the so-called good people."

—*Martin Luther King, Jr.*

POLITICAL MALPRACTICE

With the nation being sidetracked by terrorism and war, who is watching over government priorities for addressing domestic needs? In a column written by Ronald Brownstein in the *St. Petersburg Times,* he writes an article titled, "Health Care Safety Net Stretched Thin."[13] In his column, Brownstein describes a recently released study from the George Washington University School of Public Health addressing the financial strain on public hospitals' abilities to provide health care services to some 43 million uninsured Americans. Insured or not, Americans are often waiting months to be seen by specialists. One government hospital described up to a six-month wait for a neurological consult: ". . . practical steps are possible to help millions of low income families live healthier lives and receive more effective care when they need it. Ignoring that opportunity, while waiting for consensus on coverage, would be a form of political malpractice."[14]

CHAPTER REVIEW

1. This chapter presented an overview of federal statutes that were designed to protect individual rights, including the right to privacy and self-determination.

2. The Fourteenth Amendment to the Constitution of the United States provides that a state cannot act to deny any person equal protection of the laws.

3. Public policy is that principle of law which holds that no one can lawfully do that which tends to be injurious to the public or against the public good. The sources of public policy include legislation; administrative rules, regulations, or decisions; and judicial decisions. In certain instances, a professional code of ethics may contain an expression of public policy.

4. Pursuant to Title VI of the Civil Rights Act of 1964, the guidelines of HHS prohibit the practice of racial discrimination by any organization or agency receiving money under any program supported by HHS.

5. The Privacy Act of 1974, Title 5 United States Code (U.S.C.) 552, was enacted to safeguard individual privacy from the misuse of federal records, to give individuals access to records concerning them-

selves that are maintained by federal agencies, and to establish a Privacy Protection Safety Commission.

6. The HCQIA was enacted in part to provide those persons giving information to professional review bodies and those assisting in review activities limited immunity from damages that may arise as a result of adverse decisions that affect a physician's medical staff privileges.

7. In 1986, Congress passed the EMTALA, which forbids Medicare-participating hospitals from "dumping" patients out of emergency departments.

8. The Ethics in Patient Referral Act of 1989 prohibits physicians who have ownership interest or compensation arrangements with a clinical laboratory from referring Medicare patients to that laboratory.

9. The PSDA[15] was enacted to ensure that patients are informed of their rights to execute advance directives and accept or refuse medical care. Each state is required under PSDA to provide a description of the law in the state regarding advance directives to providers, whether such directives are based on state statutes or judicial decisions.

10. HIPAA (Public Law 104-191) was designed to protect the privacy, confidentiality, and security of patient information. HIPAA standards are applicable to all health information in all its formats (e.g., electronic, paper, verbal). It applies to both electronically maintained and transmitted information.

11. Practical steps are possible to help millions live healthier lives through preventative care. To ignore such an opportunity is considered by some to be a form of political malpractice.

TEST YOUR UNDERSTANDING

Terminology

public policy
Civil Rights Act
Privacy Act
EMTALA
Health Care Quality
   Improvement Act
Agency for Healthcare
   Research and Quality

Ethics in Patient Referral Act
Patient Self-Determination Act
Health Insurance Portability and
   Accountability Act
political malpractice

REVIEW QUESTIONS

1. Describe the purpose of public policy.

2. Discuss how the federal statutes discussed in this chapter protect individuals' rights (e.g., privacy and self-determination).

3. List and discuss the sources of public policy.

4. Describe the concepts of "preventative care" and "political malpractice," as discussed in this chapter.

WEB SITES

Agency for Healthcare Policy and Research
www.ahcpr.gov/clinic/cpgsix.htm

Centers for Medicare and Medicaid Services
http://www.cms.hhs.gov/default.asp

Congress
www.congress.org

Centers for Disease Control
www.cdc.gov

Centers for Medicare and Medicaid
www.cms.hhs.gov

Department of Health and Human Services
http://www.hhs.gov/

Food and Drug Administration
www.fda.com

Government Guide (government services made easy)
www.governmentguide.com

Government Manual
http://www.access.gpo.gov/nara/nara001.html

Government
www.gov.com

Health Privacy Project
http://www.healthprivacy.org

HIPAA Privacy http://www.mmmlaw.com/industry/healthcare/
surgerycenter1.ppt

Department of Health & Human Services
http://www.os.dhhs.gov/ocr/hipaa

HIPAA Summary
www.hipaaadvisory.com/regs/law/summary.htm

HIPAA Pro Supersite
http://www.himinfo.com/hipaa

HIPAA Readiness Collaborative
http://www.hhic.org/hipaa/hipaafaq.html

HIPAA
www.hipaacomply.com
HIPAA—CMS Forms
www.cms.hhs.gov/forms
MedlinePlus
www.Medlineplus.gov
National Institute on Aging
www.nih.gov/nia
National Institutes of Health
www.nih.gov
National Institutes of Standards and Technology
http://www.nist.gov/
National Library of Medicine
http://www.nlm.nih.gov/
National Institute of Medicine
www.iom.edu
Occupational Safety and Health Administration
www.osha-slc.gov
Oregon's Death with Dignity Act
http://arcweb.sos.state.or.us/
Thomas—Legislative Information of the Internet
http://thomas.loc.gov/
United States Department of Justice
http://www.usdoj.gov/
U.S. Government's Official Web Portal
http://www.firstgov.gov/

NOTES

1. Irish Politician.
2. Pierce v. Ortho Pharmaceutical Corp., 417 A.2d 505, 512 (N.J. 1980).
3. 15 U.S.C. § 1 (1982).
4. 42 U.S.C.A. § 1395dd(a) (1992).
5. 934 F.2d 1362 (5th Cir. Tex. 1991).
6. *Courts Uphold Law, Regulations against Patient Dumping*, NATION'S HEALTH, Aug. 1991, at 1.
7. *Id.* at 17.
8. Meyers v. Logan Mem. Hosp., 82 F. Supp. 2d 707 (2000).
9. 42 U.S.C. 1395cc(a)(1).
10. Public Law 101–508, November 5, 1990, sections 4206 and 4751 of the Omnibus Budget Reconciliation Act.
11. 42 U.S.C. § 1395 (1992).
12. 42 U.S.C. § 1395cc (1992).
13. *Health Care Safety Net Stretched Thin*, Ronald Brownstein, ST. PETERSBURG TIMES, June 4, 2004, Section A, at 13a.
14. *Id.*
15. 42 U.S.C. 1395cc(a)(1).

chapter eight

Organizational Ethics and the Law

LEARNING OBJECTIVES

The reader upon completion of this chapter will be able to:

- Understand the ethical and legal risks to which organizations are exposed.

- Describe corporate structure.

- Identify and discuss the duties and responsibilities of organizations as they relate to patient care.

INTRODUCTION

This chapter introduces the reader to the ethical responsibilities and legal risks to which health care organizations and their governing bodies can be exposed. An organization's code of ethics should provide guidelines for behavior that help carry out an organization's mission, vision, and values. Organizational codes of ethics build trust, increase awareness of ethical issues, guide decision making, and encourage staff to seek advice and report misconduct.

The following list provides some value statements that should be considered when preparing an organization's code of ethics.

1. All employees and staff members are expected to comply with the organization's Code of Ethics, which includes compassionate care; an understanding and acceptance of the organization's mission, vision, and values; and adherence to one's professional code of conduct.
2. Managers are expected to develop and maintain an environment that fosters the highest ethical and legal standards.
3. Patients will be provided with care that is of the highest quality regardless of the setting.
4. All patients will be treated with honesty, dignity, respect, and courtesy.
5. Patients will be informed as to the risks, benefits, and alternatives to care.
6. Each patient's culture, religion, and heritage will be respected and addressed as appropriate.
7. The organization provides assistance to patients and families through a patient advocate.
8. The organization will provide appropriate support services for those with physical disabilities (e.g., hearing and seeing impaired), language barriers, and so forth.
9. The organization and its medical staff will invoice patients or third parties only for services rendered. Assistance will be given to patients to help them better understand the costs of their care.
10. Patients will be provided with a "Patient's Bill of Rights and Responsibilities" upon admission to the hospital.
11. Each patient's rights to execute advance directives will be honored.
12. Patients will be treated in a manner that preserves their rights, dignity, autonomy, self-esteem, privacy, and involvement in their care.

ORGANIZATIONAL CONDUCT UNDER SCRUTINY

Organizational ethics in the health care setting are being carefully scrutinized across the nation by state and federal regulatory agencies. Unethical conduct that is closely being monitored includes false advertisements, fraudulent reimbursement schemes, and understatement of earnings.

Truthfulness in Advertising

On a billboard on a major highway a hospital advertised its accreditation score, which was awarded by an accrediting organization. The advertisement gave the a perception that the score was somehow an indicator of the quality of care provided by the hospital, implying that hospitals receiving lower scores delivered inferior care. Eventually this issuing of scores was discontinued because of misuse of scores as a ranking mechanism and because it could be perceived by some that organizations concentrated on scores rather than on improving patient care. From an ethical point of view, health care organizations should not advertise misleading information to encourage public confidence in the quality of care provided by the organization.

CASE: FALSE ADVERTISING

An action was filed against the defendant, Managed Care, alleging claims of false advertising in connection with Managed Care's sale, marketing, and rendering of medical services. The plaintiff alleged that he was an enrollee in Managed Care's health plan. He also alleged that through misleading and deceptive material representations and omissions, Managed Care had employed a fraudulent, unfair scheme to induce people to enroll in its plan by misrepresenting that its primary commitment was to maintain and improve the quality of health care. The plaintiff alleged that Managed Care had been aggressively engaged in implementing undisclosed systemic internal policies that were designed to discourage its primary care physicians from delivering medical services and, therefore, interfering with the medical judgment of its health care providers. The result of these policies, he alleged, was a reduction in the quality of health care that is directly contrary to Managed Care's representations.

The plaintiff claimed that Managed Care's false advertising reduced the quality of medical services available to the enrollees and decreased the monetary value of their health coverage. The plaintiff requested restitution, refund, or reimbursement of monies paid by or on behalf of enrollees, and disgorgement of the excessive and ill-gotten monies obtained by Managed Care as a result of the unlawful, fraudulent, and unfair business acts and practices and untrue and misleading advertisements.

Ethical and Legal Issues

1. Describe the ethical issues in this case.
2. Describe the value of a corporate compliance program and how it could help prevent false advertising. ■

CASE: APPEARANCE MAY NOT BE REALITY

General Hospital's staff aggregated its infection rate data for comparison purposes with four other hospitals in the community. The staff were aware that the data were flawed. They presented a false perception that General Hospital's post-operative infection rates were lower than peer hospitals. The comparison data were published in the local newspaper. The Jones family, believing the data to be correct, relied on the data in selecting General Hospital as their preferred hospital.

Ethical and Legal Issues

1. Describe the ethical principles and values violated in this case.
2. Describe what the role of an organization's ethics committee should be in addressing this or similar issues. ■

ORGANIZATIONAL STRUCTURE

The typical health care organization is incorporated under state law as a freestanding for-profit or not-for-profit corporation. The corporation has a governing body that has ultimate responsibility for the decisions made in the organization. The existence of this authority creates certain duties and liabilities. The governing body, having ultimate responsibility for the operation and management of the organization, generally delegates responsibility for the day-to-day operations of the organization to the organization's chief executive officer.

Although health care organizations may operate as sole proprietorships or partnerships, most function as corporations. Thus, an important source of law applicable to governing boards and to the duties and responsibilities of their members is found in state corporation laws. An incorporated health care organization is a legal person with recognized rights, duties, powers, and responsibilities. Because the legal "person" is in reality a "fictitious person," there is a requirement that certain people be designated to exercise the corporate powers and that they be held accountable for corporate decision making.

Health care corporations—governmental, charitable, or proprietary—have certain powers expressly or implicitly granted to them by state statutes. Generally, the authority of a corporation is expressed in the law under which the corporation is chartered and in the corporation's articles of incorporation. The existence of this authority creates certain duties and liabilities for governing bodies and their individual members. Members of the governing body have both express and implied corporate authority.

Express Corporate Authority

Express corporate authority is authority specifically delegated by statute. Health care corporations derive authority to act from the laws of the state in which they are incorporated. The articles of incorporation set forth the purposes of each corporation's existence and the powers that the corporation is authorized to exercise to carry out its purposes.

Implied Corporate Authority

Implied corporate authority is the authority to perform any and all acts necessary to exercise a corporation's expressly conferred authority and to accomplish the purposes for which it was created. Generally, implied corporate authority arises where there is a need for corporate powers not specifically granted in the articles of incorporation. A governing body, at its own discretion, may enact new bylaws, rules, and regulations; purchase or mortgage property; borrow money; purchase equipment; select personnel; adopt corporate resolutions that delineate decision-making responsibilities; and so forth. These powers can be enumerated in the articles of incorporation and, in such cases, would be categorized as express rather than implied corporate authority.

Ultra Vires Acts

A governing body can be held liable for acting beyond its scope of authority, which is either expressed (e.g., in its articles of incorporation) or implied in law. Acts of this nature are referred to as *ultra vires acts.* The state, through its attorney general, has the power to prevent the performance of an ultra vires act by injunction. Governing bodies should have their corporate charters reviewed periodically by legal counsel to make certain that their express powers are consistent with the activities in which they presently engage or plan to undertake in the future.

DOCTRINE OF RESPONDEAT SUPERIOR

Respondeat superior is a legal doctrine holding employers liable for the wrongful acts of their agents (employees). This doctrine is also referred to as *vicarious liability,* whereby an employer is answerable for the torts committed by employees. The following elements must exist in order for liability to be imputed to an employer: (1) a master–servant relationship must exist between the employer and the employee, and (2) the wrongful act of the employee must have occurred within the scope of the employee's employment.

The question of liability frequently rests on whether persons treating a patient are independent agents (responsible for their own acts) or employees of the organization. The answer to this depends on whether the organization can exercise control over the particular act that was the proximate cause of the injury. The basic rationale for imposing liability on an employer developed because the employer possesses the right to control the physical acts of its employees.

The employer is not without remedy if liability has been imposed against it for an employee's negligent act. Because the law holds negligent persons responsible for their negligent acts, employees are not absolved from liability when a health care facility is held liable through the application of *respondeat superior.* Not only may the injured party sue the employee directly, but also the employer, if sued, may seek indemnification (i.e., compensation for the financial loss caused by the employee's negligent act) from the employee.

Independent Contractor

An independent contractor relationship is established when the principal has no right of control over the manner in which the agent's work is to be performed. The independent contractor therefore is responsible for his or her own negligent acts. However, some cases indicate that an organization may be held liable for an independent contractor's negligence. For example, in *Mehlman v. Powell*[1] the court held that a hospital may be found vicariously liable for the negligence of an emergency department physician who was not a hospital employee but who worked in the emergency department in the capacity of an independent contractor. The court reasoned that the hospital had control over billing procedures, maintained an emergency department in the main hospital, and represented to the patient that the members of the emergency department staff were its employees.

CORPORATE NEGLIGENCE

There are duties that the corporation itself owes to the general public and to its patients. These duties arise from statutes, regulations, principles of law developed by the courts, and the internal operating rules of the organization. If a corporation has a duty and fails in the exercise of that duty, it has the same liability to the injured party as an individual would have.

> Corporate negligence is a doctrine under which the hospital is liable if it fails to uphold the proper standard of care owed the patient, which is to ensure the patient's safety and well-being while at the hospital. This theory of liability creates a nondelegable duty which the hospital owes directly to a patient. Therefore, an injured party does not have to rely on and establish the negligence of a third party.[2]

Corporate negligence occurs when a health care corporation fails to perform those duties it owes directly to a patient or to anyone else to whom a duty may extend. If such a duty is breached and a patient is injured as a result of that breach, the organization can be held culpable under the theory of corporate negligence.

Evolution of Corporate Negligence

Hospitals once enjoyed complete tort immunity as charitable institutions. As hospitals evolved into more sophisticated corporate entities that expected fees for their services, their tort immunity receded. Courts first recognized that hospitals could be held liable for the negligence of their employees under the theory of *respondeat superior*. Liability later extended for nonemployees who acted as a hospital's ostensible agents. In *Thompson v. Nason Hospital*,[3] a Pennsylvania court recognized that hospitals are more than mere conduits through which health care professionals are brought into contact with patients. Hospitals owe some nondelegable duties directly to their patients independent of the negligence of their employees, such as duties to use reasonable care in the maintenance of safe and adequate facilities and equipment; select and retain only competent physicians; oversee all persons who practice medicine within their walls as to patient care; and, formulate, adopt, and enforce adequate rules and policies to ensure quality care for their patients.

Darling: *Health Care's Benchmark Case*

The benchmark case in the health care field, which has had a major impact on the liability of health care organizations, was decided in 1965 in *Darling v. Charleston Community Memorial Hospital.*[4] The court here enunciated a "corporate negligence doctrine" under which hospitals have a duty to provide adequately trained medical and nursing staff. A hospital is responsible, in conjunction with its medical staff, for establishing policies and procedures for monitoring the quality of medicine practiced within the hospital.

The *Darling* case involved an 18-year-old college football player who was preparing for a career as a teacher and coach. The patient, a defensive halfback for his college football team, was injured during a play. He was rushed to the emergency department of a small, accredited community hospital where the only physician on emergency duty that day was Dr. Alexander, a general practitioner. Alexander had not treated a major leg fracture for three years.

The physician examined the patient and ordered an X-ray that revealed that the tibia and the fibula of the right leg had been fractured. The physician reduced the fracture and applied a plaster cast from a point three or four inches below the groin to the toes. Shortly after the cast had been applied, the patient began to complain continually of pain. The physician split the cast and continued to visit the patient frequently while the patient remained in the hospital. Not thinking it was necessary, the emergency department physician did not call in any specialist for consultation.

After two weeks, the student was transferred to a larger hospital and placed under the care of an orthopaedic surgeon. The specialist found a considerable amount of dead tissue in the fractured leg. During a period of two months, the specialist removed increasing amounts of tissue in a futile attempt to save the leg until it became necessary to amputate the leg eight inches below the knee. The student's father did not agree to a settlement and filed suit against the emergency department physician and the hospital. Although the physician later settled out of court for $40,000, the case continued against the hospital.

The documentary evidence relied on to establish the standard of care included the rules and regulations of the Illinois Department of Public Health under the Hospital Licensing Act; the standards for hospital accreditation, today known as the Joint Commission on Accreditation of Healthcare

Organizations; and the bylaws, rules, and regulations of Charleston Hospital. These documents were admitted into evidence without objection. No specific evidence was offered that the hospital had failed to conform to the usual and customary practices of hospitals in the community.

The trial court instructed the jury to consider those documents, along with all other evidence, in determining the hospital's liability. Under the circumstances in which the case reached the Illinois Supreme Court, it was held that the verdict against the hospital should be sustained if the evidence supported the verdict on any one or more of the 20 allegations of negligence. Allegations asserted that the hospital was negligent in its failure to: (1) provide a sufficient number of trained nurses for bedside care of all patients at all times—in this case, nurses who were capable of recognizing the progressive gangrenous condition of the plaintiff's right leg, and (2) failure of its nurses to bring the patient's condition to the attention of the hospital administration and staff so that adequate consultation could be secured and the condition rectified.

Although these generalities provided the jury with no practical guidance for determining what constitutes reasonable care, they were considered relevant to helping the jury decide what was feasible and what the hospital knew or should have known concerning hospital responsibilities for the proper care of a patient. There was no expert testimony characterizing when the professional care rendered by the attending physician should have been reviewed, who should have reviewed it, or whether the case required consultation.

Evidence relating to the hospital's failure to review Alexander's work, to require consultation or examination by specialists, and to require proper nursing care was found to be sufficient to support a verdict for the patient. Judgment was eventually returned against the hospital in the amount of $100,000.

The Illinois Supreme Court held that the hospital could not limit its liability as a charitable corporation to the amount of its liability insurance.

> [T]he doctrine of charitable immunity can no longer stand . . . a doctrine which limits the liability of charitable corporations to the amount of liability insurance that they see fit to carry permits them to determine whether or not they will be liable for their torts and the amount of that liability, if any.[5]

In effect, the hospital was liable as a corporate entity for the negligent acts of its employees and physicians. Among other things, the *Darling* case indicates the importance of instituting effective credentialing and continuing medical evaluation and review programs for all members of a professional staff.

CORPORATE DUTIES AND RESPONSIBILITIES

Along with the corporate authority that is granted to the governing body, duties are attached to its individual members. These responsibilities are considered duties because they are imposed by law and can be enforced in legal proceedings. Governing body members are considered by law to have the highest measure of accountability. They have a fiduciary duty that requires acting primarily for the benefit of the corporation. The general duties of a governing body are both implied and express. Failure of a governing body to perform its duties may constitute mismanagement of such a degree that the appointment of a receiver to manage the affairs of the corporation may be warranted.

The duty to supervise and manage is applicable to the trustees as it is to the managers of any other business corporation. In both instances, there is a duty to act as a reasonably prudent person would act under similar circumstances. The governing body must act prudently in administering the affairs of the organization and exercise its powers in good faith.

Appointment of the CEO

Members of the governing body are responsible for appointing a chief executive officer (CEO) to act as their agent in the management of the organization. The CEO is responsible for the day-to-day operations of the organization. The individual selected as CEO must possess the competence and the character necessary to maintain satisfactory standards of patient care within the organization.

The responsibilities and authority of the CEO should be expressed in an appropriate job description, as well as in any formal agreement or contract that the organization has with the CEO. Some state health codes describe the responsibilities of administrators in broad terms. They generally provide that the CEO/administrator shall be responsible for the overall management of the organization.

The general duty of a governing body is to exercise due care and diligence in supervising and managing the organization. This duty does not cease with the selection of a CEO. A governing body can be liable if the level of patient care becomes inadequate because of the governing body's failure to supervise properly the management of the organization. CEOs, as is the case with board members, can be personally liable for their own acts of negligence that injure others.

CEO Code of Ethics

The following is the Code of Ethics of the American College of Healthcare Executives (ACHE).

American College of Healthcare Executives Code of Ethics

Preamble

The purpose of the *Code of Ethics* of the American College of Healthcare Executives is to serve as a standard of conduct for affiliates. It contains standards of ethical behavior for healthcare executives in their professional relationships. These relationships include colleagues, patients, or others served;

members of the healthcare executive's organization and other organizations, the community, and society as a whole.

The *Code of Ethics* also incorporates standards of ethical behavior governing personal behavior, particularly when that conduct directly relates to the role and identity of the healthcare executive.

The fundamental objectives of the healthcare management profession are to maintain or enhance the overall quality of life, dignity, and well-being of every individual needing healthcare service; and to create a more equitable, accessible, effective, and efficient healthcare system.

Healthcare executives have an obligation to act in ways that will merit the trust, confidence, and respect of healthcare professionals and the general public. Therefore, healthcare executives should lead lives that embody an exemplary system of values and ethics.

In fulfilling their commitments and obligations to patients or others served, healthcare executives function as moral advocates and models. Since every management decision affects the health and well-being of both individuals and communities, healthcare executives must carefully evaluate the possible outcomes of their decisions. In organizations that deliver healthcare services, they must work to safeguard and foster the rights, interests, and prerogatives of patients or others served.

The role of moral advocate requires that healthcare executives take actions necessary to promote such rights, interests, and prerogatives.

Being a model means that decisions and actions will reflect personal integrity and ethical leadership that others will seek to emulate.

I. The Healthcare Executive's Responsibilities to the Profession of Healthcare Management

The healthcare executive shall:

A. Uphold the *Code of Ethics* and mission of the American College of Healthcare Executives;

B. Conduct all personal and professional activities with honesty, integrity, respect, fairness, and good faith in a manner that will reflect well upon the profession;

C. Comply with all laws and regulations pertaining to healthcare management in the jurisdictions in which the healthcare executive is located or conducts professional activities;

D. Maintain competence and proficiency in healthcare management by implementing a personal program of assessment and continuing professional education;

E. Avoid the exploitation of professional relationships for personal gain;

F. Avoid financial and other conflicts of interest;

G. Use this *Code* to further the interests of the profession and not for selfish reasons;

H. Respect professional confidences;

I. Enhance the dignity and image of the healthcare management profession through positive public information programs; and

J. Refrain from participating in any activity that demeans the credibility and dignity of the healthcare management profession.

II. The Healthcare Executive's Responsibilities to Patients or Others Served

The healthcare executive shall, within the scope of his or her authority:

A. Work to ensure the existence of a process to evaluate the quality of care or service rendered;

B. Avoid practicing or facilitating discrimination and institute safeguards to prevent discriminatory organizational practices;

C. Work to ensure the existence of a process that will advise patients or others served of the rights, opportunities, responsibilities, and risks regarding available healthcare services;

D. Work to ensure that there is a process in place to facilitate the resolution of conflicts that may arise when values of patients and their families differ from those of employees and physicians;

E. Demonstrate zero tolerance for any abuse of power that compromises patients or others served;

F. Work to provide a process that ensures the autonomy and self-determination of patients or others served; and

G. Work to ensure the existence of procedures that will safeguard the confidentiality and privacy of patients or others served.

III. The Healthcare Executive's Responsibilities to the Organization

The healthcare executive shall, within the scope of his or her authority:

A. Provide healthcare services consistent with available resources, and when there are limited resources, work to ensure the existence of a resource allocation process that considers ethical ramifications;

B. Conduct both competitive and cooperative activities in ways that improve community healthcare services;

C. Lead the organization in the use and improvement of standards of management and sound business practices;

D. Respect the customs and practices of patients or others served, consistent with the organization's philosophy;

E. Be truthful in all forms of professional and organizational communication, and avoid disseminating information that is false, misleading, or deceptive;

F. Report negative financial and other information promptly and accurately, and initiate appropriate action;

G. Prevent fraud and abuse and aggressive accounting practices that may result in disputable financial reports;

H. Create an organizational environment in which both clinical and management mistakes are minimized and, when they do occur, are disclosed and addressed effectively;

I. Implement an organizational code of ethics and monitor compliance; and

J. Provide ethics resources to staff to address organizational and clinical issues.

IV. **The Healthcare Executive's Responsibilities to Employees**
Healthcare executives have ethical and professional obligations to the employees they manage that encompass but are not limited to:

A. Creating a work environment that promotes ethical conduct by employees;

B. Ensuring that individuals may freely express ethical concerns and providing mechanisms for discussing and addressing such concerns;

C. Ensuring a work environment that is free from harassment, sexual and other; coercion of any kind, especially to perform illegal or unethical acts; and discrimination on the basis of race, ethnicity, creed, gender, sexual orientation, age, or disability;

D. Providing a work environment that promotes the proper use of employees' knowledge and skills;

E. Ensuring a safe work environment; and

F. Establishing appropriate grievance and appeals mechanisms.

V. **The Healthcare Executive's Responsibilities to Community and Society**
The healthcare executive shall:

A. Work to identify and meet the healthcare needs of the community;

B. Work to support access to healthcare services for all people;

C. Encourage and participate in public dialogue on healthcare policy issues, and advocate solutions that will improve health status and promote quality healthcare;

D. Apply short- and long-term assessments to management decisions affecting both community and society; and

E. Provide prospective patients and others with adequate and accurate information, enabling them to make enlightened decisions regarding services.

VI. **The Healthcare Executive's Responsibility to Report Violations of the Code**
An affiliate of ACHE who has reasonable grounds to believe that another affiliate has violated this *Code* has a duty to communicate such facts to the Ethics Committee.

Medical Staff Appointments

Staff privileges are both professionally and economically important to health care professionals in the practice of their chosen professions. Health care organizations must be selective in granting staff privileges to maintain quality standards.

The governing board of a hospital must therefore be given great latitude in prescribing the necessary qualifications for potential applicants. Because no court should substitute its evaluation of professional competency for that of a hospital board, a court's review should be limited to ensuring that the qualifications imposed by a board are reasonably related to the operation of the hospital and fairly administered.

Allocation of Scarce Resources

Failure of organizations to adequately staff patient care units, and provide adequate supplies and equipment for patients are questions that should be addressed by an organization's governing body and not the legal system. Although the courts do not overlook the importance of maintaining adequate levels of patient care, it is not the job of the courts to referee disagreements. For example, a disagreement between the governing body and the local community as to how to allocate limited resources is not a question for the courts to settle. Questions of this sort often involve ethical principles and values. How to spend limited resources that provide good for the many is a value judgment, not a legal decision. Hospitals are in the business of serving patients with many kinds of illnesses and disabilities. Recognizing that the medical community is best equipped to conduct the balancing that medical resource allocations inevitably require, Congress has declined to give courts a mandate to arbitrate allocation disputes.[6]

Compliance with Rules and Regulations

The governing body in general and its agents are responsible for compliance with federal, state, and local rules and regulations regarding the operation of the organization. Depending on the scope of the wrong committed and the intent of the governing body, failure to comply could subject board members and/or their agents to civil liability and, in some instances, to criminal prosecution.

Compliance with Joint Commission Standards

The governing body, if accredited by the Joint Commission on Accreditation of Healthcare Organizations (Joint Commission), is responsible for compliance with applicable standards promulgated by the Joint Commission. Noncompliance could cause an organization to lose accreditation, which in turn would provide grounds for third-party reimbursement agencies (e.g., Medicare) to deny payment for treatment rendered to patients.

Provision of Timely Treatment

Health care organizations can be held liable for delays in treatment that result in injuries to their patients. For example, the patient in *Heddinger v.*

Ashford Memorial Community Hospital[7] filed a malpractice action against a hospital and its insurer, alleging that a delay in treating her left hand resulted in the loss of her little finger. Medical testimony presented at trial indicated that if proper and timely treatment had been rendered, the finger would have been saved. The U.S. District Court entered judgment on a jury verdict for the plaintiff in the amount of $175,000. The hospital appealed, and the U.S. Court of Appeals held that even if the physicians who attended the patient were not employees of the hospital but were independent contractors, the risk of negligent treatment was clearly foreseeable by the hospital.

Professional's Incompetence

An organization owes its patients a duty of care, and this duty includes the obligation to protect them from negligent and fraudulent acts of those health care professionals it knew or should have known had a propensity to commit negligent acts. The courts will not permit organizations to hide behind a cloak of ignorance in this responsibility.

Conflict of Interest

The potential for conflict of interest exists for decision makers at all levels within an organization. Disclosure of potential conflicts of interest should be made so that appropriate action may be taken to ensure that such conflict does not inappropriately influence important organization and health care decisions. Board members, physicians, and employees are required by most organizations to submit a disclosure form that discloses potential conflicts related to decisions that may arise.

CASE: CORPORATE COVER-UP

On July 19, 1998, Mrs. Sauer, in *Advocat, Inc. v. Sauer*,[8] was a 93-year-old nursing facility patient. Her vital signs began to decline, and the nursing staff reported the developments to her treating physician, who ordered that she be taken to the emergency department at Mena. She arrived at the hospital in a semi-comatose condition and died about 16 hours later.

Nursing notes indicated that Sauer had lost 15 pounds in the last month and was in need of a feeding tube. There were signs of bedsores on her body, stemming from lying in urine and excrement. Sauer's estate sued for damages.

The trial began and lasted eight days, with 28 witnesses testifying and 24 binders of exhibits. At the trial's conclusion, the jury retired to consider four counts: ordinary negligence, medical malpractice, breach of contract, and wrongful death. The jury returned a verdict for the Sauer Estate on all counts. Total damages amounted to more than 78 million dollars. On appeal, the appellants argued that the damage awards for negligence and medical malpractice were grossly excessive.

The appellants argued that long-term care surveys conducted at the facility had been admitted into evidence over their objection. The appellants claimed that the survey results inflamed the jury, because the surveys were replete with statements that there was not enough help in the nursing home to feed, bathe, or clean residents.

Testimony submitted by witnesses that the nursing home had engaged in "false-charting" to show more staff than were actually present was prejudicial, because it suggested the appellants had staffing inadequacies that they tried to conceal from the State.

Sauer died from severe malnutrition and dehydration. There was evidence presented that she was found at times with dried feces under her fingernails from scratching herself while lying in her own excrement. At other times, staff did not get her out of her bed as they should have. Often, Sauer's food tray was found in her room, untouched, because there was no staff member at the nursing home available to feed her. She was not provided with range-of-motion assistance when the facility was short of staff.

Sauer had pressure sores on her back, lower buttock, and arms. A former staff member remembered seeing Sauer at one time with a pressure sore the size of a softball, which was open. At times, she had no water pitcher in her room, nor did she receive a bath for a week or more because of shortage of staff. Sauer was found to suffer from poor oral hygiene, having caked food and debris in her mouth.

The appellate court found that the jury verdicts were not based on passion or prejudice. There was ample testimony and evidence to demonstrate that plaintiff's decedent suffered considerably and was not properly cared for in the nursing home, that the home was short-staffed, and that the home tried to cover this up by "false-charting" and by bringing in additional employees on state inspection days. All of that serves to support the estate's case that the nursing home knew it had staffing problems and committed negligence as to decedent, because it was short-staffed due to cutbacks.

The appellate court found that the circuit court abused its discretion by not granting a new trial due to excessive damages.

Ethical and Legal Issues

1. Describe the ethical and legal issues presented this case.
2. According to a federal study, nearly 90 percent of the nation's nursing homes are poorly staffed and find it difficult to provide basic services, such as cleaning, dressing, grooming, and feeding their residents.[9] Assuming the accuracy of this number, discuss how you would distribute limited dollars to address this issue. Consider how your decision may affect the allocation of funds to other health-related programs (e.g., immunizations, prenatal care, and preventative medicine). Assume that no new dollars can be allocated for the new health care budget year. ■

Provision of a Safe Environment

It is essential that employers provide a safe environment for both patients and employees. Although one cannot guard against the unforeseeable, a health care organization is liable for injuries resulting from dangers that it knowingly failed to guard against or those that it should have known about and failed to guard against. An organization has a duty to safeguard the welfare of its patients, even from harm by third persons, and that duty is measured by the ability of the patient to provide for his or her own safety.

Fault for Patient's Accident

The patient, in *Thomas v. Sisters of Charity of the Incarnate Word*,[10] fell three stories to his death after he became locked out on the hospital roof and sat on a ledge in an apparent attempt to attract someone to get assistance. The trial court found that the fire exit configuration that allowed the patient access to the roof created an unreasonable risk of harm that was the cause-in-fact of his death.

There was testimony that the lack of signage violated both the Life Safety and 1988 Standard Building Codes. Standard Building Code required that signs direct an individual to the exit discharge or ultimate exit to the outside of the building. Lack of signage also violated hospital policy requiring that the roof should have been marked as a restricted area. The exit configuration was unsafe for either ordinary or emergency use because of the confusion encountered by an individual locked out of the building without any direction or instruction on where to go.

Given the hospital's duty regarding this exit, its breach of that duty was clear. The door to the roof contained no warning that it would lock the patient out of the building if he exited. Whether the patient exited the building voluntarily or out of momentary confusion, the hospital breached its duty to warn him that he would be locked out and to direct him across the catwalk to the fire exit stairwell.

CASE: SEXUAL ASSAULT IN THE RECOVERY ROOM

The plaintiff, a young woman, was recovering from vaginal surgery. She was sexually assaulted by a surgical resident employed by the hospital. There is no dispute about the assault or the resident's liability. The question here is whether the hospital may be liable under a theory of vicarious liability or for negligence in its duty to protect the plaintiff.

The plaintiff, under the effects of anesthesia following surgery, was placed in a small four-bed, 14 × 18-foot recovery room. Nurse R, accompanied by another nurse, admitted the plaintiff to the unit and monitored her vital signs. Minutes later, the nurses turned their attention to a second patient who had been placed on an adjacent bed two feet away. They were soon joined by Nurse G, their supervisor. Privacy curtains between the plaintiff and the second patient had not been drawn.

A surgical resident wearing hospital scrubs and an identification badge entered the recovery room and went to the plaintiff's bed. He was not one of the physicians listed on the plaintiff's chart and none of the nurses knew him. According to the plaintiff, she awoke to find the resident pulling up her hospital gown and performing an "internal pelvic exam," which was contraindicated in light of the nature of the plaintiff's surgery. The plaintiff tried to sit up and cover herself with the gown, and repeatedly asked him to stop. Upon her third plea, the physician hastily began to leave the recovery room. After the plaintiff complained to the nurses about what had taken place, the supervising nurse confronted the resident, who admitted he had examined the plaintiff without the presence of a female witness as required by hospital rules. Following an investigation, the hospital terminated the resident.

The Appellate Division Majority reasoned that a direct negligence claim must fail because the resident's misconduct was not foreseeable. The court also dismissed the vicarious liability claim against the hospital because the physician was acting outside the scope of his authority.

Two dissenting judges disagreed with the majority. They noted that the majority's holding on the direct negligence cause of action failed to consider the actual foreseeability of harm, indicated by observations the hospital staff could or should have made at the time immediately preceding the actual wrongdoing.

Nurse R had acknowledged that residents were not directly assigned to the recovery room. Her deposition testimony further indicated that she was aware of the identity of all of plaintiff's physicians and that the resident was not one of those assigned to plaintiff's care. In fact, all of the nurses in the recovery room were unacquainted with the resident. All of the nurses knew of the hospital's policy requiring the presence of a female staff member during a male physician's pelvic examination of a female patient.

Despite the nurses' assertions that they saw or heard nothing, an additional key question of credibility arises from the inference created by the undisputed close proximity of all of the nurses to the plaintiff's bed.

Contrary to the Appellate Division majority opinion, the dissenting judges considered that this confluence of factors provided a sufficient basis from which a jury could determine that the nurses unreasonably disregarded that which was readily there to be seen and heard, alerting them to the risk of misconduct against the plaintiff by the resident, which could have been prevented.

Accordingly, the Appellate Division order was modified by remitting the case to the Supreme Court (trial court in New York) for further proceedings.[11]

Ethical and Legal Issues

1. Describe the ethical and legal issues presented in this case.
2. Describe how the physician's professional code of ethics was breached. ▪

Health Care Fraud

Health care fraud is committed when a dishonest provider or consumer intentionally submits, or causes someone else to submit, false or misleading information for use in determining the amount of health care benefits payable. Some examples of provider health care fraud include:

- billing for services not performed;
- falsifying a patient's diagnosis to justify tests, surgeries, or other procedures that aren't medically necessary;
- misrepresenting procedures performed to obtain payment for noncovered services, such as cosmetic surgery;
- upcoding—billing for a more costly service than the one actually performed;
- unbundling—billing each stage of a procedure as if it were a separate procedure;
- accepting kickbacks for patient referrals; and
- waiving patient co-pays or deductibles and overbilling the insurance carrier or benefit plan.

Examples of consumer health care fraud are:

- filing claims for services or medications not received;
- forging or altering bills or receipts; and
- using someone else's coverage or insurance card.[12]

Preventing Fraud

The federal government's initiative to investigate and prosecute health care organizations for criminal wrongdoing has resulted in the establishment of corporate compliance programs for preventing, detecting, and reporting criminal conduct. An effective corporate compliance program involves:

1. developing appropriate policies and procedures;
2. appointing a compliance officer to oversee the compliance program;
3. communicating the organization's compliance program to employees;
4. providing for monitoring and auditing systems that are designed to detect criminal conduct by employees and other agents;
5. publicizing a reporting system whereby employees and other agents can report criminal conduct by others within the organization without fear of retribution;
6. taking appropriate steps to respond to criminal conduct and to prevent similar offenses;
7. periodically review and update the organization's corporate compliance program; and
8. work with state and federal law enforcement and regulatory agencies and insurance companies to detect, prevent, and prosecute health care fraud.

Healthy Dose of Fraud

Patients were allegedly brought to California where they were paid to undergo surgeries that they did not need.

> In the scam, agents say, recruiters bring "patients from across the nation to surgery centers in California where they give phony or exaggerated symptoms and doctors perform unnecessary operations on them. Then the surgery centers send inflated claims for the unnecessary procedures to the patients' insurance companies. When the insurers pay up, federal authorities say, the recruiters, the surgery centers and the patients split the proceeds.[13]

It is no wonder that the public, bombarded with such fraudulent activities, has little if any trust in the corporate world. Corporate fraud has become so rampant that the level of trust in and reputation of organizational leadership has reached an all-time low.

Organizational Culture of Safety

Organizations are expected to maintain a culture that supports patient safety and an environment that fosters respect and trust, integrity and honesty, compassionate care, privacy, confidentiality, communications between the patient and caregivers, and education.

Patient Concerns and Complaints

Organizations need to adopt policies and procedures that address patient complaints. Most organizations have a patient advocate to address patient concerns. The procedures to be followed generally are spelled out in a patient handbook. Often a telephone extension is provided to assist the patient when registering a complaint.

Management Decisions Collide with Professional Ethics

Management's financial decisions can at times be on a collision course with practice and professional codes of ethics. The principles of autonomy, beneficence, and justice, and the ability to practice what is right according to such principles, often collide when organizations have to, for example, ration scarce resources. Such rationing may require managers to cut costs at the expense of quality.

Failure to Disclose Financial Incentives

The patient, in *Shea v. Esensten*,[14] died after suffering a heart attack. Although the patient had recently visited his primary care physician and presented symptoms of cardiac problems, including a family history of cardiac trouble, the physician did not refer the patient to a cardiologist. The patient's widow sued the health management organization for failing to disclose the financial incentive system it provided to its physicians to minimize referrals to specialists. The United States Court of Appeals for the Eighth Circuit agreed that knowledge of financial incentives that affect a physician's decisions to refer patients to specialists is material information requiring disclosure, and it reversed a lower court's dismissal of the claim.

A Life Needlessly Shortened

An action filed against a health insurance company alleged that the way the insurer handled the insured's chemotherapy needlessly shortened her life, causing her last days to be more painful than they should have been. The jury awarded the plaintiff $49 million. The punitive damages award was considered excessive under Ohio law, and the trial court's failure to find as such was so unreasonable as to constitute abuse of discretion. A $30 million award was appropriate as to profits of the corporations involved and appropriate in the scheme of past punitive damages awards in Ohio.[15]

BUILDING AND RESTORING TRUST

The lack of trust is slowly demoralizing the people's faith in the nation's health care system. Lack of trust in the physician, hospital, and insurer is pervasive throughout the health care system. The horror stories in newspapers—malpractice suits, the Institute of Medicine's report on health care mistakes, among others—not only identify problems but provide a catalyst for encouraging lawsuits.

Organizations need to make a concerted effort to develop strategies to build and restore trust in the health care industry. Implementation of the following strategies would be an important step in building that trust:

- Conduct business in compliance with applicable laws, rules, and regulations.
- Adhere to the highest of ethical standards.
- Provide cost-effective care.
- Fairly and accurately represent the organization's capabilities when treating a patient's ailments.
- Maintain a uniform standard of care throughout the organization, regardless of a person's ability to pay, race, creed, color, and/or national origin.
- Consider patient values and preferences as part of recognizing the organization's legal responsibilities.
- Inform patients of their responsibilities.
- Develop and recommend guidelines that assist and support patients and their families in exercising their rights.
- Describe the process to patients by which hospital staff interact and care for them.

SUMMARY CASE

Anytown Hospital has an outstanding reputation for surgical services. Bob Right, the CEO, was told by the operating room supervisor and a surgical nurse, both considered credible employees, that Dr. Flipton, an anesthesiologist, has been abusing the use of anesthesia gases in the hospital's dental suite. He was reportedly seen by operating staff testing "laughing gas" by holding a mask against his face for short periods of time. This scene would be followed by a string of silly, seemingly meaningless jokes. Right has repeatedly discussed this matter with the medical executive committee. The medical executive committee refuses to take any action without definitive action by the department chair. Right suspects that if he pursues the matter further with the governing board, he could very well end up without a job. The governing body is generally unable to resolve disciplinary actions against a physician without support of the medical executive committee.

What do you believe the ethical issues are for Right? For Right, doing the right thing and survival are competing concerns. Which of the following would you do if you were in Right's position, with two children in college and hefty mortgage payments?

a. voluntarily leave my job
b. aggressively pursue the problem
c. secretly enlist the aid of the medical staff
d. confront Dr. Flipton
e. other option (explain) ■

CHAPTER REVIEW

1. This chapter introduces the reader to the ethical responsibilities and legal risks to which health care organizations and their governing bodies are exposed.

2. An organization's code of ethics provides guidelines for behavior that help carry out an organization's mission, vision, and values. Organizational codes of ethics build trust, increase awareness of ethical issues, guide decision making, and encourage staff to seek advice and report misconduct.

3. Organizational ethics in the health care setting are being carefully scrutinized across the nation by state and federal regulatory agencies. Unethical conduct that is closely being monitored includes, for example, false advertisements and fraudulent reimbursement schemes.

4. It is unethical for health care organizations to advertise misleading information in an effort to encourage public confidence in the quality of care that they provide.

5. Organizations are expected to maintain a culture that supports patient safety and an environment that fosters respect and trust,

integrity and honesty, compassionate care, privacy, confidentiality, communications between the patient and caregivers, and education.

6. The typical health care organization is incorporated under state law as either a freestanding for-profit or not-for-profit corporation. The corporation has a governing body that has ultimate responsibility for the decisions made in the organization.

7. Generally, the authority of a corporation is expressed in the law under which the corporation is chartered and in the corporation's articles of incorporation. Members of the governing body have both express and implied corporate authority.

8. Respondeat superior is a legal doctrine holding employers liable, in certain cases, for the wrongful acts of their agents (employees). This doctrine also has been referred to as vicarious liability, whereby an employer is answerable for the torts committed by employees.

9. Corporate negligence occurs when a health care corporation fails to perform those duties it owes directly to a patient or to anyone else to whom a duty may extend. If such a duty is breached and a patient is injured as a result of that breach, the organization can be held culpable under the theory of corporate negligence.

10. The benchmark case in the health care field, which has had a major impact on the liability of health care organizations, was decided in *Darling v. Charleston Community Memorial Hospital*.[16] The court here enunciated a "corporate negligence doctrine" under which hospitals have a duty to provide adequately trained medical and nursing staff.

11. Organizational ethics are often on a collision course with practice and professional codes of ethics. The principles of autonomy, beneficence, and justice, and the ability to practice what is right according to such principles, often collide when organizations have to, for example, ration scarce resources.

TEST YOUR UNDERSTANDING

Terminology

corporate authority
corporate negligence
respondeat superior
Darling v. Charleston Community Memorial Hospital

REVIEW QUESTIONS

1. Discuss what value statements should be included in an organization's code of ethics.

> **REVIEW QUESTIONS (continued)**
>
> 2. Discuss the importance of the *Darling* case as it relates to corporate negligence.
>
> 3. Describe how a corporate compliance program can help prevent health care fraud.
>
> 4. Describe the strategies an organization can implement to improve consumer trust.

WEB SITES

American College of Healthcare Executives
 www.ache.org/
American Medical Association Physician Select
 www.ama-assn.org/aps/amahg.htm
Best Hospitals
 www.besthospitals.com
Top Hospitals
 www.usnews.com/usnews/nycu/health/hosptl/tophosp.htm
Healthgrades.com
 www.healthgrades.com
Hospital Web
 neuro-www2.mgh.harvard.edu/hospitalwebusa.html

NOTES

1. 46 U.S.I.W.2227 (Md. 1977).
2. Thompson v. Nason Hosp., 591 A.2d 703, 707 (Pa. 1991).
3. *Id*.
4. 211 N.E.2d 253 (Ill. 1965).
5. *Id.* at 260.
6. Freilich v. Upper Chesapeake Health, Inc., 313 F.3d 205 (2002).
7. 734 F.2d 81 (1st Cir. 1984).
8. 111 S.W.3d 346 (2003).
9. Christopher Newton, *90% of Nursing Homes Providing Substandard Care–Federal Report*, Seattle Times, Feb. 20, 2002, at A1.
10. No. 38,170-CA (La. App. 2004) .
11. N.X. v. Cabrini Med. Ctr., 765 N.E.2d 844 (2002).
12. http://www.usdoj.gov/opa/pr/2003/June/03_civ_386.htm.
13. http://www.cigna.com/health/consumer/service/fraud.html.
14. ABC News, March 18, *A Healthy Dose of Fraud, Primetime Investigates a Gigantic Medical Insurance Scam*. http://www.attorneygeneral.gov/cld/articles/health.cfm.
15. 107 F.3d 625 & 8th Circuit (1997).
16. Dardinger, Exr. V. Anthem Blue Cross and Blue Shield, 2002 Ohio 7113 (Ohio 2002).

Section III

Health Care Professionals

chapter nine

Health Care Professionals' Ethical and Legal Issues

INTRODUCTION

This chapter presents an overview of how ethics and the law impact a variety of departments and health care professions. Health care professionals are governed by ethical codes, which demand a high level of integrity, honesty, and responsibility. Although this chapter reviews a sampling of ethical codes, health care professionals are encouraged to visit the pertinent Web sites that describe the various codes in more detail.

The Center for the Study of Ethics in the Professions at the Illinois Institute of Technology received a grant from the National Science Foundation to put a collection of over 850 codes of ethics on the World Wide Web. This Center's Web site includes links to the ethical codes of professional societies, corporations, government, and academic institutions (http://www.iit.edu/departments/csep/PublicWWW/codes/index.html).

Professional codes of ethics for the health care professionals have been developed to provide guidance to those faced with ethical dilemmas.

> Codes of ethics are created in response to actual or anticipated ethical conflicts. Considered in a vacuum, many codes of ethics would be difficult to comprehend or interpret. It is only in the context of real life and real ethical ambiguity that the codes take on any meaning.
>
> Codes of ethics and case studies need each other. Without guiding principles, case studies are difficult to evaluate and analyze; without context, codes of ethics are incomprehensible. The best way to use these codes is to apply them to a variety of situations and see what results. It is from the back and forth evaluation of the codes and the cases that thoughtful moral judgments can best arise.[1]

The contents of codes of ethics vary depending on the risks associated with a particular profession. For example, ethical codes for psychologists define relationships with clients in greater depth due to the personal one-to-one relationship they have with their clients. Lab technicians and technologists, on the other hand, generally have little or no personal contact with patients but can have a significant impact on their care. Lab technologists in their ethical code "pledge accuracy and reliability in the performance of tests."[2] The importance of this pledge was born out in a March 11, 2004 report by the *Baltimore Sun* whereby state health officials discovered that a hospital's laboratory personnel overrode controls in testing equipment showing results that might be in error and then mailed them to patients anyway.[3]

CHIROPRACTOR

A chiropractor is required to exercise the same degree of care, judgment, and skill exercised by other reasonable chiropractors under like or similar circumstances. He or she has a duty to determine whether a patient is treatable through chiropractic means and to refrain from chiropractic treatment when a reasonable chiropractor would or should be aware that a patient's condition will not respond to chiropractic treatment. Failure to conform to the standard of care can result in liability for any injuries suffered.

American Chiropractic Association

Code of Ethics

C. Responsibility to the Profession

C (1) Doctors of chiropractic should assist in maintaining the integrity, competency, and highest standards of the chiropractic profession.

C (2) Doctors of chiropractic should, by their behavior, avoid even the appearance of professional impropriety and should recognize that their public behavior may have an impact on the ability of the profession to serve the public. Doctors of chiropractic should promote public confidence in the chiropractic profession.

C (3) As teachers, doctors of chiropractic should recognize their obligation to help others acquire knowledge and skill in the practice of the profession. They should maintain high standards of scholarship, education, training, and objectivity in the accurate and full dissemination of information and ideas.

C (4) Doctors of chiropractic should attempt to promote and maintain cordial relationships with other members of the chiropractic profession and other professions in an effort to promote information advantageous to the public's health and well-being.[4]

CASE: POOR JUDGMENT

The chief medical officer of the Nebraska Department of Health and Human Services Regulation and Licensure entered an order revoking Poor's license to practice as a chiropractor in the State of Nebraska.[5]

Poor engaged in a conspiracy to manufacture and distribute a misbranded substance, and he introduced into interstate commerce misbranded and adulterated drugs with the intent to defraud and mislead. He was arrested for driving under the influence and was convicted of that offense. In addition, Poor did knowingly possess cocaine. He conceded that these factual determinations were understood as beyond dispute.

The district court's determination that Poor had engaged in "grossly immoral or dishonorable conduct" was not based on "trivial reasons." The appeals court found that Poor's conduct clearly fell within the plain and ordinary meaning of grossly immoral or dishonorable conduct. In its order finding Poor to be unfit, the district court relied in part on Poor's denial of conduct underlying a previous felony conviction. The court stated that Poor's denial now, after taking advantage of a plea bargain, that "he committed any of the acts he admitted to in the United States District Court is disturbing and is not consistent with the integrity and acceptance of responsibility expected by persons engaged in a professional occupation."

Chiropractic medicine is a regulated health care profession. Patients necessarily rely upon the chiropractor's honesty, integrity, sound professional judgment, and compliance with applicable governmental regulations. Poor argued that there was absolutely no testimony or evidence to the effect that anything he did constituted a threat of harm to his patients.

The Supreme Court of Nebraska determined that the seriousness of Poor's felony conviction and its underlying conduct, his subsequent lack of candor with respect to that conduct, as well as his lack of sound judgment demonstrated by his driving-under-the-influence conviction, concluded that revocation of Poor's license was an appropriate sanction.

Ethical and Legal Issues

1. Did the chiropractor violate his professional code of ethics? Explain your answer.
2. Describe ways in which your personal life can have an impact on your professional career. ■

DENTISTRY

The practice of dentistry first achieved the stature of a profession in the United States.[6] The Code of Professional Conduct for the American Dental Association is organized into five sections. Each section falls under the Principle of Ethics that predominantly applies to it. Advisory Opinions follow the section of the Code that they interpret. The following are excerpts from the code.

ADA Principles of Ethics and Professional Conduct

Section 1—Principle: Patient Autonomy ("self-governance")
The dentist has a duty to respect the patient's rights to self-determination and confidentiality.

Section 2—Principle: Nonmaleficence ("do not harm")
The dentist has a duty to refrain from harming the patient.

Section 3—Principle: Beneficence ("do good")
The dentist has a duty to promote the patient's welfare.

Section 4—Principle: Justice ("fairness")
The dentist has a duty to treat people fairly.

Section 5—Principle: Veracity ("truthfulness")
The dentist has a duty to communicate truthfully.[7]

CASE: PRACTICING OUTSIDE THE SCOPE OF PRACTICE

Practicing outside one's scope of practice involves both ethical and legal issues. For example, plaintiff Brown, in *Brown v, Belinfante*,[8] sued a dentist for performing several elective cosmetic procedures including a face-lift, eyelid revision, and facial laser resurfacing. The dentist was not a physician. He was licensed to practice dentistry in Georgia. Brown claims that after the cosmetic procedures, she could not close her eyes completely, developed chronic bilateral eye infections, and required remedial corrective surgery. Brown alleged that the dentist's performance of the cosmetic procedures constituted negligence because he exceeded the scope of the practice of dentistry.

The primary purposes of the Georgia Dental Act are to define and regulate the practice of dentistry. The statute limits the scope of the practice of dentistry. Such limitation protects the health and welfare of patients who submit themselves to the care of dentists by guarding against injuries caused by inadequate care or by unauthorized individuals. Brown falls within that class of persons the statute was intended to protect, and the harm complained of was of the type the statute was intended to guard against. In performing the elective cosmetic procedures, the dentist violated the Dental Practice Act by exceeding the statutory limits of the scope of dentistry.

Ethical and Legal Issues
1. Describe the legal issues presented here.
2. Does the professional code of ethics for dentists support the court's findings in this case? Explain your answer. ■

CASE: DENTIST'S INAPPROPRIATE SEXUAL CONDUCT

Revocation of a dentist's license on charges of professional misconduct was properly ordered in *Melone v. State Education Department*[9] on the basis of substantial evidence that while acting in a professional capacity, the dentist had engaged in physical and sexual contact with five different male patients within a three-year period. Considering the dentist's responsible position, the extended time period during which the sexual contacts occurred, the age and impressionable nature of the victims (7 to 15 years of age), and the possibility of lasting effects on the victims, the penalty was not shocking to the court's sense of fairness.

Ethical and Legal Issues
1. Describe the ethical and legal issues of this case.
2. Describe what procedures could be implemented in a dentist's office to help reduce the likelihood of sexual abuses. ■

DENTAL HYGIENIST

The following excerpts from the code of ethics of the American Dental Hygienists' Association describe *core values* for dental hygienists.

American Dental Hygienists' Association

Core Values

Individual autonomy and respect for human beings
People have the right to be treated with respect. They have the right to informed consent prior to treatment, and they have the right to full disclosure of all relevant information so that they can make informed choices about their care.

Confidentiality
We respect the confidentiality of client information and relationships as a demonstration of the value we place on individual autonomy. We acknowledge our obligation to justify any violation of a confidence.

Societal trust
We value client trust and understand that public trust in our profession is based on our actions and behavior.

Nonmaleficence
We accept our fundamental obligation to provide services in a manner that protects all clients and minimizes harm to them and others involved in their treatment.

Beneficence
We have a primary role in promoting the well-being of individuals and the public by engaging in health promotion/disease prevention activities.

Justice and fairness
We value justice and support the fair and equitable distribution of health care resources. We believe all people should have access to high-quality, affordable oral health care.

Veracity
We accept our obligation to tell the truth and assume that others will do the same. We value self-knowledge and seek truth and honesty in all relationships.[10]

CASE: DENTAL HYGIENIST'S UNLAWFUL ADMINISTRATION OF NITROUS OXIDE

This case[11] arises from a complaint by a dental hygienist against a former employer, Lowenberg and Lowenberg Corporation. The dental hygienist alleged that the defendant allowed dental hygienists to administer nitrous oxide to patients. Under state law, dental hygienists may not administer nitrous oxide. The Department of Education's Office of Professional Discipline investigated the complaint by using an undercover investigator. The investigator made an appointment for teeth cleaning. At the time of her appointment, she requested that nitrous oxide be administered. Agreeing to the investigator's request, the dental hygienist administered the nitrous oxide. There were no notations in the patient's chart indicating that she had been administered nitrous oxide.

A hearing panel found the dental hygienist guilty of administering nitrous oxide without being properly licensed. In addition, the hearing panel found that the dental hygienist had failed to accurately record in the patient's chart that she had administered nitrous oxide.

The New York Supreme Court, Appellate Division, held that the investigator's report provided sufficient evidence to support the hearing panel's determination. There is adequate evidence in the record to support a finding that the dentist's conduct was such that it could reasonably be said that he permitted the dental hygienist to perform acts that she was not licensed to perform.

Ethical and Legal Issues
1. Describe how the core values of a dental hygienist were violated in this case.
2. Describe how both ethical and legal issues are intertwined in this case. ■

DENTAL ASSISTANT

CASE: NEGLIGENT ACT

The plaintiff in *Hickman v. Sexton Dental Clinic*[12] brought a malpractice action against a dental clinic for a serious cut under her tongue. The dental assistant, without being supervised by a dentist, placed a sharp object into the patient's mouth, cutting her tongue while taking impressions for dentures. The court of common pleas entered a judgment on a jury verdict in favor of the plaintiff, and the clinic appealed. The court of appeals held that the evidence presented was sufficient to infer without the aid of expert testimony that there was a breach of duty to the patient. The testimony of Dr. Tepper, the clinic dentist, was found pertinent to the issue of the common knowledge exception in which the evidence permits the jury to recognize breach of duty without the aid of expert testimony. Tepper presented the following testimony regarding denture impressions:

Q. You also stated that you have taken, I believe, thousands?
A. Probably more than that.
Q. Of impressions?
A. Yes, sir.
Q. This never happened before?
A. No, sir, not a laceration.

Q. Would it be safe and accurate to say that if someone's mouth were to be cut during the impression process, someone did something wrong?
A. Yes, sir.[13]

Ethical and Legal Issues
1. Describe the legal issues of this case.
2. Do you see any ethical issues in this case? Explain your answer. ▪

DIETITIANS AND NUTRITIONAL CARE

American Dietetic Association

Code of Ethics

Principles
1. The dietetics practitioner conducts himself/herself with honesty, integrity, and fairness.
2. The dietetics practitioner practices dietetics based on scientific principles and current information.

•

•

•

4. The dietetics practitioner assumes responsibility and accountability for personal competence in practice. . . .
5. The dietetics practitioner recognizes and exercises professional judgment. . . .
6. The dietetics practitioner provides sufficient information to enable clients and others to make their own informed decisions.
7. The dietetics practitioner protects confidential information. . . .

•

•

•

9. The dietetics practitioner provides professional services in a manner that is sensitive to cultural differences and does not discriminate against others on the basis of race, ethnicity, creed, religion, disability, sex, age, sexual orientation, or national origin.

•

•

•

12. The dietetics practitioner is alert to situations that might cause a conflict of interest or have the appearance of a conflict. . . .

•

•

•

18. The dietetics practitioner complies with all applicable laws and regulations concerning the profession. . . .

19. The dietetics practitioner supports and promotes high standards of professional practice. . . .[14]

CASE: DIETITIANS FAILURE TO MEET DIETARY REQUIREMENTS

Health care organizations must provide each patient with a nourishing, palatable, well-balanced diet that meets the daily nutritional and special dietary needs of each patient. Failure to do so can lead to negligence suits. The daughter of the deceased in *Lambert v. Beverly Enterprises, Inc.*[15] filed an action claiming that her father had been mistreated. The notice of intent to sue indicated that the deceased suffered various injuries and malnutrition as a direct result of the acts or omissions of personnel, and that the plaintiff's father suffered actual damages that included substantial medical expenses and mental anguish due to the injuries he sustained. A motion to dismiss the case was denied.

Ethical and Legal Issues
1. Identify the ethical issues in this case.
2. How might the dietitian's professional ethical code have been violated in this case? ■

EMERGENCY DEPARTMENT

Although codes of ethics for physicians are expressed in various physicians' oaths, "emergency physicians assume more specific ethical obligations that arise out of the special features of emergency medical practice. The principles listed below express fundamental moral responsibilities of emergency physicians."[16]

American College of Emergency Physicians

Principles of Ethics

1. Embrace patient welfare as their primary professional responsibility.
2. Respond promptly and expertly, without prejudice or partiality, to the need for emergency medical care.
3. Respect the rights and strive to protect the best interests of their patients, particularly the most vulnerable and those unable to make treatment choices due to diminished decision-making capacity.
4. Communicate truthfully with patients and secure their informed consent for treatment, unless the urgency of the patient's condition demands an immediate response.
5. Respect patient privacy and disclose confidential information only with consent of the patient or when required by an overriding duty such as the duty to protect others or to obey the law.
6. Deal fairly and honestly with colleagues and take appropriate action to protect patients from health care providers who are impaired, incompetent, or who engage in fraud or deception.

7. Work cooperatively with others who care for, and about, emergency patients.

8. Engage in continuing study to maintain the knowledge and skills necessary to provide high-quality care for emergency patients.

9. Act as responsible stewards of the health care resources entrusted to them.

10. Support societal efforts to improve public health and safety, reduce the effects of injury and illness, and secure access to emergency and other basic health care for all.[17]

Federal and state statutes impose a duty on hospitals to provide emergency care. The statutes require hospitals to provide some degree of emergency service. If the public is aware that a hospital furnishes emergency services and relies on that knowledge, the hospital has a duty to provide those services to the public.

CASE: WHAT COMMON SENSE MADE EVIDENT

Hospitals are expected to notify specialty on-call physicians when their particular skills are required in the emergency department. An on-call physician who fails to respond to a request to attend a patient can be liable for injuries suffered by the patient because of his or her failure to respond. In *Thomas v. Corso*,[18] a Maryland court sustained a verdict against the hospital and physician. The patient had been brought to the hospital emergency department after he was struck by a car. A physician did not attend to him even though he had dangerously low blood pressure and was in shock. There was some telephone contact between the nurse in the emergency department and the physician who was providing on-call coverage. The physician did not act upon the hospital's call for assistance until the patient was close to death. The court reasoned that expert testimony was not even necessary to establish what common sense made evident: that a patient who had been struck by a car may have suffered internal injuries and should have been evaluated and treated by a physician. Lack of attention in such cases is not reasonable care by any standard. The concurrent negligence of the nurse, who failed to contact the on-call physician after the patient's condition had worsened, did not relieve the physician of liability for his failure to come to the emergency department at once. Rather, under the doctrine of respondeat superior, the nurse's negligence was a basis for holding the hospital liable as well.

Ethical and Legal Issues

1. Describe how both the physician and nurse failed in their ethical responsibilities to the patient.

2. Describe what actions the hospital can take to prevent future occurrences of this nature.

3. What are the legal concerns for the physician, nurse, and hospital? ▓

Failure to Respond

Treatment rendered by hospitals is expected to be commensurate with that available in the same or similar communities or in hospitals generally. In *Fjerstad v. Knutson*,[19] the South Dakota Supreme Court found that a hospital could be held liable for the failure of an on-call physician to respond to a call from the emergency department. An intern who attempted to contact the on-call physician and was unable to do so for 3½ hours treated and discharged the patient. The hospital was responsible for assigning on-call physicians and ensuring that they would be available when called. The patient died during the night in a motel room as a result of asphyxia resulting from a swelling of the larynx, tonsils, and epiglottis that blocked the trachea. Testimony from the laboratory director indicated that the emergency department's on-call physician was to be available for consultation and was assigned that duty by the hospital. Expert testimony also was offered that someone with the decedent's symptoms should have been hospitalized and that such care could have saved the decedent's life. The jury could have believed that an experienced physician would have taken the necessary steps to save the decedent's life.

Timely Response May Require a Phone Call

Hospitals are not only required to care for emergency patients, but they also are required to do so in a timely fashion. In *Marks v. Mandel*,[20] a Florida trial court was found to have erred in directing a verdict against the plaintiff. It was decided that the relevant inquiry in this case was whether the hospital and the supervisor should bear ultimate responsibility for failure of the specialty on-call system to function properly. Jury issues had been raised by evidence that the standard for on-call systems was to have a specialist attending the patient within a reasonable time of being called.

> Emergency rooms are aptly named and vital to public safety. There exists no other place to find immediate medical care. The dynamics that drive paying patients to a hospital's emergency rooms are known well. Either a sudden injury occurs, a child breaks his arm or an individual suffers a heart attack, or an existing medical condition worsens, a diabetic lapses into a coma, demanding immediate medical attention at the nearest emergency room. The catch phrase in legal nomenclature, "time is of the essence," takes on real meaning. Generally, one cannot choose to pass by the nearest emergency room, and after arrival, it would be improvident to depart in hope of finding one that provides services through employees rather than independent contractors. The patient is there and must rely on the services available and agree to pay the premium charged for those services.[21]

The public not only relies on the medical care rendered by emergency departments, but also considers the hospital as a single entity providing all of its medical services. A set of commentators observed

[T]he hospital itself has come to be perceived as the provider of medical services. According to this view, patients come to the hospital to be cured, and the doctors who practice there are the hospital's instrumentalities, regardless of the nature of the private arrangements between the hospital and the physician. Whether or not this perception is accurate seemingly matters little when weighed against the momentum of changing public perception and attendant public policy.[22]

The change in public reliance and public perceptions, as well as the regulations imposed on hospitals, has created an absolute duty for hospitals to provide competent medical care in their emergency departments.

Given the cumulative public policies surrounding the operation of emergency departments and the legal requirement that hospitals provide emergency services, hospitals must be accountable in tort for the actions of caregivers working in their emergency departments.

EMERGENCY MEDICAL TECHNICIAN

National Association of Emergency Medical Technicians

Code of Ethics

A fundamental responsibility of the Emergency Medical Technician is to conserve life, to alleviate suffering, to promote health, to do no harm, and to encourage the quality and equal availability of emergency medical care.

The Emergency Medical Technician provides services based on human need, with respect for human dignity, unrestricted by consideration of nationality, race creed, color, or status.

The Emergency Medical Technician does not use professional knowledge and skills in any enterprise detrimental to the public well-being.

The Emergency Medical Technician respects and holds in confidence all information of a confidential nature obtained in the course of professional work unless required by law to divulge such information.

The Emergency Medical Technician, as a citizen, understands and upholds the law and performs the duties of citizenship; as a professional, the Emergency Medical Technician has the never-ending responsibility to work with concerned citizens and other health care professionals in promoting a high standard of emergency medical care to all people.

The Emergency Medical Technician shall maintain professional competence and demonstrate concern for the competence of other members of the Emergency Medical Services health care team.

An Emergency Medical Technician assumes responsibility in defining and upholding standards of professional practice and education.

The Emergency Medical Technician assumes responsibility for individual professional actions and judgment, both in dependent and independent emergency functions, and knows and upholds the laws which affect the practice of the Emergency Medical Technician.

An Emergency Medical Technician has the responsibility to be aware of and participate in matters of legislation affecting the Emergency Medical Service System.

The Emergency Medical Technician, or groups of Emergency Medical Technicians, who advertise professional service, do so in conformity with the dignity of the profession.

The Emergency Medical Technician has an obligation to protect the public by not delegating to a person less qualified, any service which requires the professional competence of an Emergency Medical Technician.

The Emergency Medical Technician will work harmoniously with and sustain confidence in Emergency Medical Technician associates, the nurses, the physicians, and other members of the Emergency Medical Services health care team.

The Emergency Medical Technician refuses to participate in unethical procedures, and assumes the responsibility to expose incompetence or unethical conduct of others to the appropriate authority in a proper and professional manner.[23]

Written by Charles Gillespie, M.D. Adopted by The National Association of Emergency Medical Technicians, 1978.

Many states have enacted legislation that provides civil immunity to paramedics who render emergency life-saving services. In *Morena v. South Hills Health Systems*,[24] the Pennsylvania Supreme Court held that paramedics were not negligent in transporting a victim of a shooting to the nearest available hospital, rather than to another hospital located five or six miles farther away where a thoracic surgeon was present. The paramedics were not capable, in a medical sense, of accurately diagnosing the extent of the decedent's injury. Except for the children's center and the burn center, there were no emergency trauma centers specifically designated for the treatment of particular injuries.

The complaint, in *Riffe v. Vereb Ambulance Service, Inc.*,[25] alleged that, while responding to an emergency call, an emergency medical technician began administering lidocaine to the patient, as ordered over the telephone by the medical command physician at the defendant hospital. While in route to the hospital, the patient was administered lidocaine 44 times the normal dosage. Consequently, normal heart function was not restored and the patient was pronounced dead at the hospital shortly thereafter.

The superior court held that the liability of medical technicians could not be imputed to the hospital. The court noted the practical impossibility of the hospital carrying ultimate responsibility for the quality of care and treatment given patients by emergency medical services.

LABORATORY TECHNICIAN

As with most professional groups, there are a variety of associations and societies that laboratory professionals may join. The following are some excerpts from the American Society of Clinical Laboratory Science and the American Medical Technologists codes of ethics.

American Society of Clinical Laboratory Science

Code of Ethics

Preamble
The Code of Ethics of the American Society for Clinical Laboratory Science (ASCLS) sets forth the principles and standards by which clinical laboratory professionals practice their profession.

I. Duty to the Patient
Clinical laboratory professionals are accountable for the quality and integrity of the laboratory services they provide. This obligation includes maintaining individual competence in judgement and performance and striving to safeguard the patient from incompetent or illegal practice by others.

Clinical laboratory professionals maintain high standards of practice. They exercise sound judgment in establishing, performing, and evaluating laboratory testing.

Clinical laboratory professionals maintain strict confidentiality of patient information and test results. They safeguard the dignity and privacy of patients and provide accurate information to other health care professionals about the services they provide.

II. Duty to Colleagues and the Profession
Clinical laboratory professionals uphold and maintain the dignity and respect of our profession and strive to maintain a reputation of honesty, integrity, and reliability. They contribute to the advancement of the profession by improving the body of knowledge, adopting scientific advances that benefit the patient, maintaining high standards of practice and education, and seeking fair socioeconomic working conditions for members of the profession.

Clinical laboratory professionals actively strive to establish cooperative and respectful working relationships with other health care professionals with the primary objective of ensuring a high standard of care for the patients they serve.

III. Duty to Society

As practitioners of an autonomous profession, clinical laboratory professionals have the responsibility to contribute from their sphere of professional competence to the general well-being of the community.

Clinical laboratory professionals comply with relevant laws and regulations pertaining to the practice of clinical laboratory science and actively seek, within the dictates of their consciences, to change those which do not meet the high standards of care and practice to which the profession is committed.[26]

American Medical Technologists

Code of Ethics

While engaged in the Arts and Sciences which constitute the practice of Medical Technology, I shall practice with thorough self-restraint, always placing the welfare of the patients, entrusted to my care for tests or examinations, above all else, with full realization of my personal responsibility for the patients' best interests.

. . . I pledge myself to strive constantly to increase my technical knowledge of Medical Technology. . . .

I pledge accuracy and reliability in the performance of tests and to seek competent professional council when in doubt of my own judgment or competence in a particular test or examination.

As a further consideration for registration, I pledge myself to avoid dishonest, unethical or illegal compensation for such services as I shall render to the patients in my charge and I shall shun unwarranted professional publicity or unjust discrimination among the patients in my charge.

I pledge myself to protect the judgment of the attending physician in all cases in which I am directed to make laboratory tests or examinations, and to report the results of my findings free from all personal opinion to the attending physician only. I shall not make or offer a diagnosis or interpretation unless I be a duly licensed physician, except as the results of the report may of itself so indicate, or unless I am asked to by the attending physician.

I pledge myself to protect the identity and the integrity of all patients placed in my charge and to make only such reports public as shall be required by me by the laws of the state in which I practice or as the patient's physician shall direct. . . .[27]

An organization's laboratory provides data that are vital to a patient's treatment. Among its many functions, the laboratory monitors therapeutic ranges, measures blood levels for toxicity, places and monitors instrumentation on patient units, provides education for the nursing staff (e.g., glucose monitoring), provides valuable data used in research studies, supplies data on the most effective and economical antibiotic for treating patients, serves in a consultation role, and provides important data as to the nutritional needs of patients.

CASE: REFUSAL TO PERFORM LAB TESTS

A laboratory technician was found to have been properly dismissed from her job for refusing to perform chemical examinations on vials with AIDS warnings attached in *Stepp v. Review Board of the Indiana Employment Security Division*.[28] The court of appeals held that the employee was dismissed for just cause and that the laboratory did not waive its right to compel employees to perform assigned tasks.

Ethical and Legal Issues

1. Describe the ethical issues presented in this case.
2. Describe how the laboratory technician failed to adhere to the professional codes of ethics presented above. ■

CASE: TESTING MANIPULATED

According to the March 11, 2004 issue of the *Baltimore Sun*, a city hospital's HIV testing was manipulated. "Evidence of false results ignored by lab workers at Maryland General, state says . . . More than 400 people affected . . . Hospital president says patients will be notified to return for free re-tests.[29]

Ethical and Legal Issues

1. Describe a laboratory technician's professional responsibility to report accurate laboratory tests.
2. Should a laboratory technician report less than accurate laboratory reports if required to do so by his or her supervisor? Explain your answer. ■

MEDICAL ASSISTANT

The medical assistant is an unlicensed person who provides administrative, clerical, and/or technical support to a licensed practitioner. A licensed practitioner is generally required to be physically present in the treatment facility, medical office, or ambulatory facility when a medical assistant is performing procedures.[30]

The American Association of Medical Assistants code of ethics sets forth principles of ethical and moral conduct as they relate in particular to the practice of medical assisting.[31]

American Association of Medical Assistants

Code of Ethics

Members of AAMA . . . do pledge themselves to strive always to:

A. render service with full respect for the dignity of humanity;
B. respect confidential information obtained through employment unless legally authorized or required by responsible performance of duty to divulge such information;
C. uphold the honor and high principles of the profession and accept its disciplines;
D. seek to continually improve the knowledge and skills of medical assistants for the benefit of patients and professional colleagues;
E. participate in additional service activities aimed toward improving the health and well-being of the community.[32]

Employment of medical assistants is expected to grow much faster than the average for all occupations through the year 2012 as the health services industry expands. This growth is due in part to technological advances in medicine and a growing and aging population. Increasing use of medical assistants in the rapidly growing health care industry will most likely result in continuing employment growth for the occupation.[33]

Medical assistants work in physicians' offices, clinics, nursing homes, and ambulatory care settings. The duties of medical assistants vary from office to office, depending on the location and size of the practice and the practitioner's specialty. In small practices, medical assistants usually are generalists, handling both administrative and clinical duties. Those in large practices tend to specialize in a particular area, under supervision. Administrative duties often include answering telephones, greeting patients, updating and filing patients' medical records, filling out insurance forms, handling correspondence, scheduling appointments, arranging for hospital admission and laboratory services, and handling billing and bookkeeping. Clinical duties vary according to state law and include assisting in taking medical histories, recording vital signs, explaining treatment procedures to patients, preparing patients for examination, and assisting the practitioner during examinations. Medical assistants collect and prepare laboratory specimens or perform basic laboratory tests on the premises, dispose of contaminated supplies, and sterilize medical instruments. They instruct patients about medications and special diets, prepare and administer medications as directed by a physician, authorize drug refills as directed, telephone prescriptions to a pharmacy, prepare patients for X-rays, perform electrocardiograms, remove sutures, and change dressings.

Medical assistants who specialize have additional duties. Podiatric medical assistants make castings of feet, expose and develop X-rays, and assist podiatrists in surgery. Ophthalmic medical assistants help ophthalmologists provide eye care. They conduct diagnostic tests, measure and record vision, and test eye muscle function. They also show patients how to insert, remove, and care for contact lenses, and they apply eye dressings. Under the direction of the physician, ophthalmic medical assistants may administer eye medications. They also maintain optical and surgical instruments and may assist the ophthalmologist in surgery.[34]

Case: Looking for Help

On July 12th Mrs. Smith had severe pain in the left side of her head while at work, was not speaking coherently, and eventually lost consciousness for a few minutes. She was taken to her physician's office by a co-worker. Mrs. Smith's physician suggested that she get some imaging tests at the hospital's outpatient imaging center to rule out a transient ischemic attack (TIA).

A medical assistant at the imaging center told Mrs. Smith that her tests could not be scheduled until July 14. Upon arrival at the hospital's imaging center, Mrs. Smith was greeted by a medical assistant who said, "I am so sorry, but we cannot perform your scheduled test. Your doctor faxed us an unsigned and undated order sheet. It is confusing to us what imaging studies he wants. He checked a box on the physician's order sheet indicating that he wanted a CT scan of the head. In addition, there was a handwritten note on the form indicating that your physician wants an MRI to rule out a TIA. We are not sure if he wants one or both tests. You will have to get clarification from the physician as to exactly what procedure he wants." Mr. Smith, after having parked his wife's car, arrived at the front desk and saw his wife somewhat distressed. The medical assistant explained the problem. Mr. Smith asked the medical assistant, "Could you please contact the physician and ask him to clarify and fax back to the center exactly what tests he wants?" The medical assistant replied, "We are very busy. However, you can use our phone and ask the physician to clarify his order and have him fax us a new order." Mr. Smith replied, "What is your fax number?" The medical assistant (pointing to a wall) replied, "It is posted there on the wall by the phone. You can use that phone." The medical assistant suggested that Mrs. Smith could complete the patient intake paperwork while Mr. Smith contacted the physician. Mr. Smith was able to get a new faxed order.

Ethical and Legal Issues
1. Discuss the ethical and legal issues in this case.
2. Discuss why the medical assistant should have clarified the physician's order before the patient arrived.
3. Do you think this is an isolated incident, or might it be a common occurrence in the health care industry?
4. Describe how things could be improved at this imaging center.
5. What would you think if you learned that Mrs. Smith had to wait 48 hours before she could get her imaging studies scheduled? Would your thinking be influenced differently if it was your spouse, parent, or child?

6. How would you feel walking in the patient's shoes and learning that the imaging studies showed evidence of a minor stroke?

7. After leaving the imaging center, what do you suspect Mr. and Mrs. Smith's thoughts were after reflecting back on this scenario?

8. What advice would you give to both Mr. and Mrs. Smith if you overheard Mrs. Smith say to Mr. Smith, "I know that you would never have believed this happened unless you were there. This is how my last six years of life have been in fighting this horrendous disease."

9. Should Mrs. Smith's physician have played a different role in this situation? ■

CASE: UNTIMELY DIAGNOSIS

In 1987, the patient-plaintiff in *Follett v. Davis*[35] had her first office visit with Dr. Davis. In the spring of 1988, the plaintiff discovered a lump in her right breast and made an appointment to see Davis. The clinic had no record of her appointment. The clinic's employees directed her to radiology for a mammogram. The plaintiff was not offered an examination by Davis or any other physician at the clinic. In addition, she was not scheduled for a physician's examination as a follow-up to the mammogram. A technician examined the plaintiff's breast and confirmed the presence of a lump in her right breast. After the mammogram, clinic employees told her that she would hear from Davis if there were any problems with her mammogram.

The radiologist explained in his deposition that the mammogram was not normal. Davis received and reviewed the mammogram report and considered it to be negative for malignancy. He did not know of the new breast lump because none of the clinic employees had informed him about it. The clinic, including Davis, never contacted the plaintiff about her lump or the mammogram. On April 6, 1990, the plaintiff called the clinic and was told that there was nothing to worry about unless she heard from Davis. On September 24, 1990, the plaintiff returned to the clinic after she had developed pain associated with that same lump. A mammogram performed on that day gave results consistent with cancer. Three days later, Davis made an appointment for the plaintiff with a clinic surgeon for a biopsy and treatment. She kept her appointment with the surgeon. Nevertheless, this was her last visit with the clinic, as she subsequently transferred her care to other physicians. In October 1990, the biopsy confirmed the diagnosis of cancer.

In August 1992, the plaintiff filed a lawsuit. The evidence showed that after the patient found a lump in her breast, she went to Davis, her regular obstetrician/gynecologist, and to the clinic for aid. Davis and the clinic, through the clinic's employees and agents, undertook to treat her ailment. That undertaking ended when the clinic's surgeon performed the biopsy and therefore was continuous in nature. The evidence demonstrated that had clinic procedures been followed, Davis or another physician at the clinic would have had occasion to make a more timely diagnosis.

Ethical and Legal Issues

1. Describe the ethical and legal issues presented in this case.
2. Describe how similar incidents can be prevented in the future. ■

MEDICAL RECORDS

Health care organizations are required to maintain a medical record for each patient in accordance with accepted professional standards and practices. The main purposes of the medical record are to provide a planning tool for patient care; to record the course of a patient's treatment and the changes in a patient's condition; to document the communications between the practitioner responsible for the patient and any other health care professional who contributes to the patient's care; to assist in protecting the legal interests of the patient, the organization, and the practitioner; to provide a database for use in statistical reporting, continuing education, and research; and to provide information necessary for third-party billing and regulatory agencies. Medical records must be complete, accurate, current, readily accessible, and systematically organized.

The American Medical Record Association is now the American Health Information Management Association. The following code of ethical conduct defines the tenets necessary for carrying out the purposes of the profession. It is binding upon any member of the American Medical Record Association and any person who is certified, registered, or accredited by this Association.[36]

American Health Information Management Association

Code of Ethics

1. Place service before material gain. . . .
2. Preserve and protect the medical records.
   - •
   - •
   - •
4. Refuse to participate in or conceal unethical practices or procedures.
   - •
   - •
   - •
6. Preserve the confidential nature of professional determinations made by the staff committees.
   - •
   - •
   - •
9. Strive to advance the knowledge and practice of medical record administration, including continued self-improvement, in order to contribute to the best possible medical care.[37]

NURSING

This section provides an overview of the ethical responsibilities and legal issues of nursing practice. Although nurses traditionally have followed the instructions of attendant physicians, physicians realistically have long relied on nurses to exercise independent judgment in many situations.[38]

> When people are hospitalized, in a nursing home, having a baby, or learning to manage a chronic condition in their own home—at some of their most vulnerable moments—nurses are the health care providers they are most likely to encounter; spend the greatest amount of time with; and, along with other health care providers, depend on for their recovery.

> Research is now beginning to document what physicians, patients, other health care providers, and nurses themselves have long known: how well we are cared for by nurses affects our health, and sometimes can be a matter of life or death.[39]

Although most states have similar definitions of nursing, differences generally revolve around the scope of practice permitted.

The following two codes of ethics describe ethical principles for nurses from both a national and international perspective.

American Nurses Association

Code of Ethics for Nurses

1. The nurse, in all professional relationships, practices with compassion and respects the inherent dignity, worth and uniqueness of every individual, unrestricted by considerations of social or economic status, personal attributes, or the nature of health problems.
2. The nurse's primary commitment is to the patient, whether an individual, family, group, or community.
3. The nurse promotes, advocates for, and strives to protect the health, safety, and rights of the patient.
4. The nurse is responsible and accountable for individual nursing practice and determines the appropriate delegation of tasks consistent with the nurse's obligation to provide optimum patient care.
5. The nurse owes the same duties to self as to others, including the responsibility to preserve integrity and safety, to maintain competence, and to continue personal and professional growth.
6. The nurse participates in establishing, maintaining, and improving health care environments and conditions of employment conducive to the provision of quality health care and consistent with the values of the profession through individual and collective action.

7. The nurse participates in the advancement of the profession through contributions to practice, education, administration, and knowledge development.

8. The nurse collaborates with other health professionals and the public in promoting community, national, and international efforts to meet health needs.

9. The profession of nursing, as represented by associations and their members, is responsible for articulating nursing values, for maintaining the integrity of the profession and its practice, and for shaping social policy.

Reprinted with permission from American Nurses Association, "Code of Ethics for Nurses with Interpretive Statements," © 2001 Nursesbooks.org, American Nurses Association, Washington, DC.

International Council of Nurses

Code of Ethics for Nurses

1. Nurses and people

The nurse's primary professional responsibility is to people requiring nursing care.

In providing care, the nurse promotes an environment in which the human rights, values, customs and spiritual beliefs of the individual, family and community are respected.

The nurse ensures that the individual receives sufficient information on which to base consent for care and related treatment.

The nurse holds in confidence personal information and uses judgment in sharing this information.

The nurse shares with society the responsibility for initiating and supporting action to meet the health and social needs of the public, in particular those of vulnerable populations.

The nurse also shares responsibility to sustain and protect the natural environment from depletion, pollution, degradation and destruction.

2. Nurses and practice

The nurse carries personal responsibility and accountability for nursing practice, and maintaining competence by continual learning.

The nurse maintains a standard of personal health such that the ability to provide care is not compromised.

The nurse uses judgment regarding individual competence when accepting and delegating responsibility.

The nurse at all times maintains standards of personal conduct which reflect well on the profession and enhance public confidence.

The nurse, in providing care, ensures that the use of technology and scientific advances are compatible with the safety, dignity and rights of people.

3. **Nurses and the profession**

The nurse assumes the major role in determining and implementing acceptable standards of clinical nursing practice, management, research and education.

The nurse is active in developing a core of research-based professional knowledge.

The nurse, acting through the professional organization, participates in creating and maintaining equitable social and economic working conditions in nursing.

4. **Nurses and co-workers**

The nurse sustains a cooperative relationship with co-workers in nursing and other fields.

The nurse takes appropriate action to safeguard individuals when their care is endangered by a co-worker or any other person.

Registered Nurse

A registered nurse is one who has passed a state registration examination and has been licensed to practice nursing. The scope of practice of a registered professional nurse includes patient assessment, analyzing laboratory reports, patient teaching, health counseling, executing medical regimens, and operating medical equipment as prescribed by a physician, dentist, or other licensed health care provider. The nursing profession "is in a period of rapid and progressive change in response to the advances in technology, changes in patterns of demand for health services, and the evolution of professional relationships among nurses, physicians and other health professions."[40]

Nurse Anesthetist

Administration of anesthesia by a nurse anesthetist requires special training and certification. Nurse-administered anesthesia was the first expanded role for nurses requiring certification. Oversight and availability of an anesthesiologist are required by most organizations.

The major risks for nurse anesthetists include improper placement of an airway, failure to recognize significant changes in a patient's condition, and the improper use of anesthetics (e.g., wrong anesthetic, wrong dose, wrong route).

Nurse Midwife

Nurse midwives provide comprehensive prenatal care, including delivery for patients who are at low risk for complications. For the most part, they manage normal prenatal, intrapartum, and postpartum care. Provided that there are no complications, normal newborns are also cared for by a nurse midwife. Nurse midwives often provide primary care for women's health issues from puberty to post-menopause.

Nurse Practitioner

A nurse practitioner (NP) is a registered nurse who has completed the necessary education to engage in primary health care decision making. The NP is trained in the delivery of primary health care and the assessment of psychosocial and physical health problems, such as performing routine examinations and ordering routine diagnostic tests. The NP provides primary health care services in accordance with state nurse practice laws.

Clinical Nurse Specialist

The clinical nurse specialist is a professional registered nurse with an advanced academic degree, experience, and expertise in a clinical specialty (e.g., obstetrics, pediatrics). The clinical nurse specialist functions in a leadership capacity as a clinical role model, assisting the nursing staff to continuously evaluate patient care; acts as a resource for the management of patients with complex needs and conditions; participates in staff development activities related to his or her clinical specialty; makes recommendations to establish standards of care for patients; functions as a change agent by influencing attitudes, modifying behavior, and introducing new approaches to nursing practice; and collaborates with other members of the health care team to develop and implement the therapeutic plan of care for patients.

Special Duty Nurse

A special duty nurse is a nurse employed by a patient or patient's family to perform nursing care for the patient. An organization is generally not liable for the negligence of a special duty nurse unless a master–servant relationship can be determined to exist between the organization and the special duty nurse. If a master–servant relationship exists between the organization and the special duty nurse, the doctrine of *respondeat superior* may be applied to impose liability on the organization for the nurse's negligent acts. Although the patient employs the special duty nurse and the organization has no authority to hire or fire the nurse, the organization does have the responsibility to protect the patient from incompetent or unqualified special duty nurses.

Float Staff

There are staff members who are rotated from unit to unit based on staffing needs. Float staff can present a liability to the organization if they are assigned to work in an area outside their expertise.

Agency Personnel

Health care organizations are at risk for the negligent conduct of agency personnel. Because of this risk, it is important to ensure that agency workers have the necessary skills and competencies to carry out the duties and responsibilities assigned by the organization.

Nursing Assistants

A nursing assistant is an aide who has been certified and trained to assist patients with activities of daily living. The nursing assistant provides basic nursing care to non-acutely ill patients and assists in the maintenance of a safe and clean environment under the direction and supervision of a registered nurse or licensed practical nurse. The nursing assistant helps with positioning, turning, and lifting, and performs a variety of tests and treatments. The nursing assistant establishes and maintains interpersonal relationships with patients and other hospital personnel while ensuring confidentiality of patient information. Common areas of negligence for nursing assistants include failure to follow or improperly perform procedures, failure to assist patients and prevent falls, unsafe placement or positioning of equipment, failure to properly maintain equipment, failure to observe a patient and take vital signs at appropriate intervals, failure to chart pertinent information regarding a patient's changing condition (e.g., vital signs), and failure to respond to a patient's call for help (e.g., call bells).

Failure to Remove Endotracheal Tube

The court in *Poor Sisters of St. Francis v. Catron*[41] held that the failure of nurses and an inhalation therapist to report to the supervisor that an endotracheal tube had been left in the plaintiff longer than the customary period of three or four days was sufficient to allow the jury to reach a finding of negligence. The patient experienced difficulty speaking and underwent several operations to remove scar tissue and open her voice box. At the time of trial, she could not speak above a whisper and breathed partially through a hole in her throat created by a tracheotomy. The hospital was found liable for the negligent acts of its employees and the resulting injuries to the plaintiff.

Multiple Use of a Syringe

The respiratory therapist in *State University v. Young*[42] was suspended for using the same syringe for drawing blood from a number of critically ill patients. The therapist had been warned several times of the dangers of that practice and that it violated the state's policy of providing quality patient care.

Student Nurses

Student nurses are entrusted with the responsibility of providing nursing care to patients. When liability is being assessed, a student nurse serving at a health care facility is considered an agent of the facility. Student nurses are personally liable for their own negligent acts, and the facility is liable for their acts on the basis of *respondeat superior*.

A student nurse is held to the standard of a competent professional nurse when performing nursing duties. The courts have taken the position that anyone who performs duties customarily performed by a professional nurse is held to the standard of care required of a professional nurse. Every patient has the right to expect competent nursing services even if students provide the care as part of their clinical training.

Negligent Acts

The following cases illustrate some of the acts or omissions constituting negligence. They are by no means exhaustive and merely represent the wide range of potential legal pitfalls in which nurses might find themselves.

Nurse Assessments and Diagnosis

The defendant physicians in *Cignetti v. Camel*[43] ignored a nurse's assessment of a patient's diagnosis, which contributed to a delay in treatment and injury to the patient. The nurse had testified that she told the physician that the patient's signs and symptoms were not those associated with indigestion. The defendant physician objected to this testimony, indicating that such a statement constituted a medical diagnosis by a nurse. The trial court permitted the testimony to be entered into evidence. Section 335.01(8) of the Missouri Revised Statutes (1975) authorizes a registered nurse to make an assessment of persons who are ill and to render a *nursing diagnosis*. On appeal, the Missouri Court of Appeals affirmed the lower court's ruling, holding that evidence of negligence presented by a hospital employee, for which an obstetrician was not responsible, was admissible to show the events that occurred during the patient's hospital stay.

Ambiguous Medication Order

A nurse is responsible for making an appropriate inquiry if there is uncertainty about the accuracy of a physician's medication order in a patient's record. The medication order in *Norton v. Argonaut Insurance Co.*,[44] as entered in the medical record, was incomplete and subject to misinterpretation. Believing the order to be incorrect because of the dosage, the nurse asked two physicians present on the patient care unit whether the medication should be given as ordered. The two physicians did not interpret the order as the nurse did and therefore did not share the same concern. They advised the nurse that the attending physician's instructions did not appear out of line. The nurse did not contact the attending physician but instead administered the misinterpreted dosage of medication. As a result, the patient died from a fatal overdose of the medication.

The nurse was negligent by failing to consult with the attending physician before administering the medication. The nurse was held liable, as was the physician who wrote the ambiguous order that led to the fatal dose. In discussing the standard of care expected of a nurse who encounters an apparently erroneous order, the court stated that not only was the nurse unfamiliar with the medication in question, but she also violated the rule generally followed by members of the nursing profession in the community, which requires that the prescribing physician be called when there is doubt about an order. The court noted that it is the duty of a nurse to make absolutely certain what the physician intended, regarding both dosage and route.

Wrong Dosage of a Medication

The wrong dosage of the drug Haldol was administered by a nurse to a patient on seven occasions while she was employed at a nursing facility.[45] The patient's physician had prescribed a 0.5 mg dosage of Haldol. The patient's medication record indicated that the nurse had been administering dosages of 5 mg, which were being sent to the patient care unit by the pharmacy. The nurse had admitted that she administered the wrong dosage, and that she was aware of the facility's medication administration policy, which she breached by failing to check the dosage supplied by the pharmacy against the dosage ordered by the patient's physician. The Commissioner of the Department of Health made a determination that the administration of the wrong dosage of Haldol on seven occasions constituted patient neglect.

Medicating the Wrong Patient

A patient's identification bracelet must be checked prior to administering any medication. To ensure that the patient's identity corresponds to the name on the patient's bracelet, the nurse should address the patient by name when approaching the patient's bedside to administer any medication. Should a patient unwittingly be administered another patient's medication, the attending physician should be notified and appropriate documentation placed on the patient's chart.

Failure to Note an Order Change

Failure to review a patient's record before administering a medication to ascertain whether an order has been modified may render a nurse liable for negligence. The physician in *Larrimore v. Homeopathic Hospital Association*,[46] wrote an instruction on the patient's order sheet changing the method of administration from injection to oral medication. The nurse mistakenly gave the medication by injection. Perhaps the nurse had not reviewed the order sheet after being told by the patient that the medication was to be given orally; perhaps the nurse did not notice the physician's entry. Either way, the nurse's conduct was held to be negligent. The court went on to say that the jury could find the nurse negligent by applying ordinary common sense to establish the applicable standard of care.

Failure to Follow Instructions

Failure of a nurse to follow the instructions of a supervising nurse to wait for her assistance before performing a procedure can result in the revocation of the nurse's license. The nurse in *Cafiero v. North Carolina Board of Nursing*[47] failed to heed instructions to wait for assistance before connecting a heart monitor to an infant. The incorrect connection of the heart monitor resulted in an electrical shock to the infant. The board of nursing, under the Nursing Practice Act, revoked the nurse's license. The board had the authority to revoke the nurse's license even though her work before and after the incident had been exemplary. The dangers of electric cords are within the realm of common knowledge. The record showed that the nurse failed to exercise ordinary care in connecting the infant to the monitor.

Failure to Report Physician Negligence

An organization can be liable for the failure of nursing personnel to take appropriate action when a patient's personal physician is clearly unwilling or unable to cope with a situation that threatens the life or health of the patient. In a California case, *Goff v. Doctors General Hospital*,[48] a patient was bleeding seriously after childbirth because the physician failed to suture her properly. The nurses testified that they were aware of the patient's dangerous condition and that the physician was not present in the hospital. Both nurses knew the patient would die if nothing was done, but neither contacted anyone except the physician. The hospital was liable for the nurses' negligence in failing to notify their supervisors of the serious condition that caused the patient's death. Evidence was sufficient to sustain the finding that the nurses who attended the patient and who were aware of the excessive bleeding were negligent and that their negligence was a contributing cause of the patient's death. The measure of duty of the hospital toward its patients is the exercise of that degree of care used by hospitals generally. The court held that nurses who knew that a woman they were attending was bleeding excessively were negligent in failing to report the circumstances so that prompt and adequate measures could be taken to safeguard her life.

Failure to Question Patient Discharge

A nurse has a duty to question the discharge of a patient if he or she has reason to believe that such discharge could be injurious to the health of the patient. Jury issues were raised in *Koeniguer v. Eckrich*[49] by expert testimony that the nurses had a duty to attempt to delay the patient's discharge if her condition warranted continued hospitalization. By permissible inferences from the evidence, the delay in treatment that resulted from the premature discharge contributed to the patient's death. Summary dismissal of this case against the hospital by a trial court was found to have been improper.

Patient's Changing Condition

Failure to note changes in a patient's condition can lead to liability on the part of the nurse and the organization. The recovery room nurse in *Eyoma v. Falco*,[50] who had been assigned to monitor a post-surgical patient, left the patient and failed to recognize that the patient had stopped breathing. Nurse

Falco had been assigned to monitor the patient in the recovery room. She delegated that duty to another nurse and failed to verify that the other nurse accepted that responsibility.

> Nurse Falco admitted she never got a verbal response from the other nurse, and when she returned there was no one near the decedent. She acknowledged that Dr. Brotherton told her to watch the decedent's breathing, but claimed she was not told that decedent had been given narcotics. She maintained that upon her return she checked the decedent and observed his respirations to be eight per minute.
>
> Thereafter, Brotherton returned and inquired about the decedent's condition. Falco informed the doctor that the patient was fine. However, upon his personal observation, Brotherton realized that the decedent had stopped breathing.

• • •

> Decedent, because of oxygen deprivation, entered a comatose state and remained unconscious for over a year until his death.[51]

The jury held the nurse to be 100 percent liable for the patient's injuries. The court held that there was sufficient evidence to support the verdict.

Medical Records and the Nurse

The nurse is generally the one medical professional the patient sees more than any other. Consequently, the nurse is in a position to monitor the patient's illness, response to medication, display of pain and discomfort, and general condition. The patient's care, as well as the nurse's observations, should be recorded on a regular basis. The nurse should comply promptly and accurately with the physician orders written in the record. Should the nurse have any doubt as to the appropriateness of a particular order, he or she is expected to verify with the physician the intent of the prescribed order.

PHARMACIST

Because of the immense variety and complexity of medications now available, it is impossible for nurses or physicians to keep up with all of the information required for safe medication use. The pharmacist has become an essential resource in modern hospital practice.[52]

American Pharmacists Association

Code of Ethics

I. A pharmacist respects the covenantal relationship between the patient and pharmacist.

II.　A pharmacist promotes the good of every patient in a caring, compassionate, and confidential manner.

III.　A pharmacist respects the autonomy and dignity of each patient.

IV.　A pharmacist acts with honesty and integrity in professional relationships.

V.　A pharmacist maintains professional competence.

VI.　A pharmacist respects the values and abilities of colleagues and other health professionals.

VII.　A pharmacist serves individual, community, and societal needs.

VIII.　A pharmacist seeks justice in the distribution of health resources.[53]

Among nonoperative adverse events, medication errors are considered a leading cause of medical injury in the United States. Antibiotics, chemotherapeutic drugs, and anticoagulants are the three categories of drugs responsible for most drug-related adverse events. The prevention of medication errors requires recognition of common causes and the development of practices to help reduce the incidence of errors. With thousands of drugs, many of which look alike and sound alike, it is understandable why medication errors are so common. The more common type of medication errors include: prescription errors, transcription errors (often due to illegible handwriting and improper use of abbreviations), dispensing errors, and administration errors.

The practice of pharmacy essentially includes preparing, compounding, dispensing, and retailing medications. These activities may be carried out only by a pharmacist with a state license or by a person exempted from the provisions of a state's pharmacy statutes. The entire stock of drugs in a pharmacy is subject to strict government regulation and control. The pharmacist is responsible for developing, coordinating, and supervising all pharmacy activities and reviewing the drug regimens of each patient.

Dispensing and Administration of Drugs

The *dispensing* of medications is the processing of a drug for delivery or for administration to a patient pursuant to the order of a health care practitioner. It consists of checking the directions on the label with the directions on the prescription or order to determine accuracy; selecting the drug from stock to fill the order; counting, measuring, compounding, or preparing the drug; placing the drug in the proper container; and adding to a written prescription any required notations.

The *administration* of medications is the act of giving a single dose of a prescribed drug to a patient by an authorized person in accordance with federal and state laws and regulations. The complete act of administration includes removing an individual dose from a previously dispensed, properly labeled container (including a unit dose container); verifying it with the physician's order; giving the individual dose to the proper patient; and recording the time and dose given.

Licensed persons, in accordance with state regulations, may administer medications. Each dose of a drug administered must be recorded on the patient's clinical records. A separate record of narcotic drugs must be maintained. The record must contain a separate sheet for each narcotic of different strength or type administered to the patient. The narcotic record must contain the following information: date and time administered, physician's name, signature of person administering the dose, the balance of the narcotic drug on hand, and the proper recording of any drugs wasted/destroyed.

In the event that an emergency arises requiring the immediate administration of a particular drug, the patient's record should be documented properly, showing the necessity for administration of the drug on an emergency basis. Procedures should be in place for handling emergency situations.

Drug Substitution

Drug substitution may be defined as the dispensing of a different drug or brand in place of the drug or brand ordered. Several states prohibit this, and penal sanctions, including loss of license, are imposed for violation of the law.

Health care organizations use a "formulary system" whereby physicians and pharmacists create a formulary listing drugs used in the institution. The formulary contains the brand names and generic names of drugs. Under the formulary system, a physician agrees that his or her prescription calling for a brand name drug may be filled with the generic equivalent of that drug (i.e., a drug that contains the same active ingredients in the same proportions).

Authorization for using a generic equivalent should be given by the physician at the time of prescribing a formulary drug and should be evidenced by a written consent on the face of the prescription. When a formulary system is in use, the prescribing physician can require the use of a particular brand name drug, when he or she deems it necessary or desirable, by expressly prohibiting the use of the formulary system.

A pharmacist can be subject to liability for mishandling or misuse of drugs. Failure to meet and maintain required standards in handling drugs can lead to criminal or civil liability and even to the revocation of a pharmacist's license.

Expanding Role of the Pharmacist

Historically, the role of the pharmacist was centered on management of the pharmacy and accurate dispensing of drugs. The duties and responsibilities of pharmacists have moved well beyond the concept of filling prescriptions and dispensing drugs. Schools of pharmacy have recognized the ever-expanding role of the pharmacist into the clinical aspects of patient care, so much so that the educational requirements are getting more stringent, with emphasis on clinical education and application. Pharmacists now, among other duties, maintain patient medication profiles and monitor patient profiles, looking for incompatibilities between drugs and food-drug interactions.

Duty to Monitor Patient's Medications

In *Baker v. Arbor Drugs, Inc.,*[54] a Michigan court imposed a duty on a pharmacist to monitor a patient's medications. Three different prescriptions were prescribed by the same physician and filled at the same pharmacy. The pharmacy maintained a computer system that detected drug interactions. The pharmacy advertised to consumers that it could, through the use of a computer monitoring system, provide a medication profile of a customer for adverse drug reactions. Because the pharmacy advertised and used the computer system to monitor the medications of a customer, the pharmacist voluntarily assumed a duty of care to detect the harmful drug interaction that occurred.

The pharmacist is playing an ever-expanding interdisciplinary collaborative role on the clinical side of health care. For example, pharmacists often maintain a separate telephone line in hospitals for caregivers and practitioners to use to ask questions and discuss such issues as treatment plans for patients and proper dosing. Pharmacists are playing an important role when they respond and participate in reviving patients in cardiac arrest. Their knowledge of drugs, potential drug interactions, and proper dosing can be the difference between life and death.

Warning Patients about Potential for Overdose

A Pennsylvania court held that a pharmacy failed to exercise due care and diligence because the patient was not warned about the maximum dosage of a medication.[55] This failure resulted in an overdose, causing the patient permanent injuries. Expert testimony focused on the fact that a pharmacist who receives inadequate instructions as to the maximum recommended dosage of a medication has a duty to ascertain whether the patient is aware of the limitations concerning the use of the drug or, alternatively, to contact the prescribing physician as to the inadequacy of the prescription.

Refusal to Honor a Questionable Prescription

In *Hooks v. McLaughlin,*[56] the Indiana Supreme Court held that a pharmacist had a duty to refuse to refill prescriptions at an unreasonably faster rate than prescribed pending directions from the prescribing physician. The Indiana Code provides that a pharmacist is immune from civil prosecution or civil liability if he or she, in good faith, refuses to honor a prescription because, in his or her professional judgment, honoring of the prescription would aid or abet an addiction of habit.[57]

Billing Fraud

The court of appeals in *State v. Beatty*[58] upheld a lower court's finding that the evidence submitted against the defendant pharmacist was sufficient to sustain a conviction for Medicaid fraud. The state was billed for medications that were never dispensed, for more medications than some patients received, and, in some instances, for the more expensive trade name drugs when cheaper generic drugs were dispensed.

The pharmacists in *People v. Kendzia*[59] were convicted of selling generic drugs in vials with brand name labels. Investigators, working under-cover, were provided with Medicaid cards and fictitious prescriptions requiring brand name drugs to be dispensed as written. Between April and October 1979, the investigators had taken the prescriptions to the pharmacy where they were filled with generic substitutions in vials with the brand name labels.

PHYSICAL THERAPIST

American Physical Therapy Association

Code of Ethics

Principle 1
A physical therapist shall respect the rights and dignity of all individuals and shall provide compassionate care.

Principle 2
A physical therapist shall act in a trustworthy manner towards patients/ clients and in all other aspects of physical therapy practice.

•
•
•

Principle 11
A physical therapist shall respect the rights, knowledge, and skills of colleagues and other health care professionals.[60]

Physical therapy is the art and science of preventing and treating neuromuscular or musculoskeletal disabilities through the evaluation of an individual's disability and rehabilitation potential; the use of physical agents—heat, cold, electricity, water, and light; and neuromuscular procedures that, through their physiologic effect, improve or maintain the patient's optimum functional level. Because of different physical disabilities brought on by various injuries and medical problems, physical therapy is an extremely important component of a patient's total health care.

Ethical and Legal Concerns

There can be both ethical and legal issues when a therapist incorrectly interprets a physician's orders for physical therapy.

Incorrectly Interpreting Physician's Orders

Pontiff, in *Pontiff v. Pecot & Assoc.*,[61] filed a petition for damages against Pecot and Associates and Morris. Pontiff alleged Pecot and Associates had been negligent in failing to properly train, supervise, and monitor its employees, including Morris, and that Pecot and Associates was otherwise negligent. Pontiff alleged that employee Morris failed to exercise the degree of care and skill ordinarily exercised by physical therapists, failed to heed his protests that he could not perform physical therapy treatments she was supervising, and failed to stop performing physical therapy treatments after he began to complain he was in pain. Pontiff claimed he felt a muscle tear while he was exercising on the butterfly machine, a resistive exercise machine.

Pontiff's expert, Boulet, a licensed practicing physical therapist, testified that Pecot deviated from the standard of care of physical therapists by introducing a type of exercise that, according to her, was not prescribed by Dr. deAraujo, the treating physician. She stated that Pecot had added resistive or strengthening exercises to Pontiff's therapy and that these were not a part of the physician's prescription. Pecot argued that resistive exercises were implicitly part of the prescription, even if her interpretation of the prescription was not reasonable.

Legally, under Louisiana law, a physical therapist may not treat a patient without a written physical therapy prescription. Ethically, the Physical Therapists' Code of Ethics, Principle 3.4 states that "any alteration of a program or extension of services beyond the program should be undertaken in consultation with the referring practitioner." Because resistive exercises were not set forth in the original prescription, Boulet stated that consultation with the physician was necessary before Pontiff could be advanced to that level. Only in the case where a physician has indicated on the prescription that the therapist is to "evaluate and treat" would the therapist have such discretion. There was no such indication on the prescription written by deAraujo.

Davis, a physical therapist in private practice and Pecot's expert witness, testified that the program that Pecot designed for Pontiff was "consistent with how she interpreted the prescription for therapy that the physician wrote." Davis, however, did not at any time state that Pecot's interpretation was a reasonable one. In fact, Davis herself would not have interpreted the prescription in the manner that Pecot did. Davis testified only that Pecot's introduction of resistive exercises was reasonable based on her interpretation of the prescription.

It is clear that Pecot, as a licensed physical therapist, owed a duty to Pontiff, her client. Pecot's duty is defined by the standard of care of similar physical therapists and the Association of Physical Therapists of America. If

Pecot found the prescription to be ambiguous, she had a duty to contact the prescribing physician for clarification. The appeals court found that the trial court was correct in its determination that Pontiff presented sufficient evidence to show that this duty was breached and that Pecot's care fell below the standard of other physical therapists.

Neglect

In *Zucker v. Axelrod*,[62] a physical therapist had been charged with resident neglect for refusing to allow an 82-year-old nursing facility resident to go to the bathroom before starting his therapy treatment session. Undisputed evidence at a hearing showed that the petitioner refused to allow the resident to be excused to go to the bathroom. The petitioner claimed that her refusal was because she assumed that the resident had gone to the bathroom before going to therapy and that the resident was undergoing a bladder training program. The petitioner had not mentioned when she was interviewed after the incident or during her hearing testimony that she considered bladder training a basis for refusing to allow the resident to go to the bathroom. It is uncontroverted that the nursing facility had a policy of allowing residents to go to the bathroom whenever they wished to do so. The court held that the finding of resident neglect was supported sufficiently by the evidence.

PHYSICIAN ASSISTANT

American Academy of Physician Assistants

Statement of Values of the Physician Assistant Profession

- Physician assistants hold as their primary responsibility the health, safety, welfare, and dignity of all human beings.
- Physician assistants uphold the tenets of patient autonomy, beneficence, nonmaleficence, and justice.
- Physician assistants recognize and promote the value of diversity.
- Physician assistants treat equally all persons who seek their care.
- Physician assistants hold in confidence the information shared in the course of practicing medicine.
- Physician assistants assess their personal capabilities and limitations, striving always to improve their medical practice.
- Physician assistants actively seek to expand their knowledge and skills, keeping abreast of advances in medicine.
- Physician assistants work with other members of the health care team to provide compassionate and effective care of patients.
- Physician assistants use their knowledge and experience to contribute to an improved community.
- Physician assistants respect their personal relationship with physicians.
- Physician assistants share and expand knowledge within the profession.[63]

Physicians are increasingly employing physician assistants (PAs) as an extension of their practices. According to the American Academy, there were 46,002 PAs in the United States in the beginning of 2003, a nearly 110% increase since 1993. PAs are licensed to practice medicine under a physician's supervision and can practice only under a physician's license. They can conduct physician exams, diagnose and treat illnesses, order and interpret tests, and write prescriptions in most states.

One of the solutions to the shortage of physicians in certain rural and inner-city areas has been to train allied health professionals such as PAs to perform the more routine and repetitive medical functions. A physician may delegate to a PA such tasks as suturing minor wounds, administering injections, and performing routine history and physical examinations. A physician may not delegate a task when regulations specify that the physician must perform it personally or when the delegation is prohibited under state law or by the facility's own policies.

PAs are responsible for their own negligent acts. The employer of a PA can be held liable for the PA's negligent acts on the basis of *respondeat superior*. A physician, as an employer of a PA, also can be held liable on the basis of *respondeat superior*.

To limit the potential risk of liability for a PA's negligent acts, PAs should be monitored and supervised by a physician. Guidelines and procedures also should be established to provide a standard mechanism for reviewing a PA's performance.

PSYCHOLOGIST

American Psychological Association

General Principles

Principle A: Beneficence and Nonmaleficence

Psychologists strive to benefit those with whom they work and take care to do no harm. In their professional actions, psychologists seek to safeguard the welfare and rights of those with whom they interact professionally and other affected persons, and the welfare of animal subjects of research. . . .

Principle B: Fidelity and Responsibility

Psychologists establish relationships of trust with those with whom they work. They are aware of their professional and scientific responsibilities to society and to the specific communities in which they work. Psychologists uphold professional standards of conduct, clarify their professional roles and obligations, accept appropriate responsibility for their behavior, and seek to manage conflicts of interest that could lead to exploitation or harm. . . .

Principle C: Integrity

Psychologists seek to promote accuracy, honesty, and truthfulness in the science, teaching, and practice of psychology. In these activities psychologists do not steal, cheat, or engage in fraud, subterfuge, or intentional misrepresentation of fact. . . .

Principle D: Justice
Psychologists recognize that fairness and justice entitle all persons to access to and benefit from the contributions of psychology and to equal quality in the processes, procedures, and services being conducted by psychologists. Psychologists exercise reasonable judgment and take precautions to ensure that their potential biases, the boundaries of their competence, and the limitations of their expertise do not lead to or condone unjust practices.

Principle E: Respect for People's Rights and Dignity
Psychologists respect the dignity and worth of all people, and the rights of individuals to privacy, confidentiality, and self-determination. Psychologists are aware that special safeguards may be necessary to protect the rights and welfare of persons or communities whose vulnerabilities impair autonomous decision making. Psychologists are aware of and respect cultural, individual, and role differences, including those based on age, gender, gender identity, race, ethnicity, culture, national origin, religion, sexual orientation, disability, language, and socioeconomic status and consider these factors when working with members of such groups. . . . [64]

Unethical Conduct

Sturm, a licensed psychologist who has taught professional ethics since 1985 and who served on the ethics committee of the Oregon Psychological Association for six years, testified that testimony about the best interests of children in a custody dispute by a therapist who had not observed both parents' interactions with the children was unethical. Sturm further stated that a psychologist has an obligation to adopt an impartial stance and to avoid actions that would escalate an adversarial nature of the relationship between the parents. Sturm explained that psychologists have "an ethical responsibility to anticipate the possible purposes" behind a request to prepare an affidavit to be used in a custody dispute, in order to prevent misuse of the evaluation, and agreed that practices such as making evaluative or conclusory statements about persons or relationships not observed directly are blatantly unethical. The petitioner's affidavit made such conclusory statements, and it was not until the show-cause hearing that petitioner admitted to her bias toward her patient.[65]

American Psychological Association

Code of Ethics and Sexual Conduct

10.05. Sexual Intimacies with Current Therapy Clients/Patients
Psychologists do not engage in sexual intimacies with current therapy clients/patients.

10.06. Sexual Intimacies with Relatives or Significant Others of Current Therapy Clients/Patients

Psychologists do not engage in sexual intimacies with individuals they know to be close relatives, guardians, or significant others of current clients/patients. Psychologists do not terminate therapy to circumvent this standard.

10.07. Therapy with Former Sexual Partners
Psychologists do not accept as therapy clients/patients persons with whom they have engaged in sexual intimacies.

10.08. Sexual Intimacies with Former Therapy Clients/Patients
(a) Psychologists do not engage in sexual intimacies with former clients/patients for at least two years after cessation or termination of therapy.
(b) Psychologists do not engage in sexual intimacies with former clients/patients even after a two-year interval except in the most unusual circumstances. Psychologists who engage in such activity after the two years following cessation or termination of therapy and of having no sexual contact with the former client/patient bear the burden of demonstrating that there has been no exploitation, in light of all relevant factors, including (1) the amount of time that has passed since therapy terminated; (2) the nature, duration, and intensity of the therapy; (3) the circumstances of termination; (4) the client's/patient's personal history; (5) the client's/patient's current mental status; (6) the likelihood of adverse impact on the client/patient; and (7) any statements or actions made by the therapist during the course of therapy suggesting or inviting the possibility of a post-termination sexual or romantic relationship with the client/patient. (See also Standard 3.05, Multiple Relationships.)[66]

Psychologists Improprieties with Clients

A defense that sexual improprieties with clients did not take place during treatment sessions is unacceptable conduct. The Board of Psychologist Examiners in *Gilmore v. Board of Psychologist Examiners*[67] revoked a psychologist's license because of sexual improprieties. The psychologist petitioned for judicial review. She argued that therapy had terminated before the sexual relationships began. The court of appeals held that evidence supported the board's conclusion that the psychologist had violated an ethical standard in caring for her patients. When a psychologist's personal interests intrude into the practitioner–client relationship, the practitioner is obliged to recreate objectivity through a third party. The board's findings and conclusions indicated that the petitioner failed to maintain that objectivity.

Alleged Abuse—Immunity Provided to Psychologist

Two children were placed in the temporary custody of a foster family. One child was referred to a licensed psychologist for evaluation. After two interviews the psychologist formed the professional opinion that the child had been sexually molested. Based in part on statements made by the child, the psychologist further believed that the perpetrator of the suspected molestation was the father. At a hearing before the juvenile court, the court determined that the evidence did not support a finding that the child had been abused by his father. Custody was returned to the parents. The child's parents subsequently initiated an action for medical malpractice against the psychologist. The psychologist claimed immunity from liability as provided by a state child abuse reporting statute. The trial court and the parents appealed, arguing that the immunity provisions of the statute do not apply to the psychologist because she was not a "mandatory reporter" under that statute.[68]

The Georgia Court of Appeals held that the statute's grant of immunity from liability extended to the psychologist. The evidence did not establish bad faith on the part of the psychologist so as to deprive her of such immunity. The statute provides that any person participating in the making of a report, or participating in any judicial proceeding or any other proceeding resulting in a report of suspected child abuse, is immune from any civil or criminal liability that might otherwise be incurred or imposed, provided such participation pursuant to the statute is made in good faith. The grant of qualified immunity covers every person who, in good faith, participates over time in the making of a report to a child welfare agency. Proof of negligent reporting or bad judgment is not proof that the psychologist refused to fulfill her professional duties out of some harmful motive or that she consciously acted for some dishonest purpose. There was no competent evidence that the psychologist acted in bad faith.

RESPIRATORY THERAPIST

Respiratory care and therapy is the allied health profession responsible for the treatment, management, diagnostic testing, and control of patients with cardiopulmonary deficits. A respiratory therapist is a person employed in the practice of respiratory care who has the knowledge and skill necessary to administer respiratory care.

Respiratory therapists are responsible for their negligent acts. A respiratory therapist's employer is responsible for the negligent acts of the therapist under the legal doctrine of *respondeat suerior*.

American Association for Respiratory Care

Statement of Ethics and Professional Conduct

In the conduct of their professional activities the Respiratory Care Practitioner shall be bound by the following ethical principles. Respiratory Care Practitioners shall:

- Actively maintain and continually improve their professional competence, and represent it accurately.

- Perform only those procedures or functions in which they are individually competent and which are within the scope of accepted and responsible practice.
- Respect and protect the legal and personal rights of patients they treat, including the right to informed consent and refusal of treatment.
- Divulge no confidential information regarding any patient or family unless disclosure is required for responsible performance of duty, or required by law.
- Provide care without discrimination on any basis, with respect for the rights and dignity of all individuals.
- Promote disease prevention and wellness.
- Refuse to participate in illegal or unethical acts, and shall refuse to conceal illegal, unethical, or incompetent acts of others.
- Follow sound scientific procedures and ethical principles in research.
- Comply with state or federal laws which govern and relate to their practice.
- Avoid any form of conduct that creates a conflict of interest, and shall follow the principles of ethical business behavior.
- Promote the positive evolution of the profession, and health care in general, through improvement of the access, efficacy, and cost of patient care.
- Refrain from indiscriminate and unnecessary use of resources, both economic and natural, in their practice.[69]

CASE: RESTOCKING THE CODE CART

Dixon had been admitted to the hospital and was diagnosed with pneumonia in her right lung. [*Dixon v. Taylor*, No. 9224SC760 (Filed 20 July 1993)]. Dixon's condition began to deteriorate and she was moved to the Intensive Care Unit (ICU). A code blue was eventually called signifying that her cardiac and respiratory functions were believed to have ceased. During the code, a decision was made to intubate, insert an endotracheal tube into Dixon so that she could be given respiratory support by a mechanical ventilator.

As Dixon's condition stabilized, Dr. Taylor, Dixon's physician at that time, ordered that she be gradually weaned from the respirator. Blackham, a respiratory therapist employed by the hospital, extubated Dixon at 10:15 PM. Taylor left Dixon's room to advise her family that she had been extubated.

Blackham decided an oxygen mask would provide better oxygen to Dixon but could not locate a mask in the ICU, so he left ICU and went across the hall to the Critical Care Unit (CCU). When Blackham returned to Dixon's room with the oxygen mask and placed it on Dixon, he realized that she was not breathing properly. Blackham realized that she would have to be reintubated as quickly as possible.

A second code was called. Shackleford, a nurse in the Cardiac Critical Care Unit, responded to the code. Shackleford recorded on the code sheet that she arrived in Dixon's room at 10:30 PM. She testified that Blackham said he had too short of a blade and he needed a medium, a Number 4 Mac-

Intosh laryngoscope blade (blade), which was not on the code cart. The code cart is a cart equipped with all the medicines, supplies, and instruments needed for a code emergency. The code cart in the ICU had not been restocked after the first code that morning, so Shackleford was sent to obtain the needed blade from the CCU across the hall.

When Shackleford returned to the ICU, the blade was passed to Taylor who had responded to the code and was attempting to reintubate Dixon. Upon receiving the blade, Taylor was able to quickly intubate Dixon. Dixon was placed on a ventilator, but she never regained consciousness. After the family was informed there was no hope that Dixon would recover the use of her brain, the family requested that no extraordinary measure be taken to prolong her life.

A medical negligence claim was filed against Taylor and the hospital. The jury found that Taylor was not negligent. Evidence presented at trial established that the hospital's breach of duty in not having the code cart properly restocked resulted in a three-minute delay in the intubation of Dixon. Reasonable minds could accept from the testimony at trial that the hospital's breach of duty was a cause of Dixon's brain death, without which the injury would not have occurred. Foreseeability on the part of the hospital can be established from the evidence introduced by the plaintiff that the written standards for the hospital require every code cart be stocked with a Number 4 MacIntosh blade. This evidence permits a reasonable inference that the hospital should have foreseen that the failure to have the code cart stocked with the blade could lead to critical delays in intubating a patient. Accordingly, there was substantial evidence that the failure to have the code cart stocked with the proper blade was a proximate cause of Dixon's injuries.

Ethical and Legal Issues

1. Describe the ethical issues involved in this case.
2. Describe how this case satisfies the elements of negligence.
3. Describe how the hospital could be liable for the therapist's decision to leave the patient.
4. How can the likelihood of similar occurrences be prevented in the future? ▪

X-RAY TECHNICIAN

American Registry of Radiologic Technologists

Code of Ethics

1. The radiologic technologist conducts herself or himself in a professional manner, responds to patient needs, and supports colleagues and associates in providing quality patient care.

        •
        •
        •

3. The radiologic technologist delivers patient care and service unrestricted by the concerns of personal attributes or the nature of the disease or illness, and without discrimination on the basis of sex, race, creed, religion, or socioeconomic status.

•
•
•

5. The radiologic technologist assesses situations; exercises care, discretion, and judgment; assumes responsibility for professional decisions; and acts in the best interest of the patient.

•
•
•

9. The radiologic technologist respects confidences entrusted in the course of professional practice, respects the patient's right to privacy and reveals confidential information only as required by law or to protect the welfare of the individual or the community.[70]

Failure to Restrain Caused Patient Fall

The plaintiff in *Cockerton v. Mercy Hospital Medical Center*[71] was admitted to the hospital for the purpose of surgery. Her physician ordered post-surgical X-rays for her head and face to be taken the next day. A hospital employee took the plaintiff from her room to the X-ray department by wheelchair. A nurse had assessed her condition as slightly "oozy" and drowsy. An X-ray technician took charge of the plaintiff in the X-ray room. After the plaintiff was taken inside the X-ray room, she was transferred from a wheelchair to a portable chair for the procedure. Upon being moved, the plaintiff complained of nausea. The technician did not use the restraint straps to secure the plaintiff to the chair. At some point during the procedure, the plaintiff had a fainting seizure. The technician called for help. When another hospital employee entered the room, the technician was holding the plaintiff in an upright position. She appeared nonresponsive. The plaintiff only remembered being stood up and having a lead jacket placed across her back and shoulders. The technician maintains that the plaintiff did not fall. At the time the plaintiff left the X-ray room, her level of consciousness was poor. The plaintiff's physician noticed a deflection of the plaintiff's nose, but had difficulty assessing it because of the surgical procedure from the day before. The following day, the deflection of the plaintiff's nose was much more evident. A specialist was contacted and an attempt was made to correct the deformity. The specialist made an observation that it would require a substantial injury to the nose to deflect it to that severity.

The plaintiff instituted proceedings against the hospital, alleging that the negligence of the nurses or technicians allowed her to fall during the procedure and subsequently caused injury. The jury concluded that the hospital was negligent in leaving the plaintiff unattended or failing to restrain her, which proximately caused her fall and injury.

The X-ray technician testified that during the X-ray, the plaintiff appeared to have a "seizure episode." She also testified that she left the plaintiff unattended for a brief period of time and that she did not use the restraint straps that were attached to the portable X-ray chair. Using the restraint straps would have secured the plaintiff to the portable chair during the X-ray examination.

CERTIFICATION OF HEALTH CARE PROFESSIONALS

Certification of health care professionals is the recognition by a governmental or professional association that an individual's expertise meets the standards of that group. The standards established by professional associations generally exceed those required by government agencies. Some professional groups establish their own minimum standards for certification in those professions that are not licensed by a particular state. Certification by an association or group is a self-regulation credentialing process.

LICENSING HEALTH CARE PROFESSIONALS

Licensure can be defined as the process by which some competent authority grants permission to a qualified individual or entity to perform certain specified activities that would be illegal without a license. As it applies to health care personnel, licensure refers to the process by which licensing boards, agencies, or departments of the several states grant to individuals who meet certain predetermined standards the legal right to practice in a health care profession and to use a specified health care practitioner's title. The commonly stated objectives of licensing laws are to limit and control admission to the different health care occupations and to protect the public from unqualified practitioners by promulgating and enforcing standards of practice within the professions. Health professions commonly requiring licensure include dentists, nurses, pharmacists, physician assistants, osteopaths, physicians, and podiatrists.

The authority of states to license health care practitioners is found in their regulating power. Implicit in the power to license is the authority to collect license fees, establish standards of practice, require certain minimum qualifications and competency levels of applicants, and impose on applicants other requirements necessary to protect the general public welfare. This authority, which is vested in the legislature, may be delegated to political subdivisions or to state boards, agencies, and departments. In some instances, the scope of the delegated power is made specific in the legislation; in others, the licensing authority may have wide discretion in performing its functions. In either case, however, the authority granted by the legislature may not be exceeded.

Suspension and Revocation of License

Licensing boards have the authority to suspend or revoke the license of a health care professional who is found to have violated specified norms of conduct. Such violations may include procurement of a license by fraud;

unprofessional, dishonorable, immoral, or illegal conduct; performance of specific actions prohibited by statute; and malpractice.

Suspension and revocation procedures are most commonly contained in a state's licensing act; in some jurisdictions, however, the procedure is left to the discretion of the board or is contained in the general administrative procedure acts.

HELPFUL ADVICE FOR CAREGIVERS

- Abide by the ethical code of one's profession.
- Do not criticize the professional skills of others.
- Maintain complete and adequate medical records.
- Provide each patient with medical care comparable with national standards.
- Seek the aid of professional medical consultants when indicated.
- Obtain informed consent for diagnostic and therapeutic procedures.
- Inform the patient of the risks, benefits, and alternatives to proposed procedures.
- Do not indiscriminately prescribe medications or diagnostic tests.
- Practice the specialty in which you have been trained.
- Participate in continuing education programs.
- Keep patient information confidential.
- Check patient equipment regularly, and monitor it for safe use.
- When terminating a professional relationship with a patient, give adequate written notice to the patient.
- Authenticate all telephone orders.
- Obtain a qualified substitute when you will be absent from your practice.
- Investigate patient incidents promptly.
- Be a good listener, and allow each patient sufficient time to express fears and anxieties.
- Develop and implement an interdisciplinary plan of care for each patient.
- Safely administer patient medications.
- Closely monitor each patient's response to treatment.
- Provide education and teaching to patients.
- Foster a sense of trust and feeling of significance.
- Communicate with the patient and other caregivers.
- Provide cost-effective care without sacrificing quality.

CHAPTER REVIEW

1. Practicing outside one's scope of practice has both ethical and legal concerns.
2. Legislation in many states imposes a duty on hospitals to provide emergency care. If the public is aware that a hospital furnishes emergency services and relies on that knowledge, the hospital has a duty to provide those services to the public.

3. Hospitals are expected to notify specialty on-call physicians when their particular skills are required in the emergency department. A physician who is on call and fails to respond to a request to attend a patient can be liable for injuries suffered by the patient because of his or her failure to respond.

4. There can be both ethical and legal repercussions if a professional incorrectly interprets a physician's orders.

5. A defense that sexual improprieties with clients did not take place during treatment sessions is unacceptable conduct.

6. Scope of practice refers to the permissible boundaries of practice for health care professionals, as is often defined in state statutes, which define the actions, duties, and limits of professionals in their particular roles.

7. A professional who exceeds his or her scope of practice as defined by state practice acts can be found to have violated licensure provisions or to have performed tasks that are reserved by statute for another health care professional.

8. The power and authority to regulate drugs, their products, packaging, and distribution rest primarily with federal and state governments.

REVIEW QUESTIONS

1. Describe how ethics and the law impact on the various health care professions discussed in this chapter.

2. Discuss ethical and legal implications of practicing outside one's scope of practice.

3. Under what circumstances does a hospital have a duty to provide emergency services to the public?

4. Are sexual improprieties acceptable with clients as long as they do not take place during treatment? Explain your answer.

5. Consider under what circumstances a professional's legal responsibilities may overlap with his or her ethical duties.

6. Describe how and why the scope of practice for various professionals (e.g., nurses and pharmacists) is changing.

7. If a caregiver disagrees with a physician's written orders and is sure that he or she is right, should that caregiver violate the orders? Explain your answer.

8. Describe a professional's responsibilities if a patient's condition takes a turn for the worse.

WEB SITES

American Academy of Nurse Practitioners
www.aanp.org/default.asp
American Association of Critical Care Nurses
www.aacn.org
American Association for Respiratory Care
www.aarc.org
American Dietetic Association Foundation
www.eatright.org/Public/index.cfm
American Nurses Association
www.ana.org
American College of Nurse Practitioners
www.nurse.org/acnp
American Medical Technologists
www.amt1.com
American Occupational Therapy Association
www.aota.org
American Organization of Nurse Executives
www.aone.org
American Pharmacist Association
www.aphanet.org
American Physical Therapy Association
www.apta.org
American Registry of Radiologic Technologists
www.arrt.org/Index.htm
American Society for Clinical Laboratory Science
http://www.ascls.org/
American Speech-Hearing-Language Assoc.
www.asha.org/default.htm
Center for the Study of Ethics in the Professions
http://www.iit.edu/departments/csep/
Code of Ethics for Pharmacists
http://www.aphanet.org/pharmcare/ethics.html
College of Med Lab Tech
www.cmlto.com/government_policy/code_of_ethics
Ehealth Initiative
www.ehealthinitiative.org
Index of Ethics Codes
http://www.iit.edu/departments/csep/PublicWWW/codes/codes.html
Int'l Council of Nurses Code of Ethics
www.icn/icncode.pdf
Kennedy Institute of Ethics
http://www.georgetown.edu/research/nrebl/
Midwives Organizations
dmoz.org/Health/Professions/Midwifery/Organizations/

National Black Nurses Association, Inc.
  www.nbna.org
National Council of State Boards of Nursing
  www.ncsbn.org
National League for Nursing
  www.nln.org
Nursing Times
  www.nursingtimes.net
The Center for Ethics and Human Rights
  www.nursingworld.org/ethics/ecode.htm

NOTES

1. http://www.iit.edu/departments/csep/PublicWWW/codes/coe/Users_Guide.html.
2. http://www.iit.edu/departments/csep/PublicWWW/codes/coe/American%20Medical%20Technologists%20code%20of%20ethics.html.
3. http://www.baltimoresun.com/news/local/bal-lab0311,0,6183061.story?coll=bal-local-headlines.
4. http://www.amerchiro.org/about/ethics.shtml#public.
5. Poor v. State, No. S-02-472, 266 Neb. 183 (Neb. 2003).
6. http://www.iit.edu/departments/csep/PublicWWW/codes/coe/ada-d.html.
7. http://www.ada.org/prof/prac/law/codes/principles.asp.
8. 557 S.E.2d 339 (2001).
9. 495 N.Y.S.2d 808 (N.Y. App. Div. 1985).
10. http://www.adha.org/aboutadha/codeofethics.htm.
11. Lowenberg v. Sobol, 594 N.Y.S.2d 874 (N.Y. App. Div. 1993).
12. 367 S.E.2d 453 (S.C. 1988).
13. *Id.* at 455-456.
14. http://www.findarticles.com/p/articles/mi_m0822/is_1_99/ai_53697693/pg_1.
15. 753 F. Supp. 267 (W.D. Ark. 1990).
16. http://www.acep.org/1,1118,0.html.
17. *Id.*
18. 288 A.2d 379 (Md. 1972).
19. 271 N.W.2d 8 (S.D. 1978).
20. 477 So. 2d 1036 (Fla. Dist. Ct. App. 1985).
21. Baptist Mem'l Hosp. Sys. v. Sampson, 969 S.W.2d 945, 947 (Tex. 1998).
22. Martin C. McWilliams, Jr. & Hamilton E. Russell, III, *Hospital Liability for Torts of Independent Contractor Physicians*, 47 S.C. L. Rev. 431, 473 (1996).
23. http://www.tdh.state.tx.us/hcqs/ems/sethics.htm.
24. 462 A.2d 680 (Pa. 1983).
25. 650 A.2d 1076 (Pa. Super. 1994).
26. http://www.ascls.org/about/ethics.asp.
27. http://www.iit.edu/departments/csep/PublicWWW/codes/coe/American%20Medical%20Technologists%20code%20of%20ethics.html.
28. 521 N.E.2d 350 (Ind. Ct. App. 1988).
29. http://www.westgard.com/essay64.htm.
30. http://www.certmedassistant.com/what_is.htm.
31. http://www.aama-ntl.org/about/code_creed.aspx.

32. *Id.*
33. http://www.bls.gov/oco/ocos164.htm#outlook.
34. http://www.bls.gov/oco/ocos164.htm.
35. 636 N.E.2d 1282 (Ind. Ct. App. 1994).
36. http://www.iit.edu/departments/csep/PublicWWW/codes/coe/American%20Medical%20 Record%20Association%20Code%20of%20Ethics.html.
37. *Id.*
38. Fraijo v. Hartland Hosp., 160 Cal. Rptr. 252 (Ct. App. 1979).
39. "Keeping Patients Safe: Transforming the Work Environment of Nurses," Institute of Medicine, The National Academies Press, Washington, DC, at 2.
40. Dep't of Health, Ed. & Welfare, Pub. No. (HSM) 73-2037, "Extending the Scope of Nursing Practice: A Report of the Secretary's Committee to Study Roles for Nurses," 8 (1971).
41. 435 N.E.2d 305 (Ind. Ct. App. 1982).
42. 566 N.Y.S.2d 79 (N.Y. App. Div. 1991).
43. 692 S.W.2d 329 (Mo. Ct. App. 1985).
44. 144 So. 2d 249 (La. Ct. App. 1962).
45. Harrison v. Axelrod, 599 N.Y.S.2d 96 (N.Y. App. Div. 1993).
46. 181 A.2d 573 (Del. 1962).
47. 403 S.E.2d 582 (N.C. Ct. App. 1991).
48. 333 P.2d 29 (Cal. Ct. App. 1958).
49. 422 N.W.2d 600 (S.D. 1988).
50. 589 A.2d 653 (N.J. Super. App. Div. 1991).
51. *Id.* at 655.
52. Institute of Medicine, *To Err is Human: Building a Safer Health System*, supra note 1, at 194.
53. http://www.aphanet.org/pharmcare/ethics.html.
54. 544 N.W.2d 727 (Mich. Ct. App. 1996).
55. Riff v. Morgan Pharmacy, 508 A.2d 1247 (Pa. Super. Ct. 1986).
56. 642 N.E.2d 514 (Ind. 1994).
57. Ind. Code § 25-26-13-16(b)(3) (1993).
58. 308 S.E.2d 65 (N.C. Ct. App. 1983).
59. 478 N.Y.S.2d 209 (N.Y. App. Div. 1984).
60. http://www.apta.org/governance/HOD/policies/HoDPolicies/Section_I/ETHICS/ HOD_06001223.
61. 780 So. 2d 478 (2001).
62. 527 N.Y.S.2d 937 (N.Y. App. Div. 1988).
63. http://www.aapa.org/gandp/ethical-guidelines.pdf.
64. http://www.apa.org/ethics/.
65. Loomis v. Board of Psychologist Exam'rs, 954 P.2d 839 (1998).
66. http://www.apa.org/ethics/.
67. 725 P.2d 400 (Or. Ct. App. 1986).
68. Michaels v. Gordon, 439 S.E.2d 722 (Ga. Ct. App. 1993).
69. http://www.iit.edu/departments/csep/PublicWWW/codes/coe/aarc-d.html.
70. http://www.iit.edu/departments/csep/PublicWWW/codes/coe/American_Registry_of_ Radiologic_Technologists_0101.html.
71. 490 N.W.2d 856 (Iowa Ct. App. 1992).

chapter ten

Physicians' Ethical and Legal Issues

LEARNING OBJECTIVES

The reader upon completion of this chapter will be able to:

- Understand how ethics and the law impact on physicians.

- Identify the variety and complexity of patient care issues that physicians face daily.

- Describe how practicing one's professional code of ethics can assist in resolving the day-to-day issues that arise during the care of patients.

INTRODUCTION

The Hippocratic Oath[1]

I SWEAR by Apollo the physician, and Aesculapius, and Health, and All-heal, and all the gods and goddesses, that, according to my ability and judgment, I will keep this Oath and this stipulation—to reckon him who taught me this Art equally dear to me as my parents, to share my substance with him, and relieve his necessities if required; to look upon his offspring in the same footing as my own brothers, and to teach them this art, if they shall wish to learn it, without fee or stipulation; and that by precept, lecture, and every other mode of instruction, I will impart a knowledge of the Art to my own sons, and those of my teachers, and to disciples bound by a stipulation and oath according to the law of medicine, but to none others. I will follow that system of regimen which, according to my ability and judgment, I consider for the benefit of my patients, and abstain from whatever is deleterious and mischievous. I will give no deadly medicine to any one if asked, nor suggest any such counsel; and in like manner I will not give to a woman a pessary to produce abortion. With purity and with holiness I will pass my life and practice my Art. I will not cut persons laboring under the stone, but will leave this to be done by men who are practitioners of this work. Into whatever houses I enter, I will go into them for the benefit of the sick, and will abstain from every voluntary act of mischief and corruption; and, further from the seduction of females or males, of freemen and slaves. Whatever, in connection with my professional practice or not, in connection with it, I see or hear, in the life of men, which ought not to be spoken of abroad, I will not divulge, as reckoning that all such should be kept secret. While I continue to keep this Oath unviolated, may it be granted to me to enjoy life and the practice of the art, respected by all men, in all times! But should I trespass and violate this Oath, may the reverse be my lot!

PRINCIPLES OF MEDICAL ETHICS

The medical profession has long subscribed to a body of ethical statements developed primarily for the benefit of the patient. As a member of this profession, a physician must recognize responsibility to patients first and foremost, as well as to society, to other health professionals, and to self. The following principles adopted by the American Medical Association are not laws, but standards of conduct that define the essentials of honorable behavior for the physician.

Code of Medical Ethics

I. A physician shall be dedicated to providing competent medical care, with compassion and respect for human dignity and rights.

II. A physician shall uphold the standards of professionalism, be honest in all professional interactions, and strive to report physicians deficient in character or competence, or engaging in fraud or deception, to appropriate entities.

III. A physician shall respect the law and also recognize a responsibility to seek changes in those requirements which are contrary to the best interests of the patient.

IV. A physician shall respect the rights of patients, colleagues, and other health professionals, and shall safeguard patient confidences and privacy within the constraints of the law.

V. A physician shall continue to study, apply, and advance scientific knowledge; maintain a commitment to medical education; make relevant information available to patients, colleagues, and the public; obtain consultation; and use the talents of other health professionals when indicated.

VI. A physician shall, in the provision of appropriate patient care, except in emergencies, be free to choose whom to serve, with whom to associate, and the environment in which to provide medical care.

VII. A physician shall recognize a responsibility to participate in activities contributing to the improvement of the community and the betterment of public health.

VIII. A physician shall, while caring for a patient, regard responsibility to the patient as paramount.

IX. A physician shall support access to medical care for all people.

Source: Code of Medical Ethics, © 2001, American Medical Association.

Compassion

Compassion is a moral value expected of all caregivers. Those who lack compassion have a weakness in their moral character.

CASE: WHATEVER HAPPENED TO COMPASSION?

Mrs. Smith arranged for an appointment to see Dr. Mean, a rheumatologist, who was a specialist in her particular disease process, "systemic scleroderma." After scheduling her appointment, Mrs. Smith was asked to have her medical records faxed to Mean's office prior to her scheduled appointment on March 27. Two days prior to her scheduled appointment with Mean, Mrs. Smith called Mean's office to confirm that her records had arrived. She was told at that time that she was on Mean's calendar for March 23, not March 27. She missed her appointment by two days. Mrs. Smith had waited two months for this date and her illness had gotten progressively worse. Mrs. Smith, desperate for help, pleaded with the scheduler to reschedule her as soon as possible. The scheduler explained to Mrs.

Smith that Mean was a busy physician and that she cannot schedule a new appointment until April 27, a month later.

Ethical and Legal Issues

1. Describe how Dr. Mean violated the professional code of ethics for a physician.
2. What role, if any, should a hospital ethics committee play in addressing Dr. Mean's insensitivity to Mrs. Smith's needs? Explain your answer. ▪

CREDENTIALING PROFESSIONALS

Credentialing is a process for validating the background and assessing the qualifications of health care professionals to provide health care services in an organization. The process is an objective evaluation of a professional's current licensure, training, or experience; competence; and ability to perform the services or procedures requested. Credentialing occurs during both the initial appointment and reappointment. The process may include granting and review of specific clinical privileges. Privileges are authorizations granted by the governing body of an institution to provide specific health care services. The granting of privileges is based on a person's license, education, training, experience, and competence.

The governing body is ultimately responsible for the selection of the organization's professional staff and the delineation of clinical privileges. The duty to select members of the medical staff is legally vested in the governing body charged with managing the organization. Although cognizant of the importance of medical staff membership, the governing body must meet its obligation to maintain standards of good medical practice in dealing with matters of staff appointment, credentialing, and the disciplining of physicians for such things as disruptive behavior, incompetence, psychological problems, criminal actions, and substance abuse.

Appointment to the medical staff and medical staff privileges should be granted only after there has been a thorough investigation of the applicant. The delineation of clinical privileges should be discipline-specific and based on appropriate predetermined criteria that adhere to national standards.

A physician's right to practice medicine is subject to the licensing laws contained in the statutes of the state in which the physician resides. The right to practice medicine is not a vested right but is a condition of a right subordinate to the police power of the state to protect and preserve public health. Although a state has power to regulate the practice of medicine for the benefit of the public health and welfare, this power is restricted. Regulations must be reasonably related to the public health and welfare and must not amount to arbitrary or unreasonable interference with the right to practice one's profession.

HOSPITAL'S DUTY TO ENSURE COMPETENCY

Hospitals have a responsibility to take reasonable steps to ensure that physicians using hospital facilities are qualified for the privileges granted. Failure to properly screen a medical staff applicant's credentials can lead to liability for injuries suffered by patients as a result of that omission. Hospitals must adhere to procedures established under both its own bylaws and state statutes. The measure of quality and the degree of quality control exercised in a hospital are the direct responsibilities of the medical staff. Hospital supervision of the manner of appointment of physicians to its staff is mandatory, not optional.

Masquerading as a Physician

An action was brought against Canton (who was masquerading as a physician, Dr. LaBella), a hospital, and others in *Insinga v. LaBella*[2] for the wrongful death of a 68-year-old woman whom Canton had admitted. The patient died while she was in the hospital. Canton was found to be a fugitive from justice in Canada where he was under indictment for the manufacture and sale of illegal drugs. He fraudulently obtained a medical license from the state of Florida and staff privileges at the hospital by using the name of LaBella, a deceased physician. Canton was extradited to Canada without being served process. The U.S. District Court for the Southern District of Florida directed a verdict in favor of the hospital. On appeal, the Florida Supreme Court held that the corporate negligence doctrine imposes on hospitals an implied duty to patients to select competent physicians who, although they are independent practitioners, would be providing in-hospital care to their patients through staff privileges. Hospitals are in the best position to protect their patients and consequently have an independent duty to select competent independent physicians.

PHYSICIAN SUPERVISION AND MONITORING

The medical staff is responsible to the governing body for the quality of care rendered by members of the medical staff. The landmark decision in this area occurred in *Darling v. Charleston Community Memorial Hospital*,[3] in which it was decided that the hospital's governing body had a duty to establish a mechanism for the medical staff to evaluate, counsel, and when necessary take action against an unreasonable risk of harm to a patient arising from the patient's treatment by a physician. Physician monitoring is best accomplished through a system of peer review. Most states provide statutory protection from liability for peer review activities when they are conducted in a reasonable manner and without malice.

Standards of Ethics and Moral Commitment

A physician received a letter from a hospital informing him that his clinical privileges at the hospital had been summarily suspended. The medical executive committee reviewed the suspension and recommended that it be upheld. The hospital board ultimately revoked the physician's staff privileges. The physician received a hearing before a fair hearing panel, which recommended that he be reinstated. The board, however, upheld the revocation.

The physician alleged, among other things, wrongful termination and intentional infliction of emotional distress. The defendants argued that the courts do not have jurisdiction to review staffing decisions made by private, nonprofit hospitals.

The Court of Civil Appeals of Oklahoma, Division II, found that judicial tribunals are not equipped to review the action of hospital boards in selecting or refusing to appoint physicians to their medical staffs. The authorities of hospitals endeavor to serve in the best possible manner the sick and the afflicted. Not all professionals have identical ability, competence, experience, character, and standards of ethics. The mere fact that a physician is licensed to practice a profession does not justify any inference beyond the conclusion that a physician has met the minimum requirements for that purpose. Without regard to the absence of any legal liability, the hospital in granting a physician privileges to practice in its facilities extends a moral or official approval to him in the eyes of the public. Not all professionals have a personality that enables them to work in harmony with others, and to inspire confidence in their peers and in patients. Courts should not substitute their evaluation in such matters. It is the board, not the court, that is charged with the responsibility of providing a competent staff of physicians. The board has chosen to rely on the advice of its medical staff, and the court cannot surrogate for the medical staff in executing this responsibility. Human lives are at stake, and the board must be given discretion in its selection so that it can have confidence in the competence and moral commitment of its staff.[4]

Disruptive Physicians

Disruptive physicians can have a negative impact on an organization's staff, ultimately affecting the quality of patient care. Having the right policies in place as they relate to "conflict resolution" is imperative for an effective working environment. Criteria other than academic credentials (e.g., a physician's ability to work with others) should be considered before granting medical staff privileges. This factor was considered by the court in *Ladenheim v. Union County Hospital District*,[5] which held that the physician's inability to work with other members of the staff was in itself sufficient grounds to deny him staff privileges. The physician's record was replete with evidence of his inability to work effectively with other members of the hospital staff. As stated in *Huffaker v. Bailey*,[6] most other courts have found that the ability to work smoothly with others is reasonably related to the objective of ensuring patient welfare. The conclusion seems justified because health care professionals frequently are required to work together or in teams. A staff member who, because of personality characteristics or other problems, is incapable of getting along with others could severely hinder the effective treatment of patients. A physician's demonstrated lack of ability to work with others in the hospital setting is sufficient to support the denial of his application for admission to the medical staff.

HONORING A PATIENT'S RIGHT TO AUTONOMY

Where there are two or more medically acceptable treatment approaches to a particular medical problem, the informed consent doctrine, medical ethics, and the standard of care all provide that a competent patient has the absolute right to select from among these treatment options after being informed of the relative risks and benefits of each approach. Basic to the informed consent doctrine is that a physician has a legal, ethical, and moral duty to respect patient autonomy and to provide only authorized medical treatment. It is inappropriate for physicians to pursue a treatment alternative other than the one to which their patient has given consent. This means that unless the patient consents to the physician's recommended treatment approach, the physician may not proceed with that approach even if the physician personally believes the recommended approach to be in the patient's best interests.[7]

ABANDONMENT

Physicians have both a legal and ethical obligation to attend to their patients' needs. Physicians licensed in Illinois, for example, are specifically prohibited from abandoning their patients.[8] Further, the American Medical Association's Council on Ethical and Judicial Affairs mandates that "once having undertaken a case, the physician should not neglect the patient."[9]

The relationship between a physician and a patient, once established, continues until it is ended by the mutual consent of the parties, the patient's dismissal of the physician, the physician's withdrawal from the case, or the fact that the physician's services are no longer required. A physician who decides to withdraw his or her services must provide the patient with reasonable notice so that the services of another physician can be obtained. Premature termination of treatment is often the subject of a legal action for *abandonment*, the unilateral termination of a physician–patient relationship by the physician without notice to the patient. The following elements must be established in order for a patient to recover damages for abandonment:

- Medical care was unreasonably discontinued.
- The discontinuance of medical care was against the patient's will. Termination of the physician–patient relationship must have been brought

about by a unilateral act of the physician. There can be no issue of abandonment if the relationship is terminated by mutual consent or by dismissal of the physician by the patient.

- The physician failed to arrange for care by another physician. Refusal by a physician to enter into a physician–patient relationship by failing to respond to a call or render treatment is not considered a case of abandonment. A plaintiff will not recover for damages unless he or she can show that a physician–patient relationship had been established.
- Foresight indicated that discontinuance might result in physical harm.
- Actual harm was suffered by the patient.

Abandonment and the Hippocratic Oath

Scripps is a group medical practice governed by a group of physicians who represent Scripps's physicians. The governing physicians established a policy to terminate further medical care for all patients and their families upon the receipt of an intent to sue letter. However, Scripps would not terminate care for a patient unless it determined that another medical care system could duplicate the services Scripps had been providing and the transfer would not jeopardize the patient's care given his or her current medical state.

Scripps initiated this policy because a lawsuit compromises the physician–patient relationship, thereby potentially compromising the care rendered to the patient. Further, patient litigants' sense of what is important to communicate to other Scripps physicians could be colored by a lawsuit, making it difficult for physicians to determine what is true and unbiased. Patients may also believe that other Scripps physicians will not give them balanced care. For example, a patient may believe that a physician who does not return a telephone call in a timely manner is punishing the patient. Continuing the physician–patient relationship might also put a physician in the awkward position of testifying against a colleague.

Patricia Thompson was in a serious accident. At the time, Scripps provided medical care to the Thompsons through their health insurance provider, Health Net. Alleging negligent treatment of Patricia's broken clavicle, the Thompsons filed a medical malpractice claim against Dr. Thorne and Dr. Carpenter, both of whom were affiliated with Scripps. At the time the malpractice action was filed, Patricia was no longer being treated by Thorne and Carpenter, but was being treated by other Scripps physicians: Drs. Botte and Froenke for the broken clavicle, and Dr. Harkey for endometriosis.

Binford, a Scripps employee, sent a letter to the Thompsons notifying them that they had been notified of the legal action they had taken against the group. Because of the legal action, the Scripps Clinic requested that Health Net immediately terminate the Thompsons with the Scripps Clinic and transfer their membership to another medical group. The letter advised the Thompsons to contact Health Net's Member Services for assistance in selecting a new medical group in their area. The Thompsons were asked to transition to a new group by July 1, 2000. They were told that in the interim, the Urgent Care Center at the Torrey Pines campus was open from 7:00 AM to 10:00 PM daily and the Urgent Care Center at Rancho Bernardo was open from 9:00 AM to 9:00 PM for their urgent/emergent needs.

When Patricia received Bindford's letter, she immediately requested Health Net to reassign the couple to a new medical group. Health Net transferred the Thompsons to University of California, San Diego Medical Group, effective July 1, 2000. As the result of Scripps's actions, Patricia had to cancel a follow-up visit with Dr. Harkey that had been scheduled near the end of June even though Patricia was still suffering severe pain and bleeding. Before Patricia could be referred to a new gynecologist at UCSD, she had to schedule a visit with her new primary care physician and receive authorization. Patricia's care was also delayed until UCSD received her medical records from Scripps.

The Thompsons sued Scripps and Binford for damages arising from the termination of care.

It has long been the law in California that a physician can lawfully abandon a patient only after due notice and an ample opportunity afforded to secure the presence of other medical attendant. In the absence of the patient's consent, the physician must notify the patient he is withdrawing and allow ample opportunity to secure the presence of another physician.

Scripps contends that because it gave adequate notice to the Thompsons and because Health Net transferred them to UCSD Medical Group, the Thompsons did not raise a triable issue of fact as to breach. The court disagreed. There was a two-week hiatus between the time Scripps denied the Thompsons access to its physicians for nonemergency services and the time the Thompsons were assigned to UCSD. The Thompsons raised a triable issue of fact as to whether they were given ample time to retain other physicians.

It is of interest that the Hippocratic oath provides, "The regimen I adopt shall be for the benefit of my patients according to my ability and judgment, and not for their hurt or for any wrong."[10]

AGGRAVATION OF A PREEXISTING CONDITION

Aggravation of a preexisting condition through negligence may cause a physician to be liable for malpractice. If the original injury is aggravated, liability will be imposed only for the aggravation, rather than for both the original injury and its aggravation.

Damages were awarded in *Argus v. Scheppegrell*[11] for the wrongful death of a teenage patient with a preexisting drug addiction. It was determined that the physician had wrongfully supplied the patient with prescriptions for controlled substances in excessive amounts, with the result that the patient's preexisting drug addiction had worsened, causing her death from a drug overdose. The Louisiana Court of Appeal held that the suffering of the patient caused by drug addiction and deterioration of her mental and physical condition warranted an award of $175,000. Damages of $120,000 were to be awarded for the wrongful death claims of the parents, who not only suffered during their daughter's drug addiction caused by the physician in wrongfully supplying the prescription, but who also were forced to endure the torment of their daughter's slow death in the hospital.

ALTERNATIVE PROCEDURES: TWO SCHOOLS OF THOUGHT

The potential for liability affects the choice of treatment a physician will follow in treating his or her patient. Use of unprecedented procedures that create an untoward result may cause a physician to be found negligent even though due care was followed. A physician will not be held liable for exercising his or her judgment in applying a course of treatment supported by a reputable and respected body of medical experts even if another body of expert medical opinion would favor a different course of treatment. The *two schools of thought doctrine* is only applicable in medical malpractice cases in which there is more than one method of accepted treatment for a patient's disease or injury. Under this doctrine, a physician will not be liable for medical malpractice if he or she follows a course of treatment supported by reputable, respected, and reasonable medical experts.

A physician's efforts do not constitute negligence simply because they were unsuccessful in a particular case. A physician cannot be required to guarantee the results of his or her treatment. *The mere fact that an adverse result may occur following treatment is not in and of itself evidence of professional negligence.* Innovation in the treatment for minor ailments more likely would be questioned than would innovation in the treatment of a major disease. A physician treating a patient with a new procedure for an ordinary cold runs a greater risk of liability than does a physician treating a patient with a new procedure for an acute and painful disease.

It is assumed by law that it is unreasonable for two physicians to have differing opinions on the proper method of treating injuries or illnesses. If there is reason for the difference, the courts have held that neither side can be proven erroneous by the "proof" of the other.

CONFIDENTIAL COMMUNICATIONS

Respect for the privacy of medical information is a central feature of the physician–patient relationship. Under the Hippocratic Oath and modern principles of medical ethics derived from it, physicians are ethically bound to maintain patient confidences.

The physician–patient privilege imposes on a physician an obligation to maintain the confidentiality of each patient's communications. This obligation applies to all health care professionals. An exception to the rule of confidentiality of patient communications is the implied right to make necessary information available to others involved in the patient's care. Information received by a physician in a confidential capacity relating to a patient's health should not be disclosed without the patient's consent. Disclosure may be made under compelling circumstances (e.g., suspected child abuse) to a person with a legitimate interest in the patient's health.

The Code of Medical Ethics both requires the confidentiality of information obtained by a physician in plaintiff's position and the reporting of physicians who violate that confidentiality. Section 6530 (23) of the New York State Education Law defines professional misconduct as the "revealing of personally identifiable facts, data or information obtained in a professional capacity without the consent of the patient." The State of New York Department of Health has set forth a penalty of censure, reprimand, suspension of license, revocation of license, annulment of license, limitation on further license or fine for a person found guilty of professional misconduct (Public Health Law § 230-a), which includes revealing patient information without consent or failing to maintain accurate information. The Department of Health is responsible for maintaining standards and ethics of the profession and for enforcing those standards. In addition, the Principles of Medical Ethics of the American Medical Association states that physicians, including physicians employed by industry, have an ethical and legal duty to protect patient confidentiality.[12]

FALSIFICATION OF RECORDS

The intentional alteration, falsification, or destruction of medical records to avoid liability for one's medical negligence is generally sufficient to show actual malice, and punitive damages may be awarded whether or not the act of altering, falsifying, or destroying records directly causes compensable harm. The evidence in *Dimora v. Cleveland Clinic Foundation*[13] had showed that the patient had fallen and broken five or six ribs. Yet upon examination, the physician noted in the progress notes that the patient was smiling and laughing pleasantly, exhibiting no pain upon deep palpation of the area. Other testimony indicated that she was in pain and crying. This discrepancy between the written progress notes and the testimony of the witnesses who observed the patient was sufficient to raise a question of fact as to the possible falsification of documents by the physician to minimize the nature of the incident and the injury of the patient due to the possible negligence of the hospital personnel. The testimony of the witnesses, if believed, would have been sufficient to show that the physician falsified the record or intentionally reported the incident inaccurately in order to avoid liability for the negligent care of the patient.

The intentional alteration or destruction of medical records to avoid liability for medical negligence is sufficient to show actual malice, and punitive damages may be awarded whether or not the act of altering, falsifying, or destroying records directly causes compensable harm. Tampering with records sends the wrong signal to jurors and can shatter one's credibility. Altered records can create a presumption of negligence. The court in *Matter of Jascalevich*[14] held that "a physician's duty to a patient cannot but encompass his affirmative obligation to maintain the integrity, accuracy, truth and reliability of the patient's medical record. His obligation in this regard is no less compelling than his duties respecting diagnosis and treatment of the patient since the medical community must, of necessity, be able to rely on those records in the continuing and future care of that patient. Obviously, the rendering of that care is prejudiced by anything in those records which is false, misleading or inaccurate. A deliberate falsification by a physician of his patient's medical record, to protect his own interests at the expense of his patient's, is regarded as gross malpractice endangering the health or life of his patient."[15]

FAILURE TO RESPOND: EMERGENCY DEPARTMENT CALL

Physicians on call for a specific service in an emergency department are expected to respond to requests for emergency assistance when considered necessary. Failure to respond is grounds for negligence should a patient suffer injury as a result of no emergency assistance.

FAILURE TO PROVIDE INFORMED CONSENT

The doctrine of informed consent is a theory of professional liability independent from malpractice. A physician's duty to disclose known and existing dangers associated with a proposed course of treatment is imposed by law. The patient in *Leggett v. Kumar*[16] was awarded $675,000 for pain and disfigurement resulting from a mastectomy procedure. The physician in this case failed to advise the patient of treatment alternatives. He also failed to perform the surgery properly.

It is the physician's role to provide the necessary medical facts and the patient's role to make a subjective decision concerning treatment based on his or her understanding of those facts. Before subjecting a patient to a course of treatment, the physician has a duty to disclose information that will enable the patient to evaluate options available and the risks attendant to a specific procedure. A failure to disclose any known and existing risks of proposed treatment when such risks might affect a patient's decision to forgo treatment constitutes a *prima facie* violation of a physician's duty to disclose. If a patient can establish that a physician withheld information concerning the inherent and potential hazards of a proposed treatment, consent is abrogated. Consent for a medical procedure may be withdrawn at any time before the act consented to is accomplished.

FAILURE TO READ NURSES' NOTES

On October 17, the medical record indicated that Todd's sternotomy wound and the mid-lower left leg incision were reddened and his temperature was 99.6°. Dr. Sauls did not commonly read the nurses' notes but instead preferred to rely on his own observations of the patient. In his October 18 notes, he indicated that there was no drainage. The nurses' notes, however, show that there was drainage at the chest tube site. Contrary to the medical records showing that Todd had a temperature of 101.2°, Sauls noted that the patient was afebrile.

On October 19, Sauls noted that Todd's wounds were improving and he did not have a fever. Nurses' notes indicated redness at the surgical wounds and a temperature of 100°. No white blood count had been ordered. Again on October 20, the nurses' notes indicated a wound redness and a temperature of 100.8°. No wound culture had yet been ordered. Dr. Kamil, one of Todd's treating physicians, noted that Todd's nutritional status needed to be seriously confronted and suggested that Sauls consider supplemental feeding. Despite this, no follow-up to his recommendation appears and the record is void of any action by Sauls to obtain a nutritional consult.

Todd was transferred to the intensive care unit on October 21 because he was gravely ill with profoundly depressed ventricular function. The following day the nurses' notes describe the chest tube site as draining foul-smelling bloody purulence. The patient's temperature was recorded to have reached 100.6°. This is the first time that Sauls had the test tube site cultured. On October 23, the culture report from the laboratory indicated a staph infection, and Todd was started on antibiotics for treatment of the infection.

On October 25, at the request of family, Todd was transferred to St. Luke's Hospital. At St. Luke's, Dr. Leatherman, an internist and invasive cardiologist, treated Todd. Dr. Zeluff, an infectious disease specialist, examined Todd's surgical wounds and prescribed antibiotic treatment. Upon admission to St. Luke's, every one of Todd's surgical wounds was infected. Despite the care given at St. Luke's, Todd died on November 2, 1988. The family brought a malpractice suit against the surgeon. The District Court entered judgment on a jury verdict for the defendant, and the plaintiff appealed claiming the surgeon breached his duty of care owed to the patient by failing to: (1) aggressively treat the surgical wound infections; (2) read the nurses' observations of infections; and (3) provide adequate nourishment, allowing the patient's body weight to rapidly waste away.

Sauls committed medical malpractice when he breached the standard of care he owed to Todd. Todd was effectively ineligible for a heart transplant, which was his only chance of survival due to the infections and malnourishment caused by Sauls' malpractice. Sauls' testimony convinced the Louisiana Court of Appeals that he failed to aggressively treat the surgical wound infections, that he chose not to take advantage of the nurses' observations of infection, and that he allowed Todd's body weight to waste away, knowing that extreme vigilance was required because of Todd's already severely impaired heart.

In cases where a patient has died, the plaintiff need not demonstrate that the patient would have survived if properly treated. Rather, he need only prove that the patient had a chance of survival and that his chance of survival was lost as a result of the defendant/physician's negligence. The defendant/physician's conduct must increase the risk of a patient's harm to the extent of being a substantial factor in causing the result, but need not be the only cause. Sauls' medical malpractice exacerbated an already critical condition and "deprived Mr. Todd of a chance of survival."

FAILURE TO SEEK CONSULTATION

When a practitioner determines or should have determined that a patient's ailment is beyond his or her scope of knowledge or technical skill, or ability or capacity to treat with a likelihood of reasonable success, he or she is under a duty to disclose such determination to the patient. The patient should be advised of the necessity of other or different treatments.

A physician has a duty to consult and/or refer a patient whom he or she knows or should know needs referral to a physician familiar with and clinically capable to treat the patient's particular ailments. Whether the failure to refer constitutes negligence depends on whether referral is demanded by accepted standards of practice. To recover damages, the plaintiff must show that the physician deviated from the standard of care and that the failure to refer resulted in injury.

The California Court of Appeals found that expert testimony is not necessary where good medical practice would require a general physician to suggest a specialist's consultation.[17] The court ruled that because specialists were called in after the patient's condition grew worse, it is reasonable to assume that they could have been called in sooner. The jury was instructed by the court that a general practitioner has a duty to suggest calling in a specialist if a reasonably prudent general practitioner would do so under similar circumstances.

A physician is in a position of trust, and it is his or her duty to act in good faith. If a preferred treatment in a given situation is outside a physician's field of expertise, it is his or her duty to advise the patient. Failure to do so could constitute a breach of duty. Today, with the rapid methods of transportation and easy means of communication, the duty of a physician is not fulfilled merely by using the means at hand in a particular area of practice.

FAILURE TO OBTAIN ADEQUATE HISTORY AND PHYSICAL

Failure to obtain an adequate family history and perform an adequate physical examination violates a standard of care owed to the patient. In *Foley v. Bishop Clarkson Memorial Hospital*,[18] the spouse sued the hospital for the death of his wife. During her pregnancy, the patient was under the care of a private physician. She gave birth in the hospital on August 20, 1964, and died the following day. During July and August, her physician treated her for a sore throat. Several days after her death, one of her children was treated in the hospital for a strep throat infection. There was no evidence in the hospital record that the patient had complained about a sore throat while in the hospital. The hospital rules required a history and physical examination to be written promptly (within 24 hours of admission). No history had been taken, although the patient had been examined several times in regard to the progress of her labor. The trial judge directed a verdict in favor of the hospital. On appeal, the appellate court held that the case should have been submitted to the jury for determination. A jury might reasonably have inferred that if the patient's condition had been treated properly, the infection could have been combated successfully and her life saved. It also might have been reasonably inferred that if a history had been taken promptly when she was admitted to the hospital, the throat condition would have been discovered and hospital personnel alerted to watch for possible complications of the nature that later developed. Quite possibly, this attention also would have helped in diagnosing the patient's condition, especially if it had been apparent that she had been exposed to a strep throat infection. The court held that a hospital must guard not only against known physical and mental conditions of patients, but also against conditions that reasonable care should have uncovered.

CASE: DOCUMENTATION ISSUES

Smith was admitted to Community Hospital for surgery. The hospital's policy requires that history and physical examinations be completed prior to patients undergoing surgery. Smith's attending physician did not complete the form. He simply drew a diagonal line from the top right to the bottom left of the history and physical form, indicating that the patient had no history of/or current disease processes.

The patient's nurse, per hospital policy, completed a nursing assessment. The nurse documented on the patient admission assessment form that the patient had a history of transient ischemic attacks, diabetes, and hypothyroidism.

The anesthesiologist did not perform an anesthesia assessment prior to surgery. General anesthesia was administered without knowing the patient's previous experiences, if any, with anesthesia.

Failure of the attending physician to complete an appropriate history and physical (h & p) examination and of the anesthesiologist to perform a pre-anesthesia assessment placed the patient's life and health at risk. The physician did not complete the h & p. He merely went through the motions of completing an h & p merely because it was mandated that the patient have an h & p in his medical record prior to surgery.

Ethical and Legal Issues

1. Discuss the ethical issues and principles violated in this case.
2. What are the potential legal issues of concern in this case?
3. Discuss what actions the organization could take to improve the quality of h & p documentation. ■

INFECTION CONTROL ISSUES

Nosocomial, hospital-acquired infections are a leading cause of injury and unnecessary deaths. Such infections have been linked to unsanitary conditions in the environment and poor practices (e.g., hand-washing technique). The Centers for Disease Control and Prevention estimates that nearly two million patients annually get a hospital-acquired infection. There are estimates that as many as 90,000 of these patients die annually as a result of these infections.[19]

A district court of appeals held in *Gill v. Hartford Accident & Indemnity Co.*[20] that the physician who performed surgery on a patient in the same room as the plaintiff should have known that the infection the patient had was highly contagious. The failure of the physician to undertake steps to prevent the spread of the infection to the plaintiff and his failure to warn the plaintiff led the court to find that hospital authorities and the plaintiff's physician caused an unreasonable increase in the risk of injury. As a result, the plaintiff suffered injuries causally related to the negligence of the defendant.

MEDICATIONS

With thousands of brand and generic drugs in use, it is no surprise that medication error is one of the leading causes of patient injuries. Physicians should encourage the limited and judicious use of all medications and should document periodically the reason for their continuation. They should be alert to any contraindications and incompatibilities among prescription, over-the-counter drugs, and herbal supplements. The negligent administration of medications is often due to the following errors: the wrong medication, the wrong patient, the wrong dose, the wrong route, and/or the wrong site.

Abuse of Controlled Substances

The Board of Regents in *Moyo v. Ambach*[21] determined that a physician had prescribed methaqualone fraudulently and with gross negligence to 20 patients. The Board of Regents found that the physician did not prescribe methaqualone in good faith or for sound medical reasons. His abuse in prescribing controlled substances constituted the fraudulent practice of medicine. Expert testimony established that it was common knowledge in the medical community that methaqualone was a widely abused and addictive drug. Methaqualone should not have been used for insomnia without first trying other means of treatment. On appeal, the court found that there was sufficient evidence to support the board's finding.

MISDIAGNOSIS

Misdiagnosis is the most frequently cited injury event in malpractice suits against physicians. Although diagnosis is a medical art and not an exact science, early detection can be critical to a patient's recovery. Misdiagnosis may involve the diagnosis and treatment of a disease different from that which the patient actually suffers or the diagnosis and treatment of a disease that the patient does not have. Misdiagnosis in and of itself will not necessarily impose liability on a physician, unless deviation from the accepted standard of care and injury can be established.

In *Ramberg v. Morgan*,[22] a police department physician at the scene of an accident examined an unconscious man who had been struck by an automobile. The physician concluded that the patient's insensibility was a result of alcohol intoxication, not the accident, and ordered the police to remove him to jail instead of the hospital. The man, to the physician's knowledge, remained semiconscious for several days and finally was taken from the cell to the hospital at the insistence of his family. The patient subsequently died, and the autopsy revealed massive skull fractures. The court found that any physician should reasonably anticipate the presence of head injuries when a person is struck by a car. Failure to refer an accident victim to another physician or a hospital is actionable neglect of the physician's duty. Although a physician does not ensure the correctness of the diagnosis or treatment, a patient is entitled to such thorough and careful examination as his or her condition and attending circumstances permit, with such diligence and methods of diagnosis as usually are approved and practiced by medical people of ordinary or average learning, judgment, and skill in the community or similar localities.

OBSTETRICS AND GYNECOLOGY

One of the most vulnerable medical specialties with significant risk exposure to malpractice suits is obstetrics/gynecology. Obstetrical negligence claims often stem from errors in physician judgment, whereas gynecologic claims are often the result of inadequate technical performance. The following cases illustrate why the risks are high.

The plaintiff in *Lucchesi v. Stimmell*[23] brought an action against a physician for intentional infliction of emotional distress, claiming that the physician had failed to be present during unsuccessful attempts to deliver her premature fetus and that he thereafter had failed to disclose to her that the fetus was decapitated during attempts to achieve delivery by pulling on the hip area to free the head. The judge instructed the jury that it could conclude that the physician had been guilty of extreme and outrageous conduct for staying at home and leaving the delivery in the hands of a first-year intern and a third-year resident, neither of whom was experienced in breech deliveries.

PHYSICIAN–PATIENT RELATIONSHIP

The physician–patient relationship entails special obligations for the physician to serve the patient's health and well-being. The physician's primary commitment must always be the patient's best welfare and best interests, whether the physician is preventing or treating illness or helping the patient to cope with illness, disability, and death. It has long been recognized that the health and well-being of the patient depends upon a collaborative effort between the physician and the patient. The physician must support the dignity of all persons and respect their uniqueness.

The interests of the patient should always be promoted regardless of financial arrangements, the health care setting, and patient characteristics such as decision-making capacity or social status.

At the beginning of a physician–patient relationship, the physician must understand the patient's complaints, underlying feelings, and goals and expectations. The physician must be professionally competent, act responsively, and treat the patient with compassion and respect. The patient should understand prior to consenting to recommended treatments.

Patients enter the physician–patient relationship assuming that information acquired by the physician will be held in confidence and that the physician will not disclose confidential communications or information related to treatment unless the patient consents or disclosure is required by law. Mutual trust and confidence are essential to the physician–patient relationship, and from these elements flow the physician's obligations to fully inform the patient of his or her condition, to continue to provide medical care after the physician–patient relationship has been established, to refer the patient to a specialist if necessary, and to obtain the patient's informed consent to the medical treatment proposed.

CHAPTER REVIEW

1. The medical profession has long subscribed to a body of ethical statements developed primarily for the benefit of the patient. As a member of this profession, a physician must recognize responsibility to patients first and foremost, as well as to society, to other health professionals, and to self.

2. Credentialing is a process for validating the background and assessing the qualifications of health care professionals to provide health care services in an organization.

3. Physicians have a legal, ethical, and moral duty to respect patient autonomy and to provide only authorized medical treatment. It is inappropriate for physicians to pursue a treatment alternative other than the one to which their patient has given consent.

4. The American Medical Association's Council on Ethical and Judicial Affairs mandates that "once having undertaken a case, the physician should not neglect the patient." The relationship between a physician and a patient, once established, continues until it is ended by the mutual consent of the parties, the patient's dismissal of the physician,

the physician's withdrawal from the case, or the fact that the physician's services are no longer required.

5. A physician's efforts do not constitute negligence simply because they were unsuccessful in a particular case. A physician cannot be required to guarantee the results of his or her treatment.

6. Respect for the privacy of medical information is a central feature of the physician–patient relationship.

7. A deliberate falsification by a physician of his patient's medical record to protect his own interests at the expense of his patient's is regarded as gross malpractice endangering the health or life of his patient.

8. Physicians can be held liable for failure to order diagnostic tests, read nurses' notes, seek consultation, obtain a second opinion, obtain an adequate family history, perform an adequate physical examination, and provide an accurate diagnosis.

REVIEW QUESTIONS

1. Describe a physician's moral responsibilities to his or her patients (e.g., privacy, informed consent).

2. Discuss the ethical and legal implications of a physician who falsifies the entries on a patient's medical record.

3. When is a physician considered to have abandoned his or her patient? What are the ethical and legal implications of abandoning a patient?

4. What are the ethical and legal implications of failing to refer a patient to a specialist?

WEB SITES

American Dental Association
www.ada.org/
American Medical Association
www.ama-assn.org/
World Medical Association
www.wma.net/e/

NOTES

1. Hippocrates, written 400 B.C., translated by Francis Adams.
2. 543 So. 2d 209 (Fla. 1989).
3. 211 N.E.2d 253 (Ill. 1965).
4. Medcalf v. Coleman, No. 98906 (2003).

5. 394 N.E.2d 770 (Ill. App. Ct. 1979).
6. 540 P.2d 1398, 1400 (Or. 1975).
7. *See* Bankert v. United States, 937 F. Supp. 1169, 1173 (D. Md. 1996).
8. Bloomington Urological Associates v. Scaglia, 686 N.E.2d 389 (1997).
9. American Medical Association Code of Medical Ethics: Current Opinions with Annotations, 8.11 (1996).
10. Scripps Clinic v. Superior Ct., 134 Cal. Rptr. 2d 101 (2003).
11. 489 So. 2d 392 (La. Ct. App. 1986).
12. Horn v. New York Times, 100 N.Y.2d 85 (2003).
13. 683 N.E.2d 1175 (Ohio App. 1996).
14. 442 A.2d 635 (N.J. Super. Ct. 1982).
15. *Id.* at 644-45.
16. 570 N.E.2d 1249 (Ill. App. Ct. 1991).
17. Valentine v. Kaiser Found. Hosps., 15 Cal. Rptr. 26 (Cal. Ct. App. 1961) (dictum).
18. 173 N.W.2d 881 (Neb. 1970).
19. Burke JP. Infection Control—a problem for patient safety. NEW ENG. J. MED. 2003; 348;651-6.
20. 337 So. 2d 420 (Fla. Dist. Ct. App. 1976).
21. 523 N.Y.S.2d 645 (N.Y. App. Div. 1988).
22. 218 N.W.2d 492 (Iowa 1928).
23. 716 P.2d 1013 (Ariz. 1986).

chapter eleven

Employee Rights and Responsibilities

INTRODUCTION

This chapter prevents an overview of the rights and responsibilities of employees in the health care setting. Many of the rights and responsibilities are expressed in both federal and state laws. Health care organizations are not exempt from the impact of these laws and are required to take into account such matters as employment practices (wages, hours, and working conditions), union activity, workers' compensation laws, occupational safety and health laws, and employment discrimination laws.

EMPLOYEE RIGHTS

Employment at will does not abrogate employee rights. There are employers who treat employees as though they have no rights. Employees have experienced employers who have treated them unfairly. Many have faced discrimination involving unfair pay and benefits, wrongful termination, or any one of a host of common labor issues. There are a variety of federal and state laws that protect employee rights to be treated fairly at work. The following is a listing of but a few of the many rights that employees have.

Right to Equal Pay for Equal Work

The Equal Pay Act (EPA) of 1963 is essentially an amendment to the Federal Labor Standards Act that was passed to address wage disparities based on sex. The EPA prohibits sex discrimination in the payment of wages for women and men performing substantially equal work in the same establishment. Under the EPA, a lawsuit may be filed by the Equal Employment Opportunity Commission (EEOC) or by individuals on their own behalf. If a complainant is paid full back wages under EEOC supervision or if the EEOC takes legal action first, a private suit may not be filed.

The EPA is applicable wherever the minimum wage law is applicable and is enforced by the EEOC. The EPA requires that employees who perform equal work receive equal pay. There are situations in which wages may be unequal as long as they are based on factors other than sex, such as in the case of a formalized seniority system or a system that objectively measures earnings by the quantity or quality of production.

Right to Refuse to Participate in Care

Caregivers have a right to refuse to participate in certain aspects of patient care and treatment. This can occur when there is conflict with one's cultural, ethical, and/or religious beliefs, such as the administration of blood or blood products, participation in elective abortions, and end-of-life issues such as disconnecting a respirator. In the attempt to honor staff rights, a patient's health must not be compromised. Questionable requests not to participate in certain aspects of a patient's care should be referred to an organization's ethics committee for review and consultative advice.

CASE: RIGHT TO REFUSE TO PARTICIPATE IN ABORTIONS

Caregivers have a right to refuse to participate in abortions and can abstain from involvement in abortions as a matter of conscience, religious beliefs, or moral conviction. In a Missouri case, *Doe v. Poelker*,[1] the city was ordered to obtain the services of physicians and personnel who had no moral objections to participating in abortions. The city also was required to pay the plaintiff's attorneys' fees because of the wanton disregard of the indigent woman's rights and the continuation of a policy to disregard and/or circumvent the U.S. Supreme Court's rulings on abortion.

Ethical and Legal Issues

1. Describe the ethical issues raised in this case.
2. Should a caregiver have a right to refuse to participate in abortions? Explain your answer. ■

CASE: RIGHT TO QUESTION PATIENT'S CARE

The nurse-plaintiff in *Kirk v. Mercy Hosp. Tri-County*[2] was employed as a charge nurse with supervisory duties. A short time after one of her patients had been admitted to the hospital, the nurse diagnosed that the patient was suffering from toxic shock syndrome. The nurse believed that the physician would order antibiotics. After a period of time had passed without having received those orders from the physician, she discussed the patient's situation with the director of nursing. She was informed by the director to document and report the facts, and stay out of it.

The nurse discussed the patient's condition and lack of orders with the chief of staff. Although the chief of staff took appropriate steps to treat the patient, the patient died. After the nursing director was informed by a member of the patient's family that the plaintiff offered to obtain the medical records and was later told that the plaintiff was heard to say that the physician was "paving her way to heaven," the director terminated the plaintiff.

After her termination, the nurse received a service letter from the hospital that directed her to refrain from making any further false statements about the hospital and its staff.

The trial court entered a summary judgment for the defendant, stating that there were no triable issues of fact, and there was no public policy exception to the nurse's at-will termination. The nurse appealed.

The Missouri Court of Appeals held that the Nursing Practice Act provided a clear mandate of public policy that the nurses had a duty to provide the best possible care to patients.

Public policy clearly mandates that a nurse has an obligation to serve the best interests of patients. Therefore, if the plaintiff refused to follow her supervisor's orders to stay out of a case where the patient was dying from a lack of proper medical treatment, there would be no grounds for her discharge under the public policy exception to the employment-at-will doctrine. Pursuant to the Nursing Practice Act, the plaintiff risked discipline if she ignored improper treatment of the patient. Her persistence in attempting to get the proper treatment for the patient was her absolute duty. The hospital could not lawfully require that she stay out of a case that would have obvious injurious consequences to the patient. Public policy, as defined in case law, holds that no one can lawfully do that which tends to be injurious to the public or against the public good.

Ethical and Legal Issues

1. Describe the ethical and legal issues in this case.
2. Did the hospital violate the rights and responsibilities of the nurse? Explain your answer.
3. Would the nurse's professional code of ethics support her actions in this case? Explain your answer. ■

Right to Be Free from Sexual Harassment

Employees and staff have a right to be free from sexual harassment. Sexual harassment can be verbal or physical, and it includes a request for a sexual favor; sexual advances made as a condition of employment and unreasonably interfering with an employee's work performance, and creating an intimidating or offensive working environment. In 1980 the EEOC issued landmark sexual harassment guidelines that prohibit unwelcome sexual advances or requests that are made as a condition of employment. The guidelines also prohibit conduct that creates a hostile work environment. The U.S. Supreme Court held that a hostile work environment need not be psychologically injurious but only perceived as abusive.

Right to Suggest Changing Physician

There are circumstances in which a caregiver has a right to suggest that a patient or patient's family change their physician. The patient began losing weight and having hallucinations. A nurse documented the patient's difficulties and attempted on several occasions to call the patient's physician. The physician failed to return the nurse's calls. Because of the patient's deteriorating condition, the family contacted the nurse. After the nurse advised the patient's family as to her concerns, a member of the patient's family asked her what they should do. The nurse advised that she would reconsider their "choice of physicians." The nurse was terminated because she had advised the patient's family to consider changing physicians.

The nurse brought a lawsuit for wrongful discharge in violation of public policy. The language in the Nursing Practice Act of North Carolina and regulations of the Board of Nursing describe the practice of nursing as assessing a patient's health, which entails a responsibility to communicate, counsel, and provide accurate guidance to clients and their families. The nurse's comments that resulted in her termination were made in fulfillment of these responsibilities.

The North Carolina Court of Appeals held that the nurse stated a claim for wrongful discharge in violation of public policy. The nurse's termination for fulfilling her responsibilities as a practicing nurse violated state public policy and was a factual question for jury determination. Although there may be a right to terminate at-will employment for no reason, or for an arbitrary or irrational reason, there can be no right to terminate such employment for an unlawful reason or purpose that contravenes public policy.

Right to Be Treated with Dignity and Respect

One's dignity may be assaulted, vandalized and cruelly mocked, but it cannot be taken away unless it is surrendered

AUTHOR UNKNOWN

Each employee has the right to be treated with dignity and respect. With every right there is a corresponding duty to respect the rights of others—in this instance, the responsibility to treat others with dignity and respect.

Right to Fair Treatment in Employment

An at-will prerogative without limits could be suffered only in an anarchy, and there not for long; it certainly cannot be suffered in a society such as ours without weakening the bond of counter-balancing rights and obligations that holds such societies together.

SIDES V. DUKE HOSPITAL[3]

The common-law "employment-at-will" doctrine provides that employment is at the will of either the employer or the employee and that employment may be terminated by the employer or the employee at any time for any or no reason, unless there is a contract in place that specifies the terms and duration of employment. Historically, termination of employees for any reason was widely accepted. However, contemporary thinking does not support this concept.

> In recent years the rule that employment for an indefinite term is terminable by the employer whenever and for whatever cause he chooses without incurring liability has been the subject of considerable scholarly debate, and judicial and legislative modification. Consequently, there has been a growing trend toward a restricted application of the at-will employment rule whereby the right of an employer to discharge an at-will employee without cause is limited by either public policy considerations or an implied covenant of good faith and fair dealing.[4]

In *Sides v. Duke Hospital*, the North Carolina Court of Appeals found it to be an

> obvious and indisputable fact that in a civilized state where recipro-
> cal legal rights and duties abound, the words "at will" can never
> mean "without limit or qualification," as so much of the discussion
> and the briefs of the defendants imply; for in such a state the rights
> of each person are necessarily and inherently limited by the rights of
> others and the interests of the public. An at-will prerogative without
> limits could be suffered only in an anarchy, and there not for long; it
> certainly cannot be suffered in a society such as ours without weak-
> ening the bond of counter-balancing rights and obligations that
> holds such societies together.

• • •

> If we are to have law, those who so act against the public interest
> must be held accountable for the harm inflicted thereby; to accord
> them civil immunity would incongruously reward their lawlessness
> at the unjust expense of their innocent victims.[5]

The concept of the employment-at-will doctrine is embroiled in a combination of legislative enactments and judicial decisions. Some states have a
tendency to be more employer-oriented, such as New York, whereas others,
such as California, emerge as being much more forward thinking and in harmony with the constitutional rights of the employee.

> The employment-at-will common law doctrine is not truly applicable
> in today's society and many courts have recognized this fact. In the
> last century, the common law developed in a laissez-faire climate
> that encouraged industrial growth and improved the right of an
> employer to control his own business, including the right to fire
> without cause an employee at will. . . . The twentieth century has
> witnessed significant changes in socioeconomic values that have led
> to reassessment of the common law rule. Businesses have evolved
> from small- and medium-size firms to gigantic corporations in which
> ownership is separate from management. Formerly there was a clear
> delineation between employers, who frequently were owners of their
> own businesses, and employees. The employer in the old sense has
> been replaced by a superior in the corporate hierarchy who is him-
> self an employee.[6]

"Is it fair?" is the ultimate question that a supervisor must ask when
considering a termination. In general, bad-faith and inexplicable terminations are subject to the scrutiny of the courts. Some courts and legislative
enactments have overturned the view that employers have total discretion to

terminate workers who are not otherwise protected by collective bargaining agreements or civil service regulations. Montana legislation grants every employee the right to sue the employer for wrongful discharge. The mere fact that an employment contract is terminable at will does not give the employer an absolute right to terminate it in all cases.

Public Policy Exceptions and Employee Rights

The public policy exception to the employment-at-will doctrine provides that employees may not be terminated for reasons that are contrary to public policy. Public policy originates with legislative enactments that prohibit, for example, the discharge of employees on the basis of handicap, age, race, color, religion, sex, national origin, pregnancy, filing of safety violation complaints with various agencies (e.g., the Occupational Safety and Health Administration), or union membership. Any attempt to limit, segregate, or classify employees in any way that would tend to deprive any individual of employment opportunities on these bases is contrary to public policy.

Public policy also can arise as a result of judicial decisions that address those issues not covered by statutes, rules, and regulations. "[I]t can be said that public policy concerns what is right and just and what affects the citizens of the state collectively. It is to be found in the state's constitution and statutes and, when they are silent, in its judicial decisions."[7]

> Public policy favors the exposure of crime, and the cooperation of citizens possessing knowledge thereof is essential to effective implementation of that policy. Persons acting in good faith who have probable cause to believe crimes have been committed should not be deterred from reporting them by the fear of unfounded suits by those accused.[8]

In those instances in which state and federal laws are silent, not all courts concur with the use of judicial decisions as a means for determining public policy. A California court has determined that a public policy exception to the at-will employment doctrine must be based on constitutional or statutory provisions rather than judicial policy making.[9]

Retaliatory Discharge

There is a tendency for those in power to abuse that power through threats, abuse, intimidation, and retaliatory discharge, all of which are cause for legal action. Employees who become the targets of a vindictive supervisor often have difficulty in proving a bad-faith motive. In an effort to reduce the probability of wrongful discharge, some states, such as Connecticut,[10] Maine,[11] Michigan,[12] and Montana,[13] have enacted legislation that protects employees from terminations found to be arbitrary and capricious. The Montana Supreme Court upheld state legislation that protects workers against arbitrary discharge, while at the same time limiting the damages they can win.

> The National Labor Relations Act and other labor legislation illus-
> trate the governmental policy of preventing employers from using
> the right of discharge as a means of oppression. . . . Consistent with
> this policy, many states have recognized the need to protect employ-
> ees who are not parties to a collective bargaining agreement or other
> contract from abusive practices by the employer. . . . Those states
> have recognized a common law cause of action for employees-at-will
> who were discharged for reasons that were in some way "wrongful."
> The courts in those jurisdictions have taken various approaches:
> some recognizing the action in tort, some in contract.[14]

Dismissal of an employee shortly after a request for a grievance hearing
regarding a salary discrepancy with another employee can raise an issue of
liability for retaliatory discharge. The physician in *Jones v. Westside-Urban
Health Center*[15] was found to have established a *prima facie* case of retaliatory discharge in which the record indicated that he had been fired from the
hospital five days after his request for a grievance hearing on an alleged
salary discrepancy.

EMPLOYEE RESPONSIBILITIES

*I believe that every right implies a responsibility; every opportunity, an
obligation; every possession, a duty.*

JOHN D. ROCKEFELLER, JR.

Rights and responsibilities run parallel one to another. With every right there
is a corresponding duty to respect the rights of others. It is easy to remember
one's rights and responsibilities. The following pages describe a few of the
many responsibilities required of health care employees.

RESPONSIBILITY TO BE A PATIENT ADVOCATE

Caregivers have a responsibility to be patient advocates. Because patients are
often helpless and unable to speak for themselves, all caregivers, whether
they are volunteers or paid staff, should consider themselves as patient advocates. Many states have mandated by legislation the establishment of
ombudsman programs.

Responsibility to Be Compassionate

*How far you go in life depends on you being tender with the young,
compassionate with the aged, sympathetic with the striving and tolerant of
the weak and strong. Because someday in your life you will have been all of
these.*

GEORGE WASHINGTON CARVER

The ability to show strength of character through compassion leads this list of employee responsibilities. It is health care workers that hold in their hands the gift to be instruments of God in the healing process. Compassionate caregivers make the difference in the life of both patients and coworkers. It is the compassionate caregiver who guides the patient as he or she struggles through illness, pain, and suffering. It is the compassionate caregiver that provides hope when there seems to be no hope.

Responsibility to Honor Patient Wishes

Caregivers have a responsibility to honor a patient's right to participate in decisions regarding his or her care, including the right to formulate advance directives and have those directives honored.

Responsibility to Maintain Confidentiality

The duty of employees and staff to maintain confidentiality encompasses both verbal and written communications. This requirement also applies to consultants, contracted individuals, students, and volunteers. Information about a patient, regardless of the method in which it is acquired, is confidential and should not be disclosed without the patient's permission. Those who come into possession of the most intimate personal information about patients have both a legal and an ethical duty not to reveal confidential communications. The legal duty arises because the law recognizes a right to privacy. To protect this right, there is a corresponding duty to obey. The ethical duty is broader and applies at all times.

All health care professionals who have access to medical records have a legal, ethical, and moral obligation to protect the confidentiality of the information in the records. The communications between a physician and his or her patient and the information generated during the course of the patient's illness are generally accorded the protection of confidentiality.

Health care professionals have a clear legal and moral obligation to maintain this confidentiality. As noted previously, medical records, with proper authorization, may be used for the purposes of research, statistical evaluation, and education. The information obtained from medical records must be dealt with in a confidential manner; otherwise, an organization could incur liability.

Responsibility to Adhere to Safe Practices

Caregivers have a responsibility to adhere to safe practices in order to minimize patient injuries. This responsibility requires employees to adhere to national patient safety goals (e.g., hand washing, patient identification, verification of operative site), the purpose of which is to protect the health of the patient.

Responsibility for Infection Control

It has been well published that infections may take up to 90,000 lives on an annual basis.

> Currently, between 5 and 10 percent of patients admitted to acute care hospitals acquire one or more infections, and the risks have steadily increased during recent decades. . . . These adverse events affect approximately 2 million patients each year in the United States, result in some 90,000 deaths, and add an estimated $4.5 to $7.5 billion per year to the cost of patient care.[16]

Health care organizations must develop policies, procedures, and protocols (e.g., hand-washing techniques, cleaning of equipment and instrumentation prior to reuse) in order to reduce the likelihood of the spread of hospital-acquired infections. It is the responsibility of each staff member to protect patients, visitors, and other staff members from the spread of infection by practicing appropriate infection control techniques.

Responsibility to Exercise Judgment

Caregivers have a responsibility to exercise discretion and good judgment. This is especially true of physicians who are bound to exercise their judgment without interference from others. The Hippocratic Oath requires that the physician use his or power to help the sick to the best of his or her ability and judgment. Such discretion, however, has limits and must consider the autonomous rights of patients.

Responsibility to Adhere to Professional Standards

Caregivers have a responsibility to maintain a professional attitude in the performance of their work. Unprofessional conduct, incompatibility, and lack of cooperation in a hospital are appropriate considerations for discharging an employee or denying staff privileges. The ability to work with others is a reasonably definite standard proscribing the conduct upon which discharge or other adverse action is based. Today's health care environment has become increasingly complex. The operation of a hospital requires the coordination of numerous employees and departments, each with different responsibilities that build and depend upon each other. Thus, staff cooperation and communication are essential to ensuring a high quality of patient care. Disruptive behavior in the workplace can both affect the morale and teamwork of the staff, as well as cause actual harm to patients. A hospital's evaluation of an employee's or physician's attitude and ability to work with others is not unduly vague and is directly related to the goal of good patient care.[17]

Responsibility to Maintain Professional Relationships

Professionals are responsible for maintaining an appropriate professional relationship with their patients. They must not breach their ethical obligations by engaging in sexual affairs with their patients even if the affairs are consensual. Sexual harassment cases are often litigated in both civil and criminal arenas. Health care professionals finding themselves in such unprofessional relationships should seek help for themselves as well as refer their patients to other appropriate professionals. Besides being subject to civil and criminal litigation, health care professionals also are subject to having their licenses revoked for sexual improprieties. The following cases illustrate the pervasiveness of sexual improprieties by professionals in a variety of settings.

Organizations should take action to prevent claims of sexual improprieties by training supervisory personnel to recognize and correct questionable behavior before it becomes a problem. Policy and procedures regarding sexual harassment should be included in an organization's orientation programs.

Nurse's Relationship with Patient

A nurse's sexual relations with a patient can give rise to disciplinary action resulting in the nurse's loss of license. In *Heineche v. Department of Commerce*,[18] a male nurse lost his license after having a sexual relationship with a patient, even though she was no longer a patient at the hospital where they met. The fact that the nurse resigned from the hospital and was living with the patient was not a sufficient defense to support such behavior.

Physician's Inappropriate House Call

A hospital technologist in *Copithorne v. Framingham Union Hospital*[19] alleged that a staff physician raped her during the course of a house call. The technologist's claim against the hospital had been summarily dismissed for lack of proximate causation. On appeal, the dismissal was found to be improper when the record indicated that the hospital had received notice of allegations that the physician had assaulted patients on and off the hospital's premises. The hospital had instructed the physician to have another individual present when visiting female patients and had instructed nurses "to keep an eye on him." The physician's sexual assault was foreseeable. There was evidentiary support for the proposition that failure to withdraw the physician's privileges had caused the rape when the technologist asserted that it was the physician's good reputation in the hospital that had led her to seek his services.

Sexual Misconduct with Patient's Spouse

The sexual relationship that a psychiatrist had with the spouse of a patient was found to be improper in *Richard v. Larry*.[20] California Civil Code Section 43.5, abolishing causes of action for alienation of affection, criminal conversation, and seduction of a patient over the age of consent, did not bar damages for emotional distress caused by the alleged professional negligence of the psychiatrist who had sexual relations with the plaintiff's wife. The psychiatrist owed a special duty to use due care for his patient's health. The statute was not intended to lower the standard of care that psychiatrists owed their patients. Besides an action against the psychiatrist, allegations that the psychiatrist was an agent of the hospital stated a cause of action against the hospital.

The Bureau of Professional Medical Conduct had charged the petitioner in *Goldberg v. De Buono*,[21] a licensed physician and psychiatrist, with moral unfitness, gross negligence and incompetence, negligence on more than one occasion, and incompetence by reason of his alleged sexual relationship with a patient. Following a hearing, a Hearing Committee of the State Board for Professional Medical Conduct sustained the specifications of moral unfitness, gross negligence, and negligence, and the Committee recommended revocation of the petitioner's license.

The New York Supreme Court, Appellate Division, rejected the petitioner's assertion that the Committee erred in crediting the testimony of Patient A and her daughter. Issues of credibility, even as to witnesses with psychiatric illnesses, are exclusively for the administrative fact finder to determine. The petitioner conceded his sexual relationship with Patient A but contended that the physician–patient relationship had been terminated at the time the sexual relationship occurred. Inasmuch as the respondent's medical expert testified that the relationship was not terminated and the petitioner's relationship with Patient A constituted a serious deviation from accepted standards of practice, the court was satisfied that the Committee's determination was supported by substantial evidence.

Responsibility to Report Unethical Behavior

Caregivers have both a right and responsibility to report impaired, incompetent, and unethical colleagues in accordance with the legal requirements of each state. Unethical behavior includes conduct that threatens patient care or welfare, behavior that violates state licensing provisions, and conduct that violates criminal statutes.

Responsibility to Protect Patients from Harm

Caregivers have an ethical and legal responsibility to protect patients from harm. The rules of ethics applicable to nurses, for example, specifically recognize a nurse's obligation to safeguard not only patients' health but their safety as well. These are not duties invented by courts of equity, but rather are tenets of ethical responsibility issued by the profession itself.

Responsibility to Report Patient Abuse

Caregivers have both a right and responsibility to report patient abuse. An employer may not discharge an employee for fulfilling societal obligations or one who acts with a socially undesirable motive. Statutes protect employees against retaliation for reporting patient abuse.

Whistle-Blowing and Unethical Conduct

Employees have both a right and responsibility to report unethical conduct. Whistle-blowing has been defined as an act of someone "who, believing that the public interest overrides the interest of the organization he serves, publicly blows the whistle if the organization is involved in corrupt, illegal, fraudulent, or harmful activity."[22]

> [According] to the public policy exception, an employer may not rely on the at-will doctrine as a basis for escaping liability for discharging an employee because of the doing of, or the refusing to do, such an act. Moreover, statutes in several jurisdictions protect an employee from an employer's retaliation for engaging in certain types of protected activities, such as whistleblowing.[23]

> Given the concern of the public about ethical behavior in government, the strong policy statement of the legislature in enacting the Whistleblower statute and the explicit inclusion of the state within its reach, the Whistleblower Act operates as an implied waiver of the statutory immunity provision of Minn. Stat. § 3.736. A decision to shield potential government wrongdoing, as urged by the state, would exacerbate public cynicism about the ethics of public officials, and this we do not choose to do.[24]

CHAPTER REVIEW

Staff rights include:

- Equal pay for equal work
- Refusing to participate in care (e.g., abortions)
- Questioning a patient's care
- Being free from sexual harassment
- Suggesting that a patient change physician
- Being treated with respect and dignity
- Employment-at-will and fair treatment

Staff responsibilities include:

- Being a patient advocate
- Honoring a patient's autonomy
- Following professional codes of ethics
- Confidential communications
- Adhering to safe practices
- Exercising good judgment
- Being professional
- Reporting unethical behavior
- Protecting patients from harm
- Not sexually harassing others
- Reporting patient abuse
- Being a whistle-blower if necessary

REVIEW QUESTIONS

1. How do the rights and responsibilities of patients and employees differ, and in what ways are they similar?

2. Is the employment-at-will concept appropriate in today's society?

3. What are the pros and cons of the employment-at-will doctrine?

WEB SITES

Free Employment Law & HR Reference Center
http://ppspublishers.com/articles/resources/?c1=payperclick&source=google_ads&kw=employees

NOTES

1. 515 F.2d 541 (8th Cir. 1975).
2. 851 S.W.2d 617 (Mo. Ct. App. 1993).
3. 328 S.E.2d 818 (N.C. Ct. App. 1985).
4. 44 A.L.R. 4th 1136 (1986).
5. Sides v. Duke Hosp., 328 S.E.2d 818 (N.C. Ct. App. 1985).
6. Pierce v. Ortho Pharm. Corp., 417 A.2d 505, 509 (N.J. 1980).
7. Palmateer v. International Harvester Co., 421 N.E.2d 876, 878 (Ill. 1981).
8. Joiner v. Benton Community Bank, 411 N.E.2d 229, 231 (Ill. 1980).
9. Gantt v. Sentry Ins., 824 P.2d 680, 687–688 (Cal. 1992).
10. CONN. GEN. STAT. ANN. § 31–51m(a) (West 1987).
11. ME. REV. STAT. ANN. 26, §§ 831–840 (West 1987).
12. MICH. COMP. LAWS ANN. §§ 15.361–369 (West 1981).
13. MONT. CODE ANN. § 39-2-901 (1987).
14. Pierce v. Ortho Pharm. Corp., 417 A.2d 505, 509 (N.J. 1980).
15. 760 F. Supp. 1575 (D.C. Ga. 1991).
16. John P. Burke, M.D., *Infection Control—A Problem for Patient Safety*, NEJM, Feb. 13, 2003, at 651.
17. Freilich v. Upper Chesapeake Health, Inc., 313 F.3d 205 (2002).
18. 810 P.2d 459 (Utah 1991).
19. 520 N.E.2d 139 (Mass. 1988).
20. 243 Cal. Rptr. 807 (Cal. Ct. App. 1988).
21. 711 N.Y.S.2d 81 (N.Y. App. Div. 2000).
22. WHISTLEBLOWING: THE REPORT OF THE CONFERENCE OF PROFESSIONAL RESPONSIBILITY 6 (1972); *see also* Annotation, 99 A.L.R. Fed. 778.
23. Annotation, 99 A.L.R. Fed. 775.
24. Gambee v. State Bd. of Med. Exam'rs, 923 P.2d 679 (1996).

Section IV

The Patient

chapter *twelve*

Patient Consent

INTRODUCTION

. . . no right is held more sacred,
or is more carefully guarded, by the common law,
than the right of every individual to the possession
and control of his own person.

UNION PACIFIC RY. CO. v. BOTSFORD[1]

Consent must be obtained from the patient, or from a person authorized to consent on the patient's behalf, before any medical procedure can be performed. Every individual has a right to refuse to authorize a touching. This chapter reviews many of the issues surrounding consent in the health care setting.

Consent is the voluntary agreement by a person who possesses sufficient mental capacity to make an intelligent choice to allow something proposed by another to be performed on himself or herself. Consent changes a touching that otherwise would be nonconsensual to one that is consensual. Consent can be either express or implied.

Express consent can take the form of either a "verbal" agreement or can be accomplished through the execution of a "written" document authorizing medical care.

Implied consent is determined by some act or silence, which raises a presumption that consent has been authorized.

INFORMED CONSENT

Informed consent is a legal concept that provides that a patient has a right to know the potential risks, benefits, and alternatives of a proposed procedure. The right to be free of unwanted medical treatment has long been recognized in this country. An "individual's right to make decisions vitally affecting his private life according to his own conscience . . . is difficult to overstate . . . because it is, without exaggeration, the very bedrock on which this country was founded."[2]

The right to control the integrity of one's own body spawned the doctrine of informed consent.[3] The United States Supreme Court has held that a competent adult patient has the right to decline any and all forms of medical intervention, including lifesaving or life-prolonging treatment.[4]

Informed consent is predicated on the duty of the physician to disclose to the patient sufficient information to enable the patient to evaluate a proposed medical or surgical procedure before submitting to it. Informed consent requires that a patient have a full understanding of that to which he or she has consented. An authorization from a patient who does not understand to what he or she is consenting is not effective consent.

Hospitals generally do not have an independent duty to obtain informed consent or to warn patients of the risks of a procedure to be performed by a physician who is not an agent of the hospital. It is the treating physician who has the education, expertise, skill, and training necessary to treat a patient and determine what information a patient should have in order to give informed consent.

CASE: PATIENT AND PROVIDER OBLIGATIONS

Any glimmer of uncertainty as to a patient's desires in an emergency situation should be resolved "in favor of preserving life." The patient in *Matter of Hughes*[5] signed a standard blank hospital form entitled "Refusal to Permit Blood Transfusion." There was no indication on the form that the consequences of her refusal had been explained to her in the context of the elective surgical procedure she was about to undergo. The form should have contained an unequivocal statement that under any and all circumstances, blood is not to be used and an acknowledgment that the consequences of the refusal were fully explained. The form should fully release the physician, all medical personnel, and the hospital from liability should complications arise from the failure to administer blood, thereby resolving any doubt as to the physician's responsibility to his patient. If Hughes would have refused to sign such a form, her physician could then decide whether to continue with Hughes's treatment or to aid her in finding a physician who would carry out her wishes.

The court emphasized that this case arose in the context of elective surgery. This was not an emergency situation where the physician and patient did not have time to fully discuss the potential risks, benefits, and alternatives of the planned surgery and the conflict arising over the patient's religious beliefs. Patients have an obligation to make medical preferences known to the treating physician, including the course to follow, if life-threatening complications should arise. This protects the patient's right to freedom of religion and self-determination. In addition, it is helpful to the hospital when faced with the dilemma of trying to preserve life whenever possible and honoring the patient's wishes to forgo sustaining treatment.

Patients have an obligation to make medical preferences known to the treating physician, including the course to follow, if life-threatening complications should arise. This protects the patient's right to freedom of religion and self-determination. In addition, it is helpful to the hospital when faced with the dilemma of trying to preserve life whenever possible and honoring the patient's wishes to forgo sustaining treatment.

Ethical and Legal Issues

1. Describe the relevant ethical principles violated in this case.
2. Describe the relevant legal issues in this case.
3. What actions could the parties to this lawsuit have taken beforehand in order to have prevented this case from becoming a legal issue? ▪

CONSENT AND ETHICAL CODES

The first American Medical Association Code of Medical Ethics was written in 1847. Section One of the 1998–1999 edition, entitled "Fundamental Elements of the Patient–Physician Relationship," provides "the patient has the right to receive information from physicians and to discuss the benefits, risks, and costs of appropriate treatment alternatives." Because the American Medical Association is an organization composed of experts in the field of medicine, its code of ethics and the duties of physicians prescribed therein should be understood to reflect the standard of care of the profession on the issue of informed consent. Social policy does not accept the "paternalistic" view that the physician may remain silent, because divulgence might prompt the patient to forgo needed therapy.

The American Dental Association Code of Ethics also reflects the standard of care for the dental profession. Part III, Section 1 of the American Dental Association Code of Ethics, entitled "Principle: Patient Autonomy," provides "the dentist has a duty to respect the patient's rights to self-determination and confidentiality," and Section 1A provides "the dentist should inform the patient of the proposed treatment, and any reasonable alternatives, in a manner that allows the patient to become involved in treatment decisions." These American Medical Association and American Dental Association ethical standards embrace the doctrine of informed consent.

ASSESSING DECISION-MAKING CAPACITY

A patient is considered competent to make medical decisions regarding his or her care unless a court determines otherwise. Generally speaking, the determination of a patient's decision-making capacity is made by medical personnel. The clinical assessment of decision-making capacity should include the patient's ability to understand the risks, benefits, and alternatives of a proposed test or procedure; evaluate the information provided by the physician; express his or her treatment options/plan; and voluntarily make decisions regarding his or her treatment plan without undue influence by family, friends, or medical personnel.

Determining Incapacity

If a patient is unable to make decisions by reason of age or incapacity, a patient-appointed decision maker may "substitute his or her judgment" on behalf of the patient. Before declaring an individual incapacitated, the attending physician must find with a reasonable degree of medical certainty that the patient lacks capacity. A notation should be placed in the patient's medical record describing the cause, nature, extent, and probable duration of incapacity. Before withholding or withdrawing life-sustaining treatment, a second physician must confirm the incapacity determination and make an appropriate entry on the medical record before honoring any new decisions by a health care agent.

CASE: LACK OF CONSENT AND PATIENT DEATH

Four children, in *Riser v. American Medican Intern, Inc.*,[6] brought a medical malpractice action against Dr. Lang, a physician who performed a femoral arteriogram on their 69-year-old mother, who subsequently died following the procedure. Riser had been admitted to Hospital A experiencing impaired circulation in her lower arms and hands. She had multiple medical diagnoses, including diabetes mellitus, end-stage renal failure, and arteriosclerosis. Her physician, Dr. Sottiurai, ordered bilateral arteriograms to determine the cause of the patient's impaired circulation. Hospital A could not accommodate Sottiurai's request, and Riser was transferred to Dr. Lang, a radiologist at Hospital B. Lang performed a femoral arteriogram rather than the bilateral brachial arteriogram ordered by Sottiurai. The procedure seemed to go well, and the patient was prepared for transfer back to the hospital. However, shortly after the ambulance departed the hospital, the patient suffered a seizure in the ambulance and was returned to Hospital B. Riser's condition deteriorated and she died 11 days later. The plaintiffs claimed in their lawsuit that Riser was a poor risk for the procedure. The district court ruled for the plaintiffs, awarding damages in the amount of $50,000 for Riser's pain and suffering and $100,000 to each child. Lang appealed.

The Louisiana Court of Appeal held that Lang failed to obtain consent from the patient. Riser was under the impression that she was about to undergo a brachial arteriogram, not a femoral arteriogram. Two consent forms were signed; neither form authorized the performance of a femoral arteriogram. O'Neil, one of Riser's daughters, claimed that her mother said following the arteriogram, "Why did you let them do that to me?"[7]

Ethical and Legal Issues

1. Describe how the physician violated his professional duty to the patient.
2. Should the hospital have intervened and prevented the femoral arteriogram? Explain your answer. ∎

ADEQUACY OF CONSENT

A physician should provide as much information about treatment options as is necessary based on a patient's personal understanding of the physician's explanation of the risks of treatment and the probable consequences of the treatment. The needs of each patient can vary depending on age, maturity, and mental status.

Some courts have recognized that the condition of the patient may be taken into account to determine whether the patient has received sufficient information to give consent. The individual responsible for obtaining consent must weigh the importance of giving full disclosure to the patient against the likelihood that such disclosure will seriously and adversely affect the condition of the patient.

The operation you get often depends on where you live. One patient underwent a mastectomy only to learn that a less destructive alternative procedure was available in a region near her home. The procedure, a lumpectomy, has the same survival rate as a mastectomy. The patient claims the surgeon never informed her as to the alternative.

Ethical and Legal Issues

1. Describe the ethical and legal issues for failing to discuss alternative treatments with a patient.
2. Food for thought: Should a physician describe every possible alternative treatment procedure with his or her patient? Explain your answer. ■

When questions do arise as to whether adequate consent has been given, some courts take into consideration the information that is ordinarily provided by other physicians. A physician must reveal to his or her patient such information as a skilled practitioner of good standing would provide under similar circumstances. A physician must disclose to the patient the potential of death, serious harm, and other complications associated with a proposed procedure.

PROOF OF CONSENT

Oral Consent

Oral consent, if proved, is as binding as written consent, for there is, in general, no legal requirement that a patient's consent be in writing. However, an oral consent is more difficult to corroborate.

Written Consent

Written consent provides visible proof of a patient's wishes. Because the function of a written consent form is to preserve evidence of informed consent, the nature of the treatment, the risks, benefits, and consequences involved should be incorporated into the consent form. States have taken the view that consent, to be effective, must be "informed consent." An informed consent form should include the following elements:

- the nature of the patient's illness or injury
- the name of the proposed procedure or treatment
- the purpose of the proposed treatment
- the risks and probable consequences of the proposed treatment
- the probability that the proposed treatment will be successful
- any alternative methods of treatment along with their associated risks and benefits

- the risks and prognosis if no treatment is rendered
- an indication that the patient understands the nature of any proposed treatment, the alternatives, the risks involved, and the probable consequences of the proposed treatment
- the signatures of the patient, physician, and witnesses
- the date the consent is signed

Health care professionals have an important role in the realm of informed consent. They can be instrumental in averting major lawsuits by being observant as to a patient's doubts, changes of mind, confusion, or misunderstandings expressed by a patient regarding any proposed procedures he or she is about to undergo.

Emergency Consent

When immediate treatment is required to preserve the life of a patient or to prevent an impairment of the patient's health, and it is impossible to obtain the consent of the patient or representative legally authorized to consent for him or her, an emergency exists and consent is implied. This privilege to proceed in emergencies without consent is accorded physicians because inaction at this time may cause greater injury to the patient and would be contrary to good medical practice. However, if at all possible, consultation should be undertaken before a procedure is commenced, and every effort must be made to document the medical need for proceeding with treatment without consent. The patient's record should clearly indicate the nature of the threat to life or health, its immediacy, and its magnitude.

WHO MAY AUTHORIZE CONSENT?

Consent of the patient ordinarily is required before treatment. When a patient is either physically unable or legally incompetent to consent and no emergency exists, consent must be obtained from a person who is empowered to consent on the patient's behalf. The person who authorizes treatment of another must have sufficient information to make an intelligent judgment on behalf of the patient.

Competent Patients

A competent adult patient's wishes concerning his or her person may not be disregarded. The court in *In re Melideo*[8] held that every human being of adult years has a right to determine what shall be done with his or her own body and cannot be subjected to medical treatment without his or her consent. When there is no compelling state interest that justifies overriding an adult patient's decision, that decision should be respected. State interests include preserving life, preventing suicide, safeguarding the integrity of the medical profession, and protecting innocent third parties.

Spousal Consent

The patient in *Greynolds v. Kurman*[9] suffered from a transient ischemic attack (TIA), a sudden loss of neurological function caused by vascular impairment to the brain. He was taken to an emergency department. Because of the patient's prior medical history, which included TIAs, he was at high risk for a stroke. After receiving the results of noninvasive tests, Dr. Rafecas, a consulting physician, ordered a cerebral angiogram. Dr. Kurman performed the angiogram, and the patient suffered a stroke during the procedure that left him severely disabled.

The patient and his wife filed a medical malpractice action against Rafecas and Kurman, asserting that Rafecas had negligently recommended the procedure and that Kurman had performed the procedure without obtaining informed consent. The court of appeals held that the evidence was sufficient to support a judgment in favor of the patient and his wife.

The jury needed to determine that the risks involved in the cerebral angiogram were not disclosed, that the risks involved in the procedure materialized and caused the stroke, and that a reasonable person in the position of the patient would have decided against having the angiogram had the risks associated with the procedure been disclosed. The jury concluded that the patient did not consent to the angiogram because he "was not . . . capable of comprehending the consent form," and further noted that Kurman should have sought consent from the next of kin, specifically the spouse. Given the evidence of the patient's condition when he signed the consent forms, his past medical history, and his increased risk of suffering complications during an angiogram, the court found that evidence supported a finding of lack of informed consent.

Guardianship

A guardian is an individual who by law is invested with the power and charged with the duty of taking care of a patient by protecting the patient's rights and managing the patient's estate. Guardianship is often necessary in those instances in which a patient is incapable of managing or administering his or her private affairs because of physical and/or mental disabilities or because he or she is under the age of majority.

Temporary Guardianship

Temporary guardianship can be granted by the courts if it is determined necessary for the well-being of the patient.

Temporary guardianship was granted by the court in *In re Estate of Dorone*.[10] In this case, the physician and administrator petitioned the court on two occasions for authority to administer blood. A 22-year-old male patient brought to the Hospital Center by helicopter after an automobile accident was diagnosed as suffering from an acute subdural hematoma with a brain contusion. It was determined that the patient would die unless he underwent a cranial operation. The operation required the administration of blood to which the parents would not consent because of their religious beliefs. After a hearing by telephone, the court of common pleas appointed the hospital's administrator as temporary guardian, authorizing him to consent to the performance of blood transfusions during emergency surgery. A more formal hearing did not take place because of the emergency situation that existed. Surgery was required a second time to remove a blood clot, and the court once again granted the administrator authority to authorize administration of blood. The superior court affirmed the orders, and the parents appealed. The Pennsylvania supreme court held that the judge's failure to obtain direct testimony from the patient's parents and others concerning the patient's religious beliefs was not in error when death was likely to result from withholding blood. The judge's decisions granting guardianship and the authority to consent to the administration of blood were considered absolutely necessary in the light of the facts of this case. Nothing less than a fully conscious contemporary decision by the patient himself would have been sufficient to override the evidence of medical necessity.

Parents Refuse Transfusion for Their Child

When parents in *In re Guardianship of L.S.*[11] refused to consent to medically necessary care for their minor child based on their religious convictions, the trial court appointed the hospital as a temporary guardian to make decisions to provide medically necessary, life-saving treatment for the child. The evidence presented to the trial court in the form of an affidavit from a hospital physician stated that the parents were refusing medically necessary blood transfusions, that the child would require blood transfusions to survive, and that the child was unable to respond to this risk. The trial court reasonably concluded from this information that the child was at a risk of substantial and immediate physical harm. The trial court's decision to appoint a temporary guardian was based on the child's best interest and protected the State's interest in the welfare of children within the State.

In the midst of an emergency, the district court was confronted with the task of balancing the competing interests of the child, the parents, the hospital, and the State. Throughout the proceedings, the district court took numerous steps to protect the interests of the child and the parents, including requiring notice and a hearing within 24 hours after the original order, allowing the parents time to obtain counsel prior to reaching a final determination.

"Substantive due process guarantees that no person shall be deprived of life, liberty, or property for arbitrary reasons." The Due Process Clause of the Fourteenth Amendment protects those liberty interests that are deemed fundamental and are "deeply rooted in this Nation's history and tradition." Certain family privacy rights, including the parent–child relationship, have therefore been recognized as fundamental rights. The Nevada Supreme Court adopted a "reasonableness test" to address family privacy cases involving "competing interests within the family."

Although a parent has a fundamental liberty interest in the "care, custody, and management" of his child, that interest is not absolute. "The state also has an interest in the welfare of children and may limit parental authority," even permanently depriving parents of their children. Therefore, although the parents have a parental interest in the care of their son, both the State and L.S. have an interest in preserving the child's life. As L.S. is unable to make decisions for himself, the State's interest is heightened. The parents' liberty interest in practicing their religion must also give way to the child's welfare. Hence, the district court found that the parents' refusal to consent to treatment put L.S.'s life at substantial risk. Additionally, the State has an interest in protecting "the ethical integrity of the medical profession" and in allowing hospitals the full opportunity to care for patients under their control, especially when medical science is available to save that patient's life.

Here, the child's interest in self-preservation and the State's interests in protecting the welfare of children and the integrity of medical care outweigh the parents' interests in the care, custody, and management of their children, as well as their religious freedom. The combined weight of the interests of the child and the State are great and therefore mandate interference with parental rights.

The Supreme Court of Nevada affirmed the order of the district court appointing Valley Hospital as temporary guardian.

Consent for Minors

The courts have held, as a general proposition, that the consent of a minor to medical or surgical treatment is ineffective and that the physician must secure the consent of the minor's parent or someone standing *in loco parentis*; otherwise, he or she will risk liability. Although parental consent should be obtained before treating a minor, treatment should not be delayed to the detriment of the child.

Parental consent is not necessary when the minor is married or otherwise emancipated. Most states have enacted statutes making it valid for married and emancipated minors to provide effective consent. Several courts have held the consent of a minor to be sufficient authorization for treatment in certain situations. In any specific case, a court's determination that the consent of a minor is effective and that parental consent is unnecessary will depend on such factors as the minor's age, maturity, mental status, and emancipation and the procedure involved, as well as public policy considerations.

Incompetent Patients

The attending physician, who is in the best position to make the determination, should become familiar with his or her state's definition of legal incompetence. In any case in which a physician doubts a patient's capacity to consent, the consent of the legal guardian or next of kin should be obtained. If there are no relatives to consult, application should be made for a court order that would allow the procedure. It may be the duty of the court to assume responsibility of guardianship for a patient who is *non compos mentis*. The most frequently cited conditions indicative of incompetence are mental illness, mental retardation, senility, physical incapacity, and chronic alcohol or drug abuse.

A person who is mentally incompetent cannot legally consent to medical or surgical treatment. Therefore, consent of the patient's legal guardian must be obtained. When no legal guardian is available, a court that handles such matters must be petitioned to permit treatment.

Subject to applicable statutory provisions, when a physician doubts a patient's capacity to consent, even though the patient has not been judged legally incompetent, the consent of the nearest relative should be obtained. If a patient is conscious and mentally capable of giving consent for treatment, the consent of a relative without the consent of the competent patient would not protect the physician from liability.

IMPLIED CONSENT

Although the law requires consent for the intentional touching that involves medical or surgical procedures, exceptions do exist with respect to emergency situations. Implied consent will generally be presumed when immediate action is required to prevent death or permanent impairment of a patient's health. If it is impossible in an emergency to obtain the consent of the patient or someone legally authorized to give consent, the required procedure may be undertaken without liability for failure to procure consent.

Unconscious patients are presumed under law to approve treatment that appears to be necessary. It is assumed that such patients would have consented if they were conscious and competent. However, if a patient expressly refuses to consent to certain treatment, such treatment may not be instituted after the patient becomes unconscious. Similarly, conscious patients suffering from emergency conditions retain the right to refuse consent.

If a procedure is necessary to protect one's life or health, every effort must be made to document the medical necessity for proceeding with medical treatment without consent. It must be shown that the emergency situation constituted an immediate threat to life or health.

In *Luka v. Lowrie*,[12] involving a 15-year-old boy whose left foot had been run over and crushed by a train, consultation by the treating physician with other physicians was an important factor in determining the outcome of the case. On the boy's arrival at the hospital, the defending physician and four house surgeons decided it was necessary to amputate the foot. The court said it was inconceivable that had they been present, the parents would have refused consent in the face of a determination by five physicians that amputation would save the boy's life. Thus, despite testimony at the trial that the amputation may not have been necessary, professional consultation before the operation supported the assertion that a genuine emergency existed and could be implied consent.

Consent also can be implied in nonemergency situations. For example, a patient may voluntarily submit to a procedure, implying consent, without any explicitly spoken or written expression of consent. In the Massachusetts case of *O'Brien v. Cunard Steam Ship Co.*,[13] a ship's passenger who joined a line of people receiving injections was held to have implied his consent to a vaccination. The rationale for this decision is that individuals who observe a line of people and who notice that injections are being administered to those at the head of the line should expect that if they join and remain in the line, they will receive an injection. The voluntary act of entering the line and the plaintiff's opportunity to see what was taking place at the head of the line were accepted by the jury as manifestations of consent to the injection. The O'Brien case contains all the elements necessary to imply consent from a voluntary act: The procedure was a simple vaccination, the proceedings were visible at all times, and the plaintiff was free to withdraw up to the instant of the injection.

Whether a patient's consent can be implied is frequently asked when the condition of a patient requires some deviation from an agreed-on procedure. If a patient expressly prohibits a specific medical or surgical procedure, consent to the procedure cannot be implied. The same consent rule applies if a patient expressly prohibits a particular extension of a procedure even though the patient voluntarily submitted to the original procedure.

RIGHT TO REFUSE TREATMENT

> *"The individual's right to make decisions vitally affecting his private life according to his own conscience . . . is difficult to overstate . . . because it is, without exaggeration, the very bedrock on which this country was founded."*
>
> Wons v. Public Health Trust [14]

Patients have a right to refuse treatment and be secure from any touching, and they are free to reject recommended treatment. A competent patient's refusal to consent to a medical or surgical procedure must be adhered to, whether the refusal is grounded on lack of confidence in the physician, fear of the procedure, doubt as to the value of a particular procedure, or mere whim. The U.S. Supreme Court stated that the "notion of bodily integrity has been embodied in the requirement that informed consent is generally required for medical treatment" and the "logical corollary of the doctrine of informed consent is that the patient generally possesses the right not to consent, that is, to refuse treatment."[15] The common law doctrine of informed consent is viewed as generally encompassing the right of a competent individual to refuse medical treatment.

The question of liability for performing a medical or surgical procedure without consent is separate and distinct from any question of negligence or malpractice in performing a procedure. Liability may be imposed for a nonconsensual touching of a patient, even if the procedure improved the patient's health. The eminent Justice Cardozo, in *Schloendorff v. Society of New York Hospital*, stated:

> Every human being of adult years and sound mind has a right to determine what shall be done with his own body, and a surgeon who performs an operation without his patient's consent commits an assault, for which he is liable in damages, except in cases of emergency where the patient is unconscious and where it is necessary to operate before consent can be obtained.[16]

The courts perform a balancing test to determine whether or not to override a competent adult's decision to refuse medical treatment. The courts balance state interests, such as preservation of life, protection of third parties, prevention of suicide, and the integrity of the medical profession against a patient's rights of bodily integrity and religious freedom. The most frequently used state right to intervene in a patient's decision-making process is for the protection of third parties. In *In re Fetus Brown*,[17] the State of Illinois asserted that its interest in the well-being of a viable fetus outweighed the patient's rights to refuse medical treatment. The state argued that a balancing test should be used to weigh state interests against patient rights. The appellate court held that it could not impose a legal obligation upon a pregnant woman to consent to an invasive medical procedure for the benefit of her viable fetus.

Adult patients who are conscious and mentally competent have the right to refuse medical care to the extent permitted by law even when the best medical opinion deems it essential to life. Such a refusal must be honored whether it is grounded in religious belief or mere whim. Every person has the legal right to refuse to permit a touching of his or her body. Failure to respect this right can result in a legal action for assault and battery. If a patient refuses consent, every effort should be made to explain the importance of the procedure. Coercion through threat, duress, or intimidation must be avoided.

Case law over the past several decades has developed to a point where any person, regardless of religious beliefs, has the right to refuse any medical treatment. As part of their religious beliefs, Jehovah's Witnesses generally have refused the administration of blood, even in emergency situations.

A hospital generally has no common-law right or obligation to thrust unwanted medical care on a patient who, having been sufficiently informed of the consequences, competently and clearly declines such care. A patient's common-law right of bodily self-determination is entitled to respect and protection.

Prior to a patient leaving a health care facility against medical advice, every attempt should be made to have a release form completed and attached to the patient's chart.

All reasonable steps should be taken to: (1) inform the patient of the benefits and risks of treatment and (2) secure the patient's written informed consent to refuse examination and treatment. If the patient refuses to sign the "refusal to consent form," documentation of the refusal should be documented and maintained by the hospital.

A Mother's Right, A Child's Death

Harrell, a Jehovah's Witness, was six months pregnant when physicians discovered a life-threatening blood condition that could rapidly deteriorate, placing both her life and the life of the fetus in jeopardy. Because of her religious beliefs, Harrell objected to a blood transfusion. After an emergency hearing during which the Harrells could not summon an attorney, the court ruled that a blood transfusion could be given to Harrell if it was necessary to save the life of the fetus and that after the child was born, a blood transfusion could be given to the child if necessary to save the child's life. The Harrells appealed. The child was delivered by Caesarean section and died two days later. No blood transfusion was given to Harrell or to the child. As a result, the hospital and the state claimed that the appeal of the trial court's order is moot. Because of the hospital's serious misunderstanding about its standing to bring such proceedings, the Florida District Court of Appeal addressed the issue as capable of repetition yet evading review.

The Florida constitution guarantees that a competent person has the constitutional right to choose or refuse medical treatment, and that right extends to all relevant decisions concerning one's health. The state has a duty to ensure that a person's wishes regarding medical treatment are respected. That obligation serves to protect the rights of the individual from intrusion by the state unless the state has a compelling interest great enough to override this constitutional right (e.g., protection of innocent third parties).

Harrell argued that the hospital should not have intervened in her private decision to refuse a blood transfusion. She claimed that the state had never been a party in this action, had not asserted any interest, and that the hospital had no authority to assume the state's responsibilities.[18]

The Florida District Court of Appeal concluded that a health care provider must not be forced into the position of having to argue against the wishes of the facility's own patient. Patients do not lose their right to make decisions affecting their lives when they enter a health care facility. A health care provider's function is to provide medical treatment in accordance with the patient's wishes and best interests, not supervening the wishes of a competent adult. A health care provider must comply with the wishes of a patient to refuse medical treatment unless ordered to do otherwise by a court of competent jurisdiction. A health care provider cannot act on behalf of the state to assert state interests. When a health care provider, acting in good faith, follows the wishes of a competent and informed patient to refuse medical treatment, the health care provider is acting appropriately and cannot be subjected to civil or criminal liability.

Mother Refuses Blood, Spouse Disagrees

What would you do when the patient, a Jehovah's Witness, signs a consent form refusing a blood transfusion and the husband, who is not a Jehovah's Witness, consents to a blood transfusion to save his wife's life?

Plaintiff Perkins, in *Perkins v. Lavin*,[19] was a Jehovah's Witness. She gave birth to a baby at the defendant hospital. After going home, she began hemorrhaging and returned to the hospital. She specifically informed the defendant's employees that she was not to be provided any blood or blood derivatives, and she signed a form to that effect:

> I request that no blood or blood derivatives be administered to (plaintiff) during this hospitalization, notwithstanding that such treatment may be deemed necessary in the opinion of the attending physician or his assistants to preserve life or promote recovery. I release the attending physician, his assistants, the hospital and its personnel from any responsibility whatever for any untoward results due to my refusal to permit the use of blood or its derivatives.[20]

Due to the plaintiff's condition, it became necessary to perform an emergency dilation and curettage on her. She continued to bleed, and her condition deteriorated dramatically. Her blood count dropped, necessitating administration of blood products as a lifesaving measure. Her husband, who was not a Jehovah's Witness, consented to a blood transfusion, which was administered. The plaintiff recovered and filed an action against the defendant for assault and battery. The plaintiff's claim as to assault and battery was sustained.

The plaintiff specifically informed the defendant that she would consider a blood transfusion an offensive contact. Although both parties have noted that the plaintiff's husband provided his consent for the transfusion, the defendant has not argued that his consent was sufficient to overcome plaintiff's direction that she was not to receive a transfusion. The plaintiff submitted sufficient evidence to the trial court to establish that there was, at least, a genuine issue whether the defendant intentionally invaded her right to be free from offensive contact. Because of the plaintiff's recognition that the defendant acted to save her life, a jury may find that she is entitled to only nominal damages.

CASE: MOTHER REFUSES TREATMENT, SPOUSE AGREES

Vega, a Jehovah's Witness, executed a release requesting that no blood be administered to her during her hospitalization. Vega's husband also signed the release. She delivered a healthy baby. Following the delivery, Vega bled heavily. Her obstetrician, Dr. Sood, recommended a dilation and curettage (D&C) to stop the bleeding. Although Vega agreed to permit Sood to perform the D&C, she refused to allow a blood transfusion. Prior to undergoing the procedure, she signed a second release refusing any transfusions and releasing the hospital from liability. Despite the D&C, Vega continued to hemorrhage.

Because Sood and the other physicians involved in Vega's care believed that it was essential that she receive blood in order to survive, the hospital requested that the court issue an injunction that would permit the hospital to administer blood transfusions. The trial court convened an emergency hearing at the hospital and appointed Vega's husband as her guardian. At the hearing testimony, Vega's husband testified that, on the basis of his religious beliefs as a Jehovah's Witness, he continued to support his wife's decision to refuse transfusions and believed that she would take the same position if she were able to participate in the hearing.

The court, relying on the state's interests in preserving life and protecting innocent third parties, granted the hospital's request for an injunction permitting it to administer blood transfusions. Vega was given blood transfusions, recovered, and was discharged from the hospital.

Vega sued, arguing that if her refusal of blood transfusions interfered with certain state interests, it should be the state itself, not a private hospital, that asserts state's interests. The hospital responded that, because it was charged with Vega's care, it had a direct stake in the outcome of the controversy and was a proper party to bring the action.

The hospital had a legitimate interest in receiving official guidance in resolving the "ethical dilemma" it faced: whether to practice medicine by trying to save a patient's life despite that patient's refusal to consent to treatment, or to practice medicine in accordance with the patient's wishes and likely watch the patient die, knowing nonetheless that it had the power to save her life. The hospital had conflicting interests, and was in the role not of opposing its patient, but of a party seeking the court's guidance in determining its obligations under the circumstances.

Vega claimed that the state's interest in the welfare of her child is not sufficiently compelling as to outweigh her interest in refusing blood transfusions. Vega maintained that the trial court's injunction, issued at the behest of the hospital, violated her common-law right of self-determination, her federal constitutional right to bodily self-determination, her federal constitutional right to free exercise of religion, and her state constitutional right of religious liberty. The court concluded that, under the circumstances of this case, the issuance of the injunction, followed by the administration of blood transfusions, violated Vega's common-law right of bodily self-determination.

Although the hospital's interests are sufficient to confer standing on it in this case, they are not sufficient to take priority over Vega's common-law right to bodily integrity, even when the assertion of that right threatens her own life. The hospital had no common-law right or obligation to thrust unwanted medical care on a patient who, having been sufficiently informed of the consequences, competently and clearly declined that care. The hospital's interests were sufficiently protected by Vega's informed choice, and neither it nor the trial court was entitled to override that choice. Vega's common-law right of bodily self-determination was entitled to respect and protection.[21]

Ethical and Legal Issues

1. What would you do when a patient refuses a blood transfusion and the spouse agrees with her decision, knowing that a blood transfusion may be necessary to save her life?
2. Should a hospital challenge a patient's refusal of lifesaving blood transfusions?
3. Does the administration of a blood transfusion violate a patient's common-law right to bodily self-determination? ■

Hospitals have a legitimate interest in receiving official guidance when resolving the ethical dilemmas they face: whether to practice medicine by trying to save a patient's life despite that patient's refusal to consent to treatment, or to practice medicine in accordance with the patient's wishes and likely watch the patient die, knowing nonetheless that it had the power to save that patient's life. Hospitals often have conflicting interests, and are in the role not of opposing its patient, but of a party seeking the court's guidance in determining its obligations under the circumstances.

Patients have a common-law right of self-determination, a federal constitutional right to bodily self-determination, a federal constitutional right to free exercise of religion, and a state constitutional right of religious liberty. The administration of unwanted blood transfusions violates a patient's common-law right of bodily self-determination.

STATUTORY CONSENT

Many states have adopted legislation concerning emergency care. An emergency in most states eliminates the need for consent. When a patient is clinically unable to give consent to a lifesaving emergency treatment, the law implies consent on the presumption that a reasonable person would consent to lifesaving medical intervention.

When an emergency situation does arise, there may be little opportunity to contact the attending physician, much less a consultant. The patient's records, therefore, must be complete with respect to the description of his or her illness and condition, the attempts made to contact the physician as well as relatives, and the emergency measures taken and procedures performed. If time does not permit a court order to be obtained, a second medical opinion, when practicable, is advisable.

CHAPTER REVIEW

1. Patients have the right to make decisions regarding their own health care.
2. Consent is voluntary agreement by a person to allow something proposed by another to be performed on himself or herself. A person can consent to something only if he or she has sufficient mental capacity to make an intelligent choice.
3. The legal concept that protects a patient's right to know the potential risks, benefits, and alternatives of a proposed procedure is referred to as informed consent. Most often, the duty to inform the patient and to decide what information the patient should be given falls to the treating physician.
4. If an individual is found incompetent to give consent, and if there are no relatives or other parties from whom to obtain consent, an application should be made for a court order that would allow the procedure.
5. Implied consent is generally presumed when immediate action is required to prevent death or permanent impairment of a patient's health. In such cases, documentation justifying the need to treat before obtaining consent should be maintained.
6. Over the past few decades, case law has developed in such a way that any person, regardless of religious beliefs, has the right to refuse any medical treatment.

TEST YOUR UNDERSTANDING

Terminology

informed consent	guardianship
proof of consent	implied consent
authorization of consent	statutory consent

REVIEW QUESTIONS

1. Who should be responsible for reviewing with the patient the risks, benefits, and alternatives of a proposed diagnostic test or treatment?

2. Describe what information a patient should be provided prior to undergoing a risky procedure so that consent is "informed."

3. Why is it important to obtain consent from a patient prior to proceeding with a risky procedure?

4. Can a patient give consent and then withdraw it?

5. Can a parent refuse to consent to a lifesaving procedure for his or her child? Discuss your answer.

6. How much information is sufficient for informed consent to be effective?

7. Describe both the ethical and legal implications of consent.

NOTES

1. 141 U.S. 250, 251 (1891).
2. Wons v. Public Health Trust, 500 So. 2d 679, 687 (Fla. Dist. Ct. App. 1987), *aff'd* 541 So. 2d 96 (Fla. 1989).
3. In re Duran, 769 A.2d 497 (Pa. 2001).
4. Cruzan v. Director, Missouri Dep't of Health, 497 U.S. 261 (1990).
5. 611 A.2d 1148 (N.J. Super Ct. 1992).
6. 620 So. 2d 372 (La. Ct. App. 1993).
7. *Id.* at 380.
8. 390 N.Y.S.2d 523 (N.Y. Sup. Ct. 1976).
9. 632 N.E.2d 946 (Ohio Ct. App. 1993).
10. 534 A.2d 452 (Pa. 1987).
11. No. 38242 (Nev. 2004).
12. 136 N.W. 1106 (Mich. 1912).
13. 28 N.E. 266 (Mass. 1891).
14. 500 So. 2d 679, 687 (Fla. Dist. Ct. App. 1987), *aff'd* 541 So. 2d 96 (Fla. 1989).
15. Cruzan v. Director, Missouri Dep't of Health, 497 U.S. 261, 269 (1990).
16. 105 N.E. 92, 93 (N.Y. 1914).
17. 689 N.E.2d 397 (Ill. App. Ct. 1997).
18. Harrell v. St. Mary's Hosp., Inc., 678 So. 2d 455 (Fla. Dist. Ct. App. 1996).
19. 648 N.E.2d 839 (Ohio App. 9 Dist. 1994).
20. *Id.* at 840.
21. Stamford Hosp. v. Vega, 674 A.2d 821 (Conn. Super. Ct. 1996).

chapter thirteen

Patient Abuse

INTRODUCTION

Love and knowledge led upwards to the heavens,
But always pity brought me back to earth;
Cries of pain reverberated in my heart
Of children in famine, of victims tortured
And of old people left helpless.
I long to alleviate the evil, but I cannot,
And, I too suffer.
This has been my life;
I found it worth living.

BERTRAND RUSSELL, ADAPTED

Patient abuse refers to the mistreatment or neglect of individuals who are under the care of a health care organization. Abuse is not limited to an institutional setting and may occur in an individual's home as well as in an institution. Abuse can take many forms—physical, psychological, medical, financial, and so forth. It is not always easy to identify because injuries often can be attributed to other causes. This chapter reviews patient abuse in the health care setting.

ELDER ABUSE

A *USA Today* review of two years' of inspection records (between 2000 and 2002) for more than 5,300 assisted living facilities found that what should be havens for the elderly may in reality be exposing them to deadly risks. The study indicates that medication errors and poor staff training resulted in many of the injuries identified.[1]

Elder abuse is the harmful treatment of people and includes abandonment; emotional, financial (e.g., theft or misuse of an elder's money or property by a person in a position of trust), verbal, mental, sexual, or physical abuse; corporal punishment; and involuntary restraint and seclusion. *Neglect* is the failure to provide the care necessary to prevent physical harm (e.g., the failure of staff to turn a patient periodically to prevent pressure sores) or mental anguish.

Most states have enacted statutes mandating the reporting of elder abuse. In general, elder abuse is less likely to be reported than child abuse. Physical and emotional neglect, as well as verbal and financial abuse, are perceived as the most prevalent forms of elder abuse. Seniors often fail to report incidents of abuse because they fear retaliation and not being believed. Threats of placement in a nursing home or shame that a family member is involved often prevents the elder from seeking help.

Signs of Abuse or Neglect

Signs of abuse or neglect of a senior include the following: unexplained or unexpected death; development of pressure sores; heavy medication and sedation used in place of adequate nursing staff; occurrence of broken bones; sudden and unexpected emotional outbursts, agitation, or withdrawal; bruises, welts, discoloration, burns, and such; absence of hair and/or hemorrhaging below scalp; dehydration and/or malnourishment without illness-related cause; hesitation to talk openly; implausible stories; unusual activity in bank accounts; power of attorney given or recent changes or creation of will when the person is incapable of making such decisions; missing personal belongings; an untreated medical condition; and the senior may not be given the opportunity to speak for himself or herself, or see others, without the presence of the caregiver.

Hidden Camera

Gale . . . wasn't prepared for the rough treatment and cruel taunts she says her ailing mother suffered at the nursing home. She cried as a nurse's aide chastised her mother for failing to straighten her arthritic-stricken legs. And she watched in disbelief as an assistant jerked her mother off her rubber bed pad and pushed her into the bed's metal rails. All of these images were caught . . . by a "granny cam"—a camera hidden in her mother's room.[2]

Documentation

Caregivers who suspect abuse are expected to report their findings. Symptoms and conditions of suspected abuse should be defined clearly and objectively.

The abuse of the elderly is not a localized or isolated problem. Unfortunately, it permeates our society. *Behind Closed Doors*, a landmark book on family violence, stated that the first national study of violence in American homes estimated that one in two homes was the scene of family violence at least once a year.[3]

> We have always known that America is a violent society. . . . What is new and surprising is that the American family and the American home are perhaps as much or more violent than any other single institution or setting (with the exception of the military, and only then in the time of war). Americans run the greatest risk of assault, physical injury and even murder in their own homes by members of their own families.[4]

It is difficult to determine the extent of elder abuse, because the abused elderly are reluctant to admit that their children or loved ones have assaulted them. Unfortunately, the abuse of the elderly remains hidden from the public, and the findings of the 1990 report are as current today as when they were first published in 1990. The Senate Select Committee on Aging reported the following:

- Elder abuse is less likely to be reported than child abuse.
- Physical violence, including negligence, and financial abuse appear to be the most common forms of abuse, followed by abrogation of basic constitutional rights and psychological abuse.

- Most instances of elder abuse are recurring events rather than one-time occurrences.
- Victims are often 75 years of age or older, and women are more likely to be abused than men.
- Older people are often ashamed to admit that their children or loved ones abuse them, or they may fear reprisals if they complain.
- Many middle-aged family members, finally ready to enjoy time to themselves, are resentful of a frail and dependent elderly parent.
- Finally, the majority of the abusers are relatives.[5]

The plaintiffs in *In re Estate of Smith v. O'Halloran*[6] instituted a lawsuit in an effort to improve deplorable conditions at many nursing homes. The court concluded that

> The evidentiary record . . . supports a general finding that all is not well in the nation's nursing homes and that the enormous expenditures of public funds and the earnest efforts of public officials and public employees have not produced an equivalent return in benefits. That failure of expectations has produced frustration and anger among those who are aware of the realities of life in some nursing homes which provide so little service that they could be characterized as orphanages for the aged.[7]

Surveyors of health care organizations should look for signs of patient abuse by watching for the following: physician's order for restraints; time-limited orders; the number of patients that are physically restrained; the type of restraints being used; whether or not the restraints are applied correctly; how often restrained patients are observed by the staff; signs of overmedication; signs of mental and physical abuse of patients; signs of harassment, humiliation, or threats from staff or patients; whether patients are comfortable with the staff; the numbers of patients with bruises or other injuries; and evidence of patient neglect or patients left in urine or feces without cleaning.

Wanton Neglect of Residents

The defendant in *State v. Cunningham*,[8] the owner and administrator of a residential care facility, housed 30 to 37 mentally ill, mentally retarded, and elderly residents. The Iowa Department of Inspections and Appeals conducted various surveys at the defendant's facility between October 1989 and May 1990. All of the surveys except for one resulted in a $50 daily fine assessed against the defendant for violations of the regulations. On August 16, 1990, a grand jury filed an indictment charging the defendant with several counts of wanton neglect of a resident in violation of Iowa Code section 726.7 (1989), which provides: "A person commits wanton neglect of a resident of a health care facility when the person knowingly acts in a manner likely to be injurious to the physical, mental, or moral welfare of a resident of a health care facility. . . . Wanton neglect of a resident of a health care facility is a serious misdemeanor."

The district court held that the defendant had knowledge of the dangerous conditions that existed in the health care facility but willfully and consciously refused to provide or exercise adequate supervision to remedy or attempt to remedy the dangerous conditions. The residents were exposed to physical dangers, unhealthy and unsanitary physical conditions, and were grossly deprived of much-needed medical care and personal attention. The conditions were likely to and did cause injury to the physical and mental well-being of the facility's residents. The defendant was found guilty on five counts of wanton neglect. The district court sentenced the defendant to one year in jail for each of the five counts, to run concurrently. The district court suspended all but two days of the defendant's sentence and ordered him to pay $200 for each count, plus a surcharge and costs, and to perform community service. A motion for a new trial was denied, and the defendant appealed.

The Iowa Court of Appeals held that there was substantial evidence to support a finding that the defendant was responsible for not properly maintaining the nursing facility, which led to prosecution for wanton neglect of the facility's residents. The defendant was found guilty of knowingly acting in a manner likely to be injurious to the physical or mental welfare of the facility's residents by creating, directing, or maintaining the following hazardous conditions and unsafe practices: fire hazards and circumstances impeded safety from fire; the facility was not properly maintained (e.g., broken glass in patients' rooms, excessive hot water in faucets, dried feces on public bathroom walls and grab bars, insufficient towels and linens, cockroaches and worms in the food preparation area, no soap available in the kitchen, at one point only one bar of soap and one container of shampoo found in the entire facility); dietary facilities were unsanitary and inadequate to meet the dietary needs of the residents; there were inadequate staffing patterns and supervision in the facility; and, improper dosages of medications were administered to the residents.[9]

The defendant argued that he did not "create" the unsafe conditions at the facility. The court of appeals disagreed. The statute does not require that the defendant create the conditions at the facility to sustain a conviction. The defendant was the administrator of the facility and responsible for the conditions that existed.

Abuse and Revocation of License

The operator of a nursing facility appealed an order by the Department of Public Welfare revoking his license because of resident abuse in *Nepa v. Commonwealth Department of Public Welfare*.[10] Substantial evidence supported the department's finding. Three former employees testified that the nursing facility operator had abused residents in the following incidents:

- He unbuckled the belt of one of the residents, causing his pants to drop, and then grabbed a second resident, forcing them to kiss. (Petitioner's excuse for this behavior was to shame the resident because of his masturbating in public.)
- On two occasions he forced a resident to remove toilet paper from a commode after she had urinated and defecated in it. (Denying that there was fecal matter in the commode, petitioner's excuse was that this would stop the resident from filling the commode with toilet paper.)
- He verbally abused a resident who was experiencing difficulty in breathing and accused him of faking as he attempted to feed him liquids.[11]

The nursing facility operator claimed that the findings of fact were not based on substantial evidence and that even if they were, the incidents did not amount to abuse under the code. The defendant attempted to discredit the witnesses with allegations from a resident and another employee that one of his former employees got into bed with a resident, and that another had taken a picture of a male resident while in the shower and had placed a baby bottle and a humiliating sign around the neck of another resident. The court was not impressed. Although these incidents, if true, were reprehensible, they were collateral matters that had no bearing on the witnesses' reputation for truthfulness and therefore could not be used for impeachment purposes. The court held that there was substantial evidence supporting the department's decision and that the activities committed by the operator were sufficient to support revocation of his license.

> We believe Petitioner's treatment of these residents as found by the hearing examiner to be truly disturbing. These residents were elderly and/or mentally incapacitated and wholly dependent on Petitioner while residing in his home. As residents, they are entitled to maintain their dignity and be cared for with respect, concern, and passion.
> Petitioner testified that he did not have adequate training to deal with the patients he received who suffered from mental problems. Petitioner's lack of training in this area is absolutely no excuse for the reprehensible manner in which he treated various residents. Accordingly, DPW's order revoking Petitioner's license to operate a personal care home is affirmed.[12]

Abusive Search

A nurse in *People v. Coe*[13] was charged with a willful violation of the Public Health Law in connection with an allegedly abusive search of an 86-year-old resident at a geriatric center and with the falsification of business records in the first degree. The resident, Mr. Gersh, had heart disease and difficulty in expressing himself verbally. Another resident claimed that two $5 bills were missing. Nurse Coe assumed that Gersh had taken them because he had been known to take things in the past. The nurse proceeded to search Gersh, who resisted. A security guard was summoned, and another search was undertaken. When Gersh again resisted, the security guard slammed a chair down in front of him and pinned his arms while the defendant nurse searched his pockets, failing to retrieve the two $5 bills. Five minutes later, Gersh collapsed in a chair gasping for air. Coe administered cardiopulmonary resuscitation but was unsuccessful, and Gersh died.

Coe was charged with violation of the New York Penal Law for falsifying records, because of the defendant's "omission" of the facts relating to the search of Gersh. These facts were considered relevant and should have been included in the nurse's notes regarding this incident. "The first sentence states, 'Observed resident was extremely confused and talks incoherently. Suddenly became unresponsive. . . .' This statement is simply false. It could only be true if some reference to the search and the loud noise was included."[14] A motion was made to dismiss the indictment at the end of the trial.

The court held that the search became an act of physical abuse and mistreatment, the evidence was sufficient to warrant a finding of guilt on both charges, and the fact that searches took place frequently did not excuse an otherwise illegal procedure.

> It may well be that this incident reached the attention of the criminal justice system only because, in the end, a man had died. In those instances which are equally violative of residents' rights and equally contrary to standards of common decency but which do not result in visible harm to a patient, the acts are nevertheless illegal and subject to prosecution. A criminal act is not legitimized by the fact that others have, with impunity, engaged in that act.[15]

Forcible Administration of Medications

The medical employee in *In re Axelrod*[16] sought review of a determination by the commissioner of health that she was guilty of resident abuse. Evidence showed that the employee, after a resident refused medication, "held the patient's chin and poured the medication down her throat."[17] There was no indication or convincing evidence that an emergency existed that would have required the forced administration of the medication. The court held that substantial evidence supported the commissioner's finding that the employee had been guilty of resident abuse.

Intimidation of Abusive Resident/Disciplinary Overkill

A difficult and abusive 80-year-old resident of a veterans home in *Beasley v. State Personnel Board*[18] slapped the face of an aide who was assisting him. The resident, referring to his inability to have sex, said that he might as well have it cut off. The aide, Beasley, responded by indicating that if he did not behave then she might accommodate him. A nursing supervisor who passed by at that moment noted that a nursing assistant and a hospital aide who were standing nearby laughed and did nothing to intervene. Beasley was fired and the other two employees were suspended for 10 days. After the State Board upheld the overkill, the three employees went by mandate to the superior court where Beasley's dismissal was ruled too severe. The trial court found that action against the nursing assistant and hospital aide, although harsh, was within discretion.

On appeal, the court held that Beasley's comments did not constitute misconduct, and the veterans home nursing assistant and hospital aide did not commit actionable conduct by "sort of laughing." When this incident was viewed in its context and in light of the whole record, it did not support the state personnel board's finding that Beasley's attitude toward patients was poor.

Care Given Deceased Deficient

In *Montgomery Health Care Facility v. Ballard*,[19] three nurses testified that the facility was understaffed. "One nurse testified that she asked her supervisor for more help but that she did not get it."[20] The estate of a nursing home resident, who had expired as the result of multiple infected bedsores, brought a malpractice action against the nursing home. First American Health Care, Inc. is the parent corporation of the Montgomery Health Care Facility, a nursing home. The trial court entered a judgment on a jury verdict against the home, and an appeal was taken. The Alabama Supreme Court held that reports compiled by the Alabama Department of Public Health concerning deficiencies found in the nursing home were admissible as evidence. Evidence showed that the care given to the deceased was deficient in the same ways as noted in the survey and complaint reports, which indicated that deficiencies in the home included:

> [I]nadequate documentation of treatment given for decubitus ulcers; 23 patients found with decubitus ulcers, 10 of whom developed those ulcers in the facility; dressings on the sores were not changed as ordered; nursing progress notes did not describe patients' ongoing conditions, particularly with respect to descriptions of decubitus ulcers; ineffective policies and procedures with respect to sterile dressing supplies; lack of nursing assessments; incomplete patient care plans; inadequate documentation of doctor's visits, orders or progress notes; a.m. care not consistently documented; inadequate documentation of turning of patients; incomplete "activities of daily living" sheets; "range of motion" exercises not documented; patients found wet and soiled with dried fecal matter; lack of bowel and bladder retaining programs; incomplete documentation of ordered force fluids. . . .[21]

From a corporate standpoint, the parent corporation of the nursing facility could be held liable for the nursing facility's negligence, where the parent company controlled or retained the right to control the day-to-day operations of the home. The defendants had argued that the punitive damage award of $2 million against the home was greater than what was necessary to meet society's goal of punishing them. The Alabama Supreme Court, however, found the award not to be excessive. "The trial court also found that because of the large number of nursing home residents vulnerable to the type of neglect found in Mrs. Stovall's case, the verdict would further the goal of discouraging others from similar conduct in the future."[22]

CHILD ABUSE

The physically abused or neglected child presents a medical, social, and legal problem. What constitutes an abused child is difficult to determine, because it is often impossible to ascertain whether a child was injured intentionally or accidentally.

Definition

An abused child is one who has suffered intentional serious mental, emotional, sexual, and/or physical injury inflicted by a parent or other person responsible for the child's care. Some states extend the definition to include a child suffering from starvation. Other states include moral neglect in the definition of abuse. Others mention immoral associations; endangering a child's morals; and the location of a child in a disreputable place or in association with vagrant, vicious, or immoral persons. Sexual abuse also is enumerated as an element of neglect in the statutes of some states.

An abused child is generally defined as a person younger than 18 years of age whose parent or other person legally responsible for his or her care does any of the following: inflicts, or allows to be inflicted, upon that child, physical injury by nonaccidental means that causes or creates a substantial risk of death, serious or protracted disfigurement, protracted impairment of physical or emotional health, or protracted loss or impairment of the function of any bodily organ; commits, or allows to be committed, a sex offense against that child; and/or allows, permits, or encourages the child to engage in an act considered unlawful.

Child abuse statutes have been enacted in most states to provide civil immunity for those making or participating in good-faith reports of suspected child abuse. Most states also provide immunity from criminal liability. The New York State Social Services Law provides that "[a]ny person, official, or institution participating in good faith in the making of a report, the taking of photographs, or the removal or keeping of a child pursuant to this title shall have immunity from any liability, civil or criminal, that might otherwise result by reason of such actions."[23] Even in states that do not provide immunity, it is unlikely that anyone making a good-faith report of suspected child abuse would be subject to criminal liability. State laws generally specify what persons (e.g., physicians, nurses, and social workers) are required to report suspected child abuse that comes before them in their official capacities. In some states, failure to report a case of suspected child abuse carries criminal penalties as well as civil liability for the damages resulting from such failure.[24]

Reporting Abuse

Presently, all states have enacted laws to protect abused children. Most states protect the persons required to report cases of child abuse. In a few states, certain identified individuals who are not required to report instances of child abuse, but who do so, are protected. Child abuse laws may or may not provide penalties for failure to report. Those in the health care setting who are required to report or cause a report to be made when they have reasonable cause to suspect that a child has been abused include the following: administrators, physicians, interns, registered nurses, chiropractors, social service workers, psychologists, dentists, osteopaths, optometrists, podiatrists, mental health professionals, and volunteers in residential facilities.

Detecting Abuse

An individual who reports child abuse should be aware of the physical and behavioral indicators of abuse and maltreatment that appear to be part of a pattern (e.g., bruises, burns, and broken bones). In reviewing the indicators of abuse and maltreatment, the reporter does not have to be absolutely certain that abuse or maltreatment exists before reporting. Rather, abuse and maltreatment should be reported whenever they are suspected, based on the existence of the signs of abuse and maltreatment and in light of the reporter's training and experience. Behavioral indicators include, but are not limited to, substantially diminished psychological or intellectual functioning, failure to thrive, no control of aggression, self-destructive impulses, decreased ability to think and reason, acting out and misbehavior, or habitual truancy. Such impairment must be clearly attributable to the unwillingness or inability of the person responsible for the child's care to exercise a minimum degree of care toward the child.

Good-Faith Reporting

Any report of suspected child abuse must be made with a good-faith belief that the facts reported are true. The definition of *good faith* as used in a child abuse statute may vary from state to state. However, when a health care practitioner's medical evaluation indicates reasonable cause to believe a child's injuries were not accidental and when the health care practitioner is not acting from his or her desire to harass, injure, or embarrass the child's parents, making the report will not result in liability.

Statutes generally require that when a person covered by a statute is attending a child and suspects child abuse, the staff member must report such concerns. Typical statutes provide that an oral report be made immediately, followed by a written report.

The criminal and civil risks for health care professionals do not lie in good-faith reporting of suspected incidents of child abuse, but in failing to report such incidents. Most states have legislated a variety of civil and criminal penalties for failure to report suspected child abuse incidents. New York, for example, provides:

1. Any person, official, or institution required by this title to report a case of suspected child abuse or maltreatment who willfully fails to do so shall be guilty of a class A misdemeanor.
2. Any person, official, or institution required by this title to report a case of suspected child abuse or maltreatment who knowingly and willfully fails to do so shall be civilly liable for the damages proximately caused by such failure.[25]

Immunity and Good-Faith Reporting

A minor child and his mother brought an action for damages against physicians for failing to diagnose disease and filing erroneous child abuse reports in *Awkerman v. Tri-County Orthopedic Group*.[26] The Wayne County Circuit Court granted the physicians' motions for partial summary judgment, and the plaintiffs appealed. The Michigan Court of Appeals held that the child abuse reporting statute provides immunity to persons who file child abuse reports in good faith even if the reports were filed because of negligent diagnosis of the cause of the child's frequent bone fractures, which eventually was diagnosed as osteogenesis imperfecta. The court of appeals also held that damages for shame and humiliation were not recoverable pursuant to Michigan statute. Immunity from liability did not extend to damages for malpractice that may have resulted from the failure to diagnose the child's disease as long as all the elements of negligence were present.

CHAPTER REVIEW

1. Patient abuse is the mistreatment or neglect of individuals who are under the care of a health care organization. Abuse is not limited to an institutional setting and may occur in an individual's home as well as in an institution.
2. Abuse can take many forms. It can be physical, psychological, medical, financial, or otherwise. It is not always easy to identify because injuries often can be attributed to other causes.
3. Seniors often fail to report incidents of abuse because they fear retaliation and not being believed.

4. Signs of abuse include unexplained or unexpected death; broken bones; sudden and unexpected emotional outbursts, agitation, or withdrawal; bruises, welts, discoloration, or burns; absence of hair; dehydration and malnourishment without an illness-related cause; hesitation to talk openly; implausible stories; and unusual or inappropriate bank account activity.

5. Caregivers who suspect abuse are expected to report their findings. Symptoms and conditions of suspected abuse should be defined clearly and objectively.

6. Elder abuse is less likely to be reported than child abuse.

7. An abused child is one who has suffered intentional serious mental, emotional, sexual, and/or physical injury inflicted by a parent or other person responsible for the child's care.

8. The various states have enacted various child abuse statutes to provide civil immunity for those making or participating in good-faith reports of suspected child abuse.

9. An individual who reports child abuse should be aware of the physical and behavioral indicators of abuse and maltreatment that appear to be part of a pattern (e.g., bruises, burns, and broken bones).

REVIEW QUESTIONS

1. Based on the cases reviewed in this chapter, discuss why patients are often reluctant to complain about their health care.

2. When a health care provider reports abuse, should the accuser be able to know the identity of his or her accuser? Explain your answer.

3. Should a health care provider be sanctioned for reporting abuse if it proves to be false?

4. Discuss both the ethical and legal issues of abuse.

NOTES

1. "Havens for Elderly May Expose Them to Deadly Risks," USA TODAY, May 25, 2004, at 1.
2. USA Today, September 14, 1999.
3. RICHARD J. GELLES, MURRAY A. STRAUSS, & SUZANNE K. STEINMETZ, BEHIND CLOSED DOORS: VIOLENCE IN THE AMERICAN FAMILY (1980).
4. Id.
5. SENATE SUBCOMM. ON HEALTH AND LONG-TERM CARE, supra note 53.
6. 557 F. Supp. 289 (D. Colo. 1983).
7. Id. at 293.
8. State v. Cunningham, 493 N.W.2d 884 (Iowa Ct. App. 1992).

9. *Id.* at 887–888.
10. 551 A.2d 354 (Pa. Commw. Ct. 1988).
11. *Id.* at 355.
12. *Id.* at 357.
13. 501 N.Y.S.2d 997 (N.Y. Sup. Ct. 1986).
14. *Id.* at 1001.
15. *Id.*
16. 560 N.Y.S.2d 573 (N.Y. App. Div. 1990).
17. *Id.*
18. 178 Cal. Rptr. 564 (Cal. Ct. App. 1981).
19. 565 So. 2d 221, 224 (Ala. 1990).
20. *Id.* at 224.
21. *Id.* at 223–224.
22. *Id.* at 226.
23. N.Y. Soc. Serv. Law § 419 (McKinney 1992).
24. N.Y. Soc. Serv. Law § 420 (McKinney 1992).
25. N.Y. Soc. Serv. Law § 420 (McKinney 1992).
26. 373 N.W.2d 204 (Mich. Ct. App. 1985).

chapter fourteen

Patient Rights and Responsibilities

INTRODUCTION

Every person possesses certain rights guaranteed by the Constitution of the United States and its Amendments, including freedom of speech, religion, and association and the right not to be discriminated against on the grounds of race, creed, color, or national origin. The Supreme Court has interpreted the Constitution as also guaranteeing certain other rights not expressly mentioned, such as the right to privacy and self-determination and the right to accept or reject medical treatment. This chapter provides a brief overview of both the rights and responsibilities of all patients.

PATIENT RIGHTS

Patients of the various states have certain rights and protections guaranteed by state and federal laws and regulations. Patient rights include the right to participate in health care decisions and to understand treatment options. Patients have a right to receive a clear explanation of tests, diagnoses, treatment options, prescribed medications, and prognosis.[1]

It is recognized that a professional relationship between the physician and the patient is essential for the provision of proper medical care. The traditional physician/patient relationship takes on a new dimension when care is rendered within an organizational structure. Legal precedent has established that not only does the institution have responsibility to the patient, but that the patient also has responsibility to the institution.

Patients have the right to choose the medical care they wish to receive. As medical technology becomes more advanced, these decisions become increasingly difficult to decide. Should I have the surgery? Do I want to be maintained on a respirator? Frequently, these decisions involve not only medical questions, but moral and ethical dilemmas as well. What has the greater value, the length of life or the quality of life? What is the right choice for the patient? Although patients have a right to make their own care and treatment decisions, they often face conflicting religious and moral values. Often, it is difficult to make a choice when two roads may seem equally desirable.

Help! I'm Wrestling with My Values!

- Should I accept a blood transfusion if it will save my life?
- Should I refuse a blood transfusion and risk death because it is against my religious beliefs?
- Did I do a bad thing by refusing blood to save my life?
- Was I immoral to accept death over life?

Patient rights may be classified as either legal, those emanating from law, or human statements of desirable ethical principles, such as the right to health care or the right to be treated with human dignity. Both staff and patients should be aware and understand not only their own rights and responsibilities but also the rights and responsibilities of each other.

Right to Know Patient Rights

Upon admission for care, patients have a right to receive a copy of an organization's patient's bill of rights and responsibilities. It is expected that observing a patient's bill of rights will contribute to more effective patient care and greater satisfaction for patients, caregivers, and health care organizations alike.

Right to Explanation of Patient Rights

Patients have a right to receive an explanation of their rights and responsibilities. An organization's description of patient rights and responsibilities should be viewed as a document with legal significance whether or not the state in question has adopted a similar code. The rights of patients must be respected at all times. Each patient is an individual with unique health care needs. The patient has a right to make decisions regarding his or her medical care, including the decision to discontinue treatment, to the extent permitted by law.

Organization policy should provide that upon admission, each patient will be provided with a written statement of his or her rights, responsibilities, and a privacy notice. This statement includes the rights of the patient to make decisions regarding medical care and information regarding protected health information. Patients have a right to receive an explanation of the patient's bill of rights.

Right to Participate in Care Decisions

Patients have a right to participate in all aspects of their care and should be encouraged to do so. They have a right to know their treatment options and to accept or refuse care.

Right to Informed Consent

Patients have a right to receive all the information necessary to make an informed decision prior to consenting to a proposed procedure or treatment. This information should include the possible risks and benefits of the procedure or treatment. The right to receive information from the physician includes information about the illness, the suggested course of treatment, the prospects of recovery in terms that can be understood, risks of treatment, benefits of treatment, alternative care options, and proof of consent.

Right to Ask Questions

Patients have the right and should be encouraged to ask questions regarding their care ("I saw blood in my IV tubing. Is this OK? Is it infiltrating?" and "My wound dressing seems wet. Is this OK? Should the dressing be changed?").

Reducing medical errors requires that the patient actively participate in his or her care. Patients should not hesitate to ask for the following:

- Clarification of the caregiver's instructions.
- Interpretation of a caregiver's illegible handwriting.
- Instructions for medication usage (e.g., frequency, dosing, drug–drug, drug–food interactions, contraindications, side effects).
- Clarification of the physician's diet orders (e.g., "Does my iced tea contain sugar-free substitutes?").
- Explanation of the treatment plan.
- A copy of the organization's hand-washing policy.
- A description of the hospital's procedures to prevent wrong site surgery (e.g., the surgical site has been appropriately marked. If the site cannot be directly marked, have the surgeon draw an arrow pointing to the surgical site.
- The opportunity to provide the organization with a copy of any advance directives that may have been executed (e.g., living will).
- The right to appoint a surrogate decision maker should you become incapacitated.
- A second opinion.

Right to Refuse Treatment

Patients have a right to refuse treatment and be told what effect such a decision could have on his or her health. The responsibility of caregivers requires balancing risks and benefits. This balancing can lead to situations where health care professionals view their obligations to a patient different from the patient's own assessment. The patient may refuse a certain procedure, for example, and forcing the patient to undergo an unwanted procedure would result in a failure to respect the patient's right of self-determination.

Right to Execute Advance Directives

Patients must be informed of their right to execute advance directives. The advance directives must be honored within the limits of the law and the organization's mission, philosophy, and capabilities.

Right to Designate a Decision Maker

Patients have a right to appoint a health care decision maker to make health care decisions when the patient becomes incapacitated or is unable to make decisions on his or her behalf.

Right to Privacy and Confidentiality

Patients have a right to expect that information regarding their care and treatment will be kept confidential. *Confidentiality* requires that the caregiver safeguard a patient's confidences within the constraints of law. Caregivers must be careful not to discuss any aspect of a patient's case with others not involved in the case.

Written permission must be obtained before a patient's medical record can be made available to anyone not associated with the patient's care.

The limitations of space and financial restraints make it difficult to continuously preserve a patient's right to privacy in many hospital settings (e.g., emergency departments). Nevertheless, health care organizations have a responsibility to provide for a reasonable amount of privacy for patients.

The issues of confidentiality and privacy are both ethical and legal. Caregivers must safeguard each patient's right to privacy and the right to have information pertaining to his or her care to be kept confidential.

Patients have a right to receive "Notice of Privacy Standards," a requirement under the Health Insurance Portability and Accountability Act.

Disclosures Permitted without Authorization

The following list describes some of the ways a health care provider may disclose medical information about a patient without his or her written consent.

- Patient information (e.g., diagnoses, anesthesia history, surgical and other invasive procedures, drug allergies, medication usage, lab test results, and imaging studies) may be disclosed to other providers who may be caring for the patient in order to provide safe health care treatment.
- Disclosure of patient information to third-party payers so that providers can obtain payment for services rendered.
- Disclosure of patient information for health care operations.
- Disclosure of patient information as may be required by a law enforcement agency.
- Disclosure of patient information as may be required to avert a serious threat to public health or safety.
- Disclosure of patient information as required by military command authorities for their medical records.
- Disclosure of patient information to worker's compensation or similar programs for processing of claims.
- Disclosure of patient information in response to a subpoena for a legal proceeding.
- Disclosure of patient information to a coroner or medical examiner for purposes of identification.

Right to Limit Disclosures

Some of the individual rights a patient has regarding disclosure of access to his or her medical information are as follows:

- Right to request restrictions or limitations regarding information used or disclosed about one's treatment.
- Right to an accounting of nonstandard disclosures: The patient has a right to request a list of the disclosures made of information released regarding his or her care.

- Right to amend: If you believe that medical information regarding your care is incorrect or incomplete, you have a right to request that the information be corrected.
- Right to inspect and copy medical information that may be used to make decisions about your care.
- Right to file a complaint with the provider, or the Secretary of the Department of Health and Human Services in Washington, DC, if you believe your privacy rights have been violated.
- Right to a paper copy of a notice pertaining to patient.

Right to Know of Restrictions on Rights

Any restrictions on a patient's visitors, mail, telephone, or other communications must be evaluated for their therapeutic effectiveness and fully explained to and agreed upon by the patient or patient representative.

Right to Have Special Needs Addressed

Patients have a right to an interpreter whenever possible. Patients who have physical or mental disabilities, or are hearing or vision impaired, have a right to special help, such as an interpreter.

Right to Emergency Care

Patients have a right to receive emergency care in a hospital's emergency department. At the time of admission, each patient has the right to be informed in writing of his or her rights and responsibilities, including any explanations if needed.

Health care organizations must not discriminate by reason of race, creed, color, sex, religion, or national origin. Those that do discriminate violate constitutionally guaranteed rights. They also may be in violation of federal, state, and local laws. Discrimination in some states can be considered a misdemeanor and also may carry a civil penalty. Federal and state funds may be withheld from those institutions that practice discrimination.

Most federal, state, and local programs specifically require, as a condition for receiving funds under such programs, an affirmative statement on the part of the organization that it will not discriminate. For example, the Medicare and Medicaid programs specifically require affirmative assurances by health care organizations that no discrimination will be practiced.

Right to Discharge

Patients have a right to be discharged and not be detained in a health care setting merely because of an inability to pay for services rendered. An unauthorized detention of this nature could subject the offending organization to charges of false imprisonment. Although patients have a right not to be held against their will, there are circumstances where reasonable detainment can be justified (e.g., a minor's release only to a parent or authorized guardian).

Right to Transfer

Patients have a right to be transferred to an appropriate facility when the admitting facility is unable to meet a patient's particular needs. This will at times necessitate the transfer of the patient to another health care organization that has the special services the patient requires. For this reason, it is important for each organization to execute transfer agreements with other health care organizations.

Patients also have a right to choose a receiving facility, whenever possible. The Medicaid patient in *Macleod v. Miller*[2] was entitled to an injunction preventing his involuntary transfer from the nursing home. The patient had not been accorded a pre-transfer hearing as was required by applicable regulations. In addition, it was determined that the trauma of transfer might result in irreparable harm to the patient. The appeals court remanded the case to the trial court with directions to enter an order prohibiting the defendants from transferring the plaintiff pending exhaustion of his administrative remedies.

Health care organizations should have a written transfer agreement in effect with other organizations to help ensure the smooth transfer of patients from one facility to another when such is determined appropriate by the attending physician(s). Generally speaking, a transfer agreement is a written document that sets forth the terms and conditions under which a patient may be transferred to a facility that more appropriately provides the kind of care required by the patient. It also establishes procedures to admit patients of one facility to another when their condition warrants a transfer.

Transfer agreements should be written in compliance with and reflect the provisions of the many federal and state laws, regulations, and standards affecting health care organizations. The parties to a transfer agreement should be particularly aware of applicable federal and state regulations.

Right to Access Medical Records

The courts have taken the view that patients have a legally enforceable interest in the information contained in their medical records and, therefore, have a right to access their records. Some states have enacted legislation permitting patients access to their records. Patients may generally have access to review and/or obtain copies of their records, X-rays, and laboratory and diagnostic tests. Access to information includes that maintained or possessed by a health care organization and/or a health care practitioner who has treated or is treating a patient. Organizations and physicians can withhold records if it is determined that the information could reasonably be expected to cause substantial and identifiable harm to the patient (e.g., patients in psychiatric hospitals, institutions for the mentally disabled, or alcohol- and drug-treatment programs).

Right to Know of Third-Party Care Relationships

Patients have a right to know the hospital's relationships with outside parties that may influence their care and treatment. These relationships may be with educational institutions, insurers, and other health care caregivers.

Right to Know the Caregivers

Patients have a right to be informed of the names, qualifications, and positions of the caregivers who will be in charge of their care in the hospital. Patients have a right to know the functions of any hospital staff involved in their care and to refuse treatment, examination, or observation by any of them. These rights include:

- Patients should know who is treating them by name, discipline, and role and responsibility in their care plan.
- Patients should know the names of all consulting physicians and hospital-designated caregivers.
- Caregivers should identify themselves to patients by name, discipline, specialty, and identification badge of the treatment team.

Right to Sensitive and Compassionate Care

Patients have a right to be free from harassment, including verbal and physical abuse. They should receive considerate and respectful care given from competent caregivers who respect the patient's personal belief systems.

Right to a Timely Response to Care Needs

Patients have a right to have their care needs responded to within a reasonable time frame. Delay in responding to patient needs can put patients' lives at risk.

Right to Pain Management

I am locked in a prison of pain,
Where doctors hold the key,
Why can't they think beyond the box,
And develop a cure for me?

Ns

Pain management is the process whereby caregivers work with the patient to develop a pain control treatment plan. The process involves educating the patient as to the importance of pain management in the healing process. With current treatments, pain can often be prevented or at least be controlled. Patients have a right to have a pain assessment and management of any pain identified. These rights include the right to:

- Have pain managed to the best of existing medical knowledge
- Ask questions (e.g., "How much pain can I expect?" "How severe will my pain be?" "How long will my pain last?" "Will my pain ever go away?")
- Be believed when they describe their pain
- Have their pain assessed using an appropriate pain scale [(e.g., 0 (no pain) to 10 (worst possible pain)] to measure and assess the degree of pain.

A pain rating scale is a visual tool used to help patients measure their pain. It helps the caregiver know how well treatment is working and whether changes in the treatment plan are necessary. An example of a pain scale is shown here.

A patient has the right to the following with regard to pain management:

- A pain control treatment plan should be developed with the caregiver.
- Alternative and or complementary strategies should be included in the pain management treatment plan that might help improve the efficacy of traditional treatment options (e.g., pain medications), for example, acupuncture).
- Spouse, significant other, family, and caregivers should be involved in the decision-making process.
- The patient should know what medications, anesthesia, or other treatments are planned.
- The risks, benefits, and side effects of suggested treatment(s) should be explained.
- Alternative pain treatments available should be discussed.
- The patient should ask for changes in treatment if pain persists.
- It is acceptable to refuse the pain treatment(s) recommended.
- Finally, pain medication should be administered on a timely basis.

What's Wrong with This Picture?

The following is a letter that a frustrated patient with complex medical issues wrote to her consulting physician. After reviewing the contents of this letter, describe the ethical and patient rights issues that appear in the correspondence.

> When I went to your office, it was with great hopes that someone was finally going to piece together all of the bizarre symptoms I have been experiencing over the last several months and get to the cause of my pain.
>
> I was quite frankly shocked by how I was treated as a patient— especially one experiencing a health crisis.
>
> I was examined by a medical student who wrote my history and current health problems on the pages of a small "yellow sticky pad." You were not in the room when he examined me, and then I saw you for approximately 10 minutes.

You took the card of my New York doctor and said you were going to call him, and then call me regarding what you thought the next steps should be.

I called you on Friday because my local doctor said that you had not called, and I was told you were on vacation until yesterday. I had asked that you call me. You never did. I called you yesterday again, but you did not answer nor did you return my call.

On Monday, I received a letter from a medical student, I assume. Although I empathize with the demands on your time, I have never seen a handwritten letter, which I received, informing me of test results I provided to you prior to my appointment with you. You never mentioned the liver enzyme elevations or my February test from New York. Moreover, no mention was made regarding any plan to help me alleviate immediate problems.

Doctor, I am not a complainer or a person with a low pain tolerance. Since moving here, I've had fainting episodes, severe chest pain and pressure, leg and arm pain and stiffness, congestion on the left side when the pain kicks in, and by 3 o'clock I have to go home and lie down because I'm so weak and tired. I cannot continue to exist like this. It is not normal. If you're too busy and don't want to take me as a patient, you will not offend me. Frankly, I need attention now to get these things resolved. Testing my cholesterol in a month will not address the problem. I've been treated for that for three years.

Please call or write to me so I can get another doctor if I have to.

The physician never responded.

PATIENT RESPONSIBILITIES

Patients have responsibilities as well as rights. Patients have a responsibility to:

- Ask questions if they do not understand what the caregiver is describing about how to best manage their pain
- Report their pain to their caregivers
- Discuss pain relief treatment options with their caregivers
- Work with their health care caregivers to develop a treatment plan for pain control
- Adhere to the pain control plan
- Remind those who care for them that pain management is an important part of their health care treatment
- Inform health care caregivers about any other prescriptions or over-the-counter medicines they are taking to control their pain
- Provide caregivers with information about pain control methods that have worked, or not worked, for them
- Discuss concerns about taking pain medication
- Alert caregivers of any allergies they have to any medications

- Ask caregivers about the side effects associated with their pain management program
- Maintain a record of the effects of medications or other pain relief measures
- Participate with caregivers in setting a pain control goal, including their pain ratings and activities that are important to them

A Historical Perspective

The following is an excerpt from Cornwall General Hospital of Connecticut's "Rules for Patients," which were posted in the hospital in 1897:

1. Patients on admission to the Hospital must have a bath, unless orders to the contrary are given by the Attending Medical Attendant.

•
•
•

6. Patients must be quiet and exemplary in their behavior and conform strictly to the rules and regulations of the Hospital, and carry out all orders and prescriptions of the various officers of the establishment.

•
•
•

8. No male patient shall, under any pretense whatever, enter the apartments or wards for the females, nor shall a female patient enter the apartments or wards for males, without express orders from the Medical Attendant or Lady Superintendent.

•
•
•

10. Every patient shall retire to bed at 9 pm from First May to First November, and at 8 pm from November to May; and those who are able shall rise at 6 am in the Summer and 7 am in the Winter.
11. Such patients as are able, in the opinion of the physicians and surgeons, shall assist in nursing others, or in such services as the Lady Superintendent may require.

•
•
•

13. Patients must not take away bottles, labels or appliances when leaving the Hospital.
14. No patients shall enter into the basement story, operating theater, or any of the officers' or attendants' rooms, except by permission of an officer of the Hospital.

•
•
•

17. Any patient bringing spirituous liquors into the Hospital or the grounds, or found intoxicated, will be discharged.

18. Whenever patients misbehave or violate any of the standing rules of the Hospital, the Attending Physician may remove or discharge them, as provided by clauses 91 and 93 of Rules for Medical Staff.

A Contemporary Perspective

Today, patient responsibilities are stated somewhat differently than they were in 1897. A current perspective of patient responsibilities includes:

- Providing caregivers with information relevant to medical complaints, symptoms, past illnesses, treatments, surgical procedures, hospitalizations, and medications. Information provided must be accurate, timely, and complete. (The court of appeal in *Fall v. White*[3] affirmed the superior court's ruling that the patient had a duty to provide the physician with accurate and complete information and to follow the physician's instructions for further care or tests.)
- Reporting unexpected changes in condition to caregivers
- Making it known whether one clearly understands the plan of care
- Following the treatment plan recommended (which may include following the instructions of nurses and allied health personnel)
- Following an institution's rules and regulations
- Refraining from the self-administration of medications not prescribed by the physician
- Accepting responsibility for the consequences of refusing treatment or not following instructions
- Being considerate of the rights of others, including health care personnel, in the control of noise, smoking, and limitation on number of visitors
- Being respectful of the property of others
- Recognizing the effect of lifestyle on one's health
- Keeping appointments (Patients have a responsibility to promptly notify caregivers whenever they are unable to keep a scheduled appointment. Failure to notify caregivers of a cancellation means longer delays for other patients who may already be finding it difficult to schedule appointments with specialists.)
- Speaking up and asking questions (Patients have a responsibility to ask questions and understand explanations. Such questions include those regarding medications, diet, and infection control-related issues.)
- Requesting a second opinion
- Describing the location and severity of your pain
- With your surgeon, making sure that staff accurately mark the site of your surgical procedure to avoid confusion in the operating suite
- Making sure that the staff are aware of your preferences for care, including who your decision maker will be in the event that you become incapacitated
- Making sure that you understand caregiver instructions

CHAPTER REVIEW

1. Patients should be informed of their rights and responsibilities at the time of admission. If a patient does not understand these rights and responsibilities, they should be explained to the patient.
2. Patients have rights, but they also have responsibilities. These responsibilities help health care providers treat patients in the most appropriate way possible and help maintain order within the facility.

REVIEW QUESTIONS

1. List and discuss the importance of patient rights from both an ethical and legal point of view.

2. Describe why a patient's responsibilities are as important as his or her rights.

WEB SITES

Home Care Provider & Patient Rights
http://www.nahc.org/Consumer/wamraap.html
Mental Health Patient Rights
http://www.athealth.com/Practitioner/Newsletter/FPN_3_11.html
Protect Your Healthcare
http://www.protectyourhealth care.org
Patient Rights in New York
http://www.health.state.ny.us/
Patient Rights & Responsibilities
http://www.consumer.gov/qualityhealth/rights.htm
20 Tips to Help Prevent Medical Errors
http://www.ahrq.gov/consumer/20tips.htm
The California Patient's Guide
http://www.calpatientguide.org/
University of Michigan Hospitals' Patient Rights
http://www.med.umich.edu/1toolbar/visinfo/umh11.htm
Veterans—Patients Rights and Responsibilities
http://www.palo-alto.med.va.gov/PatientRights.htm

NOTES

1. *Your Rights as a Hospital Patient in New York State*, State of New York, Department of Health.
2. 612 P.2d 1158 (Colo. Ct. App. 1980).
3. 449 N.E.2d 628 (Ind. Ct. App. 1983).

Glossary

Abandonment: Unilateral severance by the physician of the professional relationship between himself or herself and the patient without reasonable notice at a time when the patient still needs continuing care.

Abortion: Premature termination of pregnancy at a time when the fetus is incapable of sustaining life independent of the mother.

Admissibility (of evidence): Refers to the issue of whether a court, applying the rules of evidence, is bound to receive or permit introduction of a particular piece of evidence.

Advance directives: Written instructions expressing an individual's health care wishes in the event that he or she becomes incapacitated and is unable to make such decisions for himself or herself.

Agent: An individual who has been designated by a legal document to make decisions on behalf of another individual; a substitute decision maker.

Appellant: Party who appeals the decision of a lower court to a court of higher jurisdiction.

Appellee: Party against whom an appeal to a higher court is taken.

Artificial nutrition and hydration: Providing food and liquids when a patient is unable to eat or drink, such as intravenous feedings.

Assault: Intentional act that is designed to make the victim fearful and produces reasonable apprehension of harm.

Autonomy: Right of an individual to make his or her own independent decisions.

Battery: Intentional touching of one person by another without the consent of the person being touched.

Beneficence: Describes the principle of doing good, demonstrating kindness, and helping others.

Borrowed servant doctrine: Refers to a situation in which an employee is temporarily under the control of someone other than his or her primary employer. It may involve a situation where an employee is carrying out the specific instructions of a physician. The traditional example is that of a nurse employed by a hospital who is "borrowed" and under the control of the attending surgeon during a procedure in the operating room. The temporary employer of the borrowed servant can be held responsible for the negligent acts of the borrowed servant under the doctrine of *respondeat superior*. This rule is not easily applied, especially if the acts of the employee are for the furtherance of the objectives of the employer. The courts apply a narrow application if the employee is fulfilling the requirement of his or her position.

Captain of the ship doctrine: A doctrine making the physician responsible for the negligent acts of other professionals because he or she had the right to control and oversee the totality of care provided to the patient.

Cardiopulmonary resuscitation: A lifesaving method used by caregivers to restore heartbeat and breathing.

Case citation: Describes where a court's opinion in a particular case can be located. It identifies the parties in the case, the text in which the case can be found, the court writing the opinion, and the year in which the case was decided. For example, the citation *"Bouvia v. Superior Court (Glenchur)*, 225 Cal. Rptr. 297 (Ct. App. 1986)" is described as follows:
- *"Bouvia v. Superior Court (Glenchu)"* identifies the basic parties involved in the lawsuit.
- "225 Cal. Rptr. 297" identifies the case as being reported in volume 225 of the California Reporter at page 297.
- "Ct. App. 1986" identifies the case as being in the California Court of Appeals in 1986.

Case law: Aggregate of reported cases on a particular legal subject as formed by the decisions of those cases.

Civil law: Body of law that describes the private rights and responsibilities of individuals. The part of law that does not deal with crimes, it involves actions filed by one individual against another (e.g., actions in tort and contract).

Clinical privileges: On qualification, the diagnostic and therapeutic procedures that an institution allows a physician to perform on a specified patient population. Qualification includes a review of a physician's credentials, such as medical school diploma, state licensure, and residency training.

Common law: Body of principles that has evolved and continues to evolve and expand from court decisions. Many of the legal principles and rules applied by courts in the United States had their origins in English common law.

Complaint: In a negligence action, the first pleading that is filed by the plaintiff's attorney. It is the first statement of a case by the plaintiff against the defendant and states a cause of action, notifying the defendant as to the basis for the suit.

Congressional Record: Document in which the proceedings of Congress are published. It is the first record of debate officially reported, printed, and published directly by the federal government. Publication of the *Record* began March 4, 1873.

Consent: *See* Informed consent.

Consequentialism: An ethical theory that determines good or bad, right or wrong, based on outcomes.

Contextualism: An ethical doctrine that considers the rightness or wrongness of an action, such as lying, to be based on the particular circumstances of a given situation. The implication is that lying is acceptable in one situation but not in another, even though the situation may be similar. In other words, it depends on the context within which something occurs.

Criminal negligence: Reckless disregard for the safety of others; the willful indifference to an injury following an act.

Defamation: Injury of a person's reputation or character caused by the false statements of another made to a third person. Defamation includes both libel and slander.

Defendant: In a criminal case, the person accused of committing a crime. In a civil suit, the party against whom the suit is brought, demanding that he or she pay the other party legal relief.

Deontological ethics: An ethical approach that focuses on duty, rather than the consequences, when determining the right conduct to be followed.

Deposition: A method of pretrial discovery that consists of statements of fact taken by a witness under oath in a question-and-answer format, as it would be in a court of law with opportunity given to the adversary to be present for cross-examination. Such statements may be admitted into evidence if it is impossible for a witness to attend a trial in person.

Determinism: The view that nothing happens without a cause.

Directed verdict: When a trial judge decides either that the evidence and/or law is clearly in favor of one party or that the plaintiff has failed to establish a case, and that it is pointless for the trial to proceed further, the judge may direct the jury to return a verdict for the appropriate party. The conclusion of the judge must be so clear and obvious that reasonable minds could not arrive at a different conclusion.

Discovery: To ascertain that which was previously unknown through a pretrial investigation; it includes testimony and documents that may be under the exclusive control of the other party. Discovery facilitates out-of-court settlements.

Dogmatic: Stubborn refusal to consider challenges to your own ethical point of view.

Do-not-resuscitate order (DNR): Directive of a physician to withhold cardiopulmonary resuscitation in the event a patient experiences cardiac or respiratory arrest.

Durable power of attorney: A legal instrument enabling an individual to act on another's behalf. In the health care setting, a *durable power of attorney for health care* is a legal instrument that designates and grants authority to an agent, for example, to make health care decisions for another.

Ethical conduct: Conducting oneself in a manner consistent with acceptable principles of right and wrong. Such conduct may relate to one's community, country, profession, and so on.

Ethical dilemma: A situation that forces us to make a decision that involves breaking some ethical norm or contradicting some ethical value. The effect of an action may put others at risk, harm others, or violate another person's rights.

Ethicist: One who specializes in ethics.

Ethics: A set of principles of right and wrong conduct. A theory or system of moral values, of what is right and what is wrong. Ethics is a system of values that guides behavior in relationships among people in accordance with certain social roles.

Ethics committee: A committee created to deal with ethical problems and dilemmas in the delivery of patient care.

Euthanasia: A Greek word meaning "the good death." It is an act conducted for the purpose of causing the merciful death of a person who is suffering from an incurable condition, such as providing a patient with medications to hasten his or her death.

Evidence: Proof of a fact, which is legally presented in a manner prescribed by law, at trial.

Expert witness: Person who has special training, experience, skill, and/or knowledge in a relevant area and who is allowed to offer an opinion as testimony in court.

Futility: Having no useful result. Futility of treatment, as it relates to medical care, occurs when the physician recognizes that the effect of treatment will be of no benefit to the patient. Morally, the physician has a duty to inform the patient when there is little likelihood of success.

Good Samaritan laws: Laws designed to protect those who stop to render aid in an emergency. These laws generally provide immunity for specified persons from any civil suit arising out of care rendered at the scene of an emergency, provided that the one rendering assistance has not done so in a grossly negligent manner.

Guardian: Person appointed by a court to protect the interests of and make decisions for a person who is incapable of making his or her own decisions.

Health: According to the World Health Organization, "[a] state of complete physical, mental, and social well-being and not merely the absence of disease or infirmity."

Health care proxy: Document that delegates the authority to make one's own health care decisions to another adult, known as the health care agent, when one has become incapacitated or is unable to make his or her own decisions.

Hearsay rule: Rule of evidence that restricts the admissibility of evidence that is not the personal knowledge of the witness. Hearsay evidence is admissible only under strict rules.

Hospice: Long-term care for terminally ill persons, provided in a setting more economical than that of a hospital or nursing home. Hospice care generally is sought after a decision has been made to discontinue aggressive efforts to prolong life. A hospice program includes such characteristics as support services by trained individuals, family involvement, and control of pain and discomfort.

Hydration: Intravenous addition of fluids to the circulatory system.

Incapacity: An individual's lack of ability to make decisions for himself or herself.

Incompetent: Individual determined by a court to be incapable of making rational decisions on his or her own behalf.

Independent contractor: One who agrees to undertake work without being under the direct control or direction of the employer.

Informed consent: Legal concept providing that a patient has the right to know the potential risks, benefits, and alternatives of a medical procedure or treatment prior to consenting to the procedure or treatment. Informed consent implies that a patient understands a particular procedure or treatment, including the risks, benefits, and alternatives; is capable of making a decision; and gives consent voluntarily.

Injunction: Court order requiring a person to perform, or prohibiting a person from performing, a particular act.

In loco parentis: Legal doctrine that permits the courts to assign a person to stand in the place of parents and possess their legal rights, duties, and responsibilities toward a child.

Joint Commission on Accreditation of Healthcare Organizations: A not-for-profit independent organization dedicated to improving the quality of health care in organized health care settings. The major functions of the

Joint Commission include the development of organizational standards, awarding accreditation decisions, and providing education and consultation to health care organizations.

Judicial notice: Act by which a court, in conducting a trial or forming a decision, will of its own motion and without evidence recognize the existence and truth of certain facts bearing on the controversy at bar (e.g., serious falls require X-rays).

Jurisdiction: Right of a court to administer justice by hearing and deciding controversies.

Jurisprudence: Philosophy or science of law on which a particular legal system is built.

Justice: The obligation to be fair in the distribution of benefits and risks.

Legal wrong: Invasion of a protected right.

Liability: As it relates to damages, an obligation one has incurred or might incur through a negligent act.

Libel: False or malicious writing intended to defame or dishonor another person and is published so that someone other than the one defamed will observe it.

Life Support: Medical intervention(s) designed to prolong life (e.g., respirator, kidney dialysis machine, tube feedings).

Living will: A document in which an individual expresses in advance his or her wishes regarding the application of life-sustaining treatment in the event that he or she is incapable of doing so at some future time. A living will describes in advance the kind of care one wants to receive or does not wish to receive in the event that he or she is unable to make decisions for himself or herself. A living will takes effect when a person is in a terminal condition or permanent state of unconsciousness.

Malfeasance: Execution of an unlawful or improper act.

Malpractice: Professional misconduct, improper discharge of professional duties, or failure to meet the standard of care of a professional that results in harm to another. The negligence or carelessness of a professional person, such as a nurse, pharmacist, physician, or accountant.

Misfeasance: Improper performance of an act.

Nasogastric tube, insertion of: Involves placing a tube through the patient's nose, down the back of the throat into the esophagus, and then into the stomach. Its purpose is to suction out the contents of the stomach.

Negligence: Omission or commission of an act that a reasonably prudent person would or would not do under given circumstances. It is a form of heedlessness or carelessness that constitutes a departure from the standard of care generally imposed on members of society.

Nonfeasance: Failure to act, when there is a duty to act, as a reasonably prudent person would in similar circumstances.

Norms: Accepted rules and ways of doing things. Without norms, society would be chaotic and unpredictable.

Objectivism: The belief that morality is based on some universal, external, and unchangeable fact. For example, murder is always wrong.

Ombudsman: Person who is designated to speak and act on behalf of a patient/resident, especially in regard to his or her daily needs.

Paternalism: A doctrine that literally means "rule by the father." In health care it is the concept of physicians making decisions for their patients, whereas the more acceptable approach is *autonomy*, whereby the physician informs the patient as to the risks, benefits, and alternatives to care and treatment, and then the patient makes the final choice as to what is best.

Plaintiff: Party who brings a civil suit seeking damages or other legal relief.

Privileged communication: Statement made to an attorney, physician, spouse, or anyone else in a position of trust. Because of the confidential nature of such information, the law protects it from being revealed even in court. The term is applied in two distinct situations. First, the communications between certain persons, such as physician and patient, cannot be divulged without the consent of the patient. Second, in some situations the law provides an exemption from liability for disclosing information where there is a higher duty to speak, such as statutory reporting requirements.

Probate: Judicial proceeding that determines the existence and validity of a will.

Process: A series of related actions to achieve a defined outcome. Ordering and/or administering medications are processes.

Prognosis: Informed judgment regarding the likely course and probable outcome of a disease.

Proximate: In immediate relation with something else. In negligence cases, the careless act must be the proximate cause of injury.

Rational: Having the capacity to think logically.

Real evidence: Evidence furnished by tangible things (e.g., medical records and equipment).

Rebuttal: Giving of evidence to contradict the effect of evidence introduced by the opposing party.

Relativism: The belief that morality is relative to each individual culture. What is right in one culture may be wrong in another culture. In ethics, it is a theory that conceptions of truth and moral values are not absolute but are relative to the persons or groups holding them.

Relativist: A person who is a proponent of relativism.

Release: Statement signed by one person relinquishing a right or claim against another.

Remand: Referral of a case by an appeals court back to the original court, out of which it came, for the purpose of having some action taken there.

Res gestae: "The thing done." All the surrounding events that become part of an incident. If statements are made as part of the incident, they are admissible in court as *res gestae* despite the hearsay rule.

Res ipsa loquitur: "The thing speaks for itself." A doctrine of law applicable to cases where the defendant had exclusive control over the thing that caused the harm and where the harm ordinarily could not have occurred without negligent conduct.

Res judicata: "The thing is decided." That which has been acted on or decided by the courts.

Respirator: A machine used to assist to keep a patient breathing.

Respondeat superior: "Let the master answer." An aphorism meaning that the employer is responsible for the legal consequences of the acts of the servant or employee who is acting within the scope of his or her employment.

Restraint: Restraints can be either "physical" or "chemical" (medication). A physical restraint involves a device (e.g., safety belts, safety bars, geriatric chairs, and bed rails) that restricts or limits voluntary movement and that cannot be removed by the patient.

Slander: False oral statement, made in the presence of a third person, that injures the character or reputation of another.

Standard of care: Description of the conduct that is expected of an individual in a given situation. It is a measure against which a defendant's conduct is compared.

Stare decisis: "Let the decision stand." The legal doctrine that prescribes adherence to those precedents set forth in cases that have been decided.

Statute of limitations: Legal limit on the time allowed for filing suit in civil matters, usually measured from the time of the wrong or from the time when a reasonable person would have discovered the wrong.

Statutory law: Law that is prescribed by legislative enactments.

Subjectivism: A doctrine that says moral judgments are based on personal preferences.

Subpoena ad testificandum: Court order requiring one to appear in court to give testimony.

Subpoena duces tecum: Court order that commands a person to come to court and to produce whatever documents are named in the order.

Summons: Court order directed to the sheriff or other appropriate official to notify the defendant in a civil suit that a suit has been filed and when and where to appear.

Surrogate decision maker: An individual who has been designated to make decisions on behalf of another person determined incapable of making his or her own decisions.

Terminal condition: A medical condition that is incurable and in which death will occur.

Theodicy: A vindication of God's goodness and justice in the face of the existence of evil. We often wonder why God allows bad things to happen to good people. The answer often given is that what God allows to happen in the lives of good people is often mysterious to us. We often have difficulty understanding this, and it often provokes anger in us.

Tort: Civil wrong committed by one individual against another. Torts may be classified as either intentional or unintentional. When a tort is classified as a criminal wrong (e.g., assault, battery, and false imprisonment), the wrong-doer can be held liable in a criminal and/or civil action.

Tort-feasor: Person who commits a tort.

Utilitarianism: A moral theory that treats pleasure and happiness as the only absolute moral good. Acts that bring about happiness and pleasure are good, and acts that bring about pain and suffering are morally bad.

Value: Worth or usefulness. Intrinsic values are those goods that are valuable in their own right. Instrumental values are those goods that help us achieve another good,

Value judgment: A judgment that assigns value to an action.

Virtue: A moral trait that refers to excellence and righteousness.

Waiver: Intentional giving up of a right, such as allowing another person to testify to information that ordinarily would be protected as a privileged communication.

Will: Legal declaration of the intentions a person wishes to have carried out after death concerning property, children, or estate. A will designates a person or persons to serve as the executor(s) responsible for carrying out the instructions of the will.

Wrongful birth: Applies to the cause of action of parents who claim that negligent advice or treatment deprived them of the choice of aborting conception or of terminating the pregnancy.

Wrongful life: Refers to a cause of action brought by or on behalf of a defective child who claims that but for the defendant (e.g., a laboratory's negligent testing procedures or a physician's negligent advice or treatment of the child's parents), the child would not have been born.

Index

A